Kindly donated by

Mr Lewis

ATLAS OF

Gynecologic Endoscopy

Second Edition

ALAN G GORDON
MB FRCS FRCOG
Consultant Obstetrician and Gynaecologist
Hull and East Riding Hospital
Hull, UK

B VICTOR LEWIS
MD FRCS FRCOG
Consultant Obstetrician and Gynaecologist
Watford General Hospital
Watford, UK

ALAN H DECHERNEY
MD
Louis E Phaneuf, Professor and Chairman
Department of Obstetrics and Gynecology
Tufts University School of Medicine
New England Medical Center Hospital
Boston, USA

Foreword by
John J Sciarra
MD PhD
Thomas J Watkins Professor and Chairman
Department of Obstetrics and Gynecology
Northwestern University Medical School
Chicago, USA

ℳ Mosby-Wolfe

London Baltimore Barcelona Bogotá Boston Buenos Aires Caracas Carlsbad, CA Chicago Madrid Mexico City Milan Naples, FL New York Philadelphia St. Louis Seoul Singapore Sydney Taipei Tokyo Toronto Wiesbaden

Project Manager: Alison Taylor

Developmental Editor: Jennifer Prast

Designer: Lara Last

Layout Artist and Illustrator: Jenni Miller

Production: Jane Tozer

Indexer: Kathy Croom

Publisher: Richard Furn

CONTENTS

FOREWORD

The fields of gynecology and obstetrics have undergone some truly revolutionary changes in our time. In gynecology, two of the most significant events have been the explosive development and acceptance of gynecologic endoscopy.

In the foreword to the first edition of *Gynecologic Endoscopy* by Alan Gordon and Victor Lewis, published in 1988, Patrick Steptoe, a great pioneer in the introduction of endoscopy into gynecologic practice, wrote: 'Many operative procedures can now be carried out under endoscopic vision safely and swiftly with little disturbance to the patient. Biopsy of tissues can be performed without undue risk. Moreover, permanent records of the pathology can be made by photography, films and videotapes in full color'.

Little did Steptoe, or indeed any of us, realise the impact that endoscopic procedures would have on the practice of obstetrics and gynecology in just seven short years. Endoscopy has now secured its place as an indispensable technology in the practice of gynecologic surgery. It is now clear that the future direction of gynecologic surgery will in large part be guided by the evolution of gynecologic endoscopy. This is the reason why the second edition of the *Atlas of Gynecologic Endoscopy* is so welcome. The new volume has been greatly expanded and covers in depth all of the significant advances in diagnostic and operative laparoscopy and hysteroscopy that have occurred during the past decade. In a highly readable and lavishly illustrated format, it provides the reader with comprehensive information on all pertinent applications of gynecologic endosopy, and brings the reader totally up-to-date on this exciting and rapidly changing technology. This is a superb atlas with nearly 600 pictures, 500 of which are in wonderful full color, making it easy for both the beginner and the seasoned professional to visualize the pathology and the operative procedures described. The text contains the latest information available, and the references are highly selective and pertinent.

The editors and authors who have contributed to this volume are among the international leaders in gynecologic endoscopy and represent a true European-American alliance. They provide a detailed and well illustrated description of the standard procedures as well as some more controversial issues and also of new operations which are on the 'cutting edge' of technology. Laparoscopic surgery for endometriosis and ectopic pregnancy, hysteroscopic myomectomy and endometrial ablation are given informative and complete coverage by experts. Less common and occasionally now controversial procedures such as the laparoscopic management of ovarian cysts, intratubal surgery and hysteroscopic sterilization are discussed by international authorities whose leadership and clinical research form the basis of the information they are imparting in their chapters. Newer and more advanced procedures such as laparoscopic hysterectomy, pelvic lymphadenectomy, and pelvic reconstructive surgery are discussed by some of the pioneers of these operations. Their extensive and invaluable experience makes this a truly unique text and atlas.

Surgeons rarely like to discuss complications, but any contemporary text must address the reality that on occasion, complications do occur. The strength of the chapters on complications of operative laparoscopy and hysteroscopy is that they give us insights into how to avoid and minimise complications of endoscopic surgery. This information is of particular value to those entering the field, but is also extremely useful to heighten the awareness of regular practitioners.

The beauty of the *Atlas of Gynecologic Endoscopy* lies in the profuse, accurate, clearly labelled and detailed color illustrations. Illustrations are essential in the study and practice of endoscopy, and this volume succeeds and builds upon the information presented in the first edition by providing a wealth of visual information to the reader. I am certain that these illustrations will be referred to time and time again.

The future of gynecologic surgery lies with gynecologic endoscopy. Alan Gordon, Victor Lewis and Alan deCherney, in this beautiful volume, have given us an exciting glimpse of this future. This volume will provide the student and practitioner alike a thorough, thoughtfully-written, and informative atlas that will be an invaluable guide for the contemporary practice of gynecology. The second edition of the *Atlas of Gynecologic Endoscopy* is destined to become a classic publication, and belongs in the library of every gynecologic surgeon.

John J Sciarra MD PhD
Thomas J Watkins Professor and Chairman
Department of Obstetrics and Gynecology
Northwestern University Medical School
Chicago, IL
USA

In the preface to the first edition of *Gynaecological Endoscopy*, published just seven years ago, we discussed the place of conservative laparoscopic surgery, intrauterine and intratubal endoscopy and laser endometrial ablation. As Dr Sciarra has observed in his elegant foreword to this edition, we did not realize then the enormous changes in surgical philosophy and the major technical advances that would occur in such a short time.

In this edition we have built on our past experience and now include almost all current thought. The field of endoscopy is changing so fast that it is impossible to produce a completely up-to-date text book or atlas. The chapters on instrumentation and diagnostic techniques give an overview of the current range of instruments and a practical guide to basic surgical technique. The overwhelming emphasis is now centered less on diagnostic procedures and more on the techniques of endoscopic surgery.

The laparoscopic management of ectopic pregnancy has proved to be superior to conventional laparotomy and is now the 'gold standard'. Other operations such as laparoscopic ovariotomy, are more controversial. Surgery for tubal pregnancy should be within the compass of all practising gynecologists and all trainees should be given the opportunity to develop expertise in performing these relatively simple procedures and be taught the appropriate clinical indication for their use.

Laparoscopic hysterectomy may soon replace open surgery for many abdominal hysterectomies except for the very large uterus with extensive adhesions. From its start in 1989 the procedure has gained in popularity and is now the operation which is in greatest demand in training courses for gynecologic surgeons. Although training in simple laparoscopic surgery should be part of the basic training for all gynecologists, operations such as hysterectomy should be taught in dedicated postgraduate training courses followed by supervision in the operating room until competence is gained.

The chapters on more advanced operations such as pelvic reconstruction and oncologic surgery are especially interesting because, even more than in conventional surgery, specialist training is vitally important. A urogynecologist or oncologist who is also a laparoscopic surgeon can provide women with all the benefits of minimal access surgery without compromising the standard of care. This relatively small number of expert gynecologic surgeons will form a subgroup of physicians with special expertise and experience.

Hysteroscopic surgery has also advanced in complexity in the last seven years. Ablative operations provide minimally invasive treatment for disordered uterine bleeding although even simpler therapy with hormonal intrauterine devices may soon be more widely available. We have included chapters on less common operations such as hysteroscopic sterilization, but the main place of hysteroscopic surgery seems to be in the treatment of submucous fibroids, septa and synechia. These techniques are described by some of the foremost exponents in the world.

In 1988 we singled out two names for special thanks – not only for their help in producing the first edition but for their pioneering work in endoscopy. The names of Professors Hans Frangenheim from Konstanz and Kurt Semm from Kiel still command the greatest respect and we are in their debt for their help and advice.

It is becoming more difficult to publish an atlas with high quality pictures. In the 1970's and 1980's many of us used still photography to record the operations and illustrate our work but now we use video cameras. We have included an updated chapter on documentation but the availability of high quality 'frame grabbing' facilities to transfer from video to slide is far from uniform.

No book of this size and breadth can be produced by a small group of authors. We would like to thank all our colleagues and friends in Europe and North America who have given freely of their time and expertise. We hope that they consider the finished work has been worth the effort.

Finally, we would like to thank our publishers, Mosby-Wolfe, and especially Jennifer Prast and Alison Taylor for their help and courtesy during the production and design of *Atlas of Gynecologic Endoscopy*.

Alan G Gordon
B Victor Lewis
Alan H DeCherney

CONTRIBUTING AUTHORS

Ediberto de Araujo, Jr. MD
Research Fellow
Division of Reproductive Endocrinology and
Infertility
University of California
Irvine, CA
USA

Santiago Dexeus MD
Head of Obstetrics and Gynecology
Department
Institut Universitari Dexeus
Barcelona
Spain

Alain J M Audebert MD
Ancien Chef de Clinique à la Facultié de
Médicine de Bordeaux
Ancien Assistant de Gynécologie-Obstétriques
des Hôpitaux
Gynaecological Endoscopy
Polyclinique de Bordeaux
Bordeaux
France

Jose P Balmaceda MD
Professor and Director
Division of Reproductive Endocrinology
and Infertility
Department of Obstetrics and Gynecology
University of California
Irvine, CA
USA

Ivo A Brosens MD
Director
Centre for Surgical Technology
Catholic University of Leuven
Leuven
Belgium

Jan Brundin, MD PhD
Associate Professor
Karolinska Institutet
Division of Obstetrics and Gynaecology
Danderyd Hospital
Danderyd
Sweden

Maurice A Bruhat MD
Chairman, Department of Obstetrics,
Gynaecology and Reproductive Medicine
Polyclinique de l'Hôtel-Dieu
Clermont Ferrand
Université d'Auvergne
Clermont Ferrand
France

Françoise Casanas-Roux BS
Department of Gynaecology
Catholic University of Louvain
Cliniques Universitaires St. Luc
Brussels
Belgium

Françoise Clerckx BS
Department of Gynaecology
Catholic University of Louvain
Cliniques Universitaires St. Luc
Brussels
Belgium

Joel M Childers MD
Associate Professor of Clinical Obstetrics and
Gynecology
Division of Gynecologic Oncology
University of Arizona
Tucson, AZ
USA

Ian D Cooke MB BS DGO MRCOG FRCOG
Professor of Obstetrics and Gynaecology
Jessop Hospital for Women
Sheffield
England, UK

James F Daniell MD FACOG
Clinical Professor of Obstetrics and
Gynecology
Vanderbilt University
Nashville, TN
USA

Alan H DeCherney, MD
Louis E Phaneuf, Professor and Chairman
Department of Obstetrics and Gynecology
Tufts University School of Medicine
New England Medical Center Hospital
Boston
USA

Michael P Diamond, MD
Professor of Obstetrics and Gynecology
Director, Reproductive Endocrinology and
Infertility
Hutzel Hospital/Wayne State University
Detroit, MI
USA

Jacques Donnez MD PhD
Department of Gynaecology
Catholic University of Louvain
Cliniques Universitaires St. Luc
Brussels
Belgium

Ray Garry, MD FRCOG
Vice President of the British Society of
Gynaecological Endoscopy
Consultant Gynaecologist
South Cleveland Hospital
Middlesborough
Director of Minimal Access Gynaecological
Surgery, St James's University Hospital, Leeds
Medical Director of the Womens' Endoscopic
Laser Foundation
Middlesborough and Leeds
England, UK

Victor Gomel MD FRCS(C)
Professor
Faculty of Medicine
University of British Columbia
Vancouver, B.C.
Canada

Alan G Gordon, FRCS FRCOG
Consultant Obstetrician and Gynaecologist
Hull and East Riding Hospital
Hull
England, UK

Jacques E Hamou MD
Hôpital Antoine Béclére
Clamart
Paris
France

Robert JS Hawthorn MD MRCOG
Consultant Gynaecologist
Southern General Hospital NHS Trust
Southern General Hospital
Glasgow
Scotland, UK

Bradley S Hurst MD
Assistant Professor
Reproductive Endocrinology and Infertility
Department of Obstetrics and Gynecology
University of Colorado Health Science Center
Denver, CO
USA

Salil Khandwala MD
Clinical Associate
Division of Gynaecological Endoscopy
Polyclinique de L'Hotel Dieu
University of Clermont Ferrand
Clermont Ferrand
France

Ramón Labastida MD
Head of Gynecologic Oncology Unit
Institut Universitari Dexeus
Barcelona
Spain

C Terence Lee MD
Clinical Instructor
Division of Reproductive Endocrinology and
Infertility
University of California
Los Angeles, CA
USA

John M Leventhal MD FACS FACOG
Department of Obstetrics and Gynecology
Harvard Medical School
Boston. MA
USA

B Victor Lewis MD FRCS FRCOG
Senior Consultant Gynaecologist
Mount Vernon and Watford Hospitals
NHS Trust
Watford General Hospital
Watford
England, UK

Adam L Magos BSc MD MRCOG
Consultant Obstetrician and Gynaecologist
Minimally Invasive Therapy Unit and
Endoscopy Training Centre
Royal Free Hospital
London
England, UK

Patricia E Munday MD FRCOG
Consultant Genitourinary Physician
Mount Vernon and Watford Hospitals
NHS Trust
Watford General Hospital
Watford
England, UK

Hubert Manhès MD
Diplômé du CES de Gynécologie-obstétrique
Président du Groupe de Recherche pour
l'Avancement de la Laparoscopie
Ancien externe des hôpitaux de Montpellier
Polyclinique La Pergola
Vichy
France

Amir Nasseri MD
Chief Resident
Division of Gynecologic Oncology
University of Arizona
Tucson, AZ
USA

Robert S Neuwirth MD
Director of Hysteroscopic Surgery
St Luke's-Roosevelt Hospital Center
Babcock Professor of Obstetrics and Gynecology
College of Physicians and Surgeons
Columbia University
New York
USA

Michelle Nisolle MD
Department of Gynaecology
Catholic University of Louvain
Cliniques Universitaires St. Luc
Brussels
Belgium

Jeffrey H Phipps BSc MD MRCOG
Consultant Gynaecologist and Director,
George Elliot Minimal Access Gynaecological
Surgery Unit
George Elliot Hospital
Nuneaton,
England, UK

Ian F Russell B.Med.Biol(Hons) MBChB FSARCS
Consultant Anaesthetist
Royal Hull Hospital Trust
Hull Royal Infirmary
Hull
England, UK

John A Rock MD
James Robert McCord Professor and Chairman
Department of Gynecology and Obstetrics
Emory University School of Medicine
Atlanta GA
USA

Ian W Scudamore MB BS MRACOG MRCOG
Lecturer, Department of Obstetrics and
Gynaecology
Jessop Hospital for Women
Sheffield
England

Patrick J Taylor MD
Chairman, Professor of Obstetrics and
Gynaecology
University of British Columbia
Vancouver. B.C.
Canada

Alicia Ubeda MD
Head of Gynaecologic Endoscopy Unit
Institut Universitari Dexeus
Barcelona
Spain

Jaime M Vasquez MD
Assistant Professor
Division of Reproductive Endocrinology
and Infertility
Department of Obstetrics and Gynecology
Vanderbilt University Medical School
Nashville, TN
USA

Arnaud Wattiez MD
Département de Gynécologie et Obstétrique
Université de Clermont-Ferrand 1
Clermont Ferrand
France

Rafael F Valle MD
Professor, Department of Obstetrics and
Gynecology
Northwestern University Medical School
Chicago, IL
USA

Jeremy T Wright MB.BS FRCOG
Consultant Gynaecologist
St Peter's Hospital
Chertsey
England, UK

INSTRUMENTS FOR DIAGNOSTIC AND OPERATIVE LAPAROSCOPY

1

Alan G Gordon

INTRODUCTION

It is not necessary to have a large range of instruments to perform diagnostic or operative laparoscopy; it is, however, necessary to have the correct instruments. Failure to do so may compromise the operation making it difficult to perform or impossible to complete with safety.

Laparoscopy has become widely accepted not only as a diagnostic tool but also as a means of access to the abdominal and pelvic cavities to perform surgical procedures. Instruments have been developed to allow a wide range of operations to be performed. These operations vary from simple procedures such as tubal sterilization and lysis of minor adhesions to complex operations such as the treatment of advanced endometriosis, conservative tubal surgery, pelvic lymphadenectomy and laparoscopically assisted vaginal hysterectomy. Many of the instruments in current use have been adapted from those used in other specialties. Others have been developed for the specific needs of endoscopic surgery. The main developments in the past 25 years in the latter instruments have been automated pneumoflators for safe distension of the abdomen, fiberoptic cables for transmission of light and telescopes with rod lens systems which provide a clear, undistorted view. The safety of laparoscopic surgery has been helped by better control of bleeding by electrocoagulation, hemostatic clips and ligatures. The scope has been increased by the development of forceps for effective and gentle tissue handling and electrical and laser instruments for precise tissue dissection. The essential equipment for performing diagnostic or operative laparoscopy is as follows:

1. pneumoperitoneum apparatus and insufflating needles
2. laparoscope
3. light source
4. trocars
5. forceps and scissors
6. electro- and thermocoagulation
7. instruments for introduction of laser
8. needle holders
9. flushing cannula
10. clips and rings for tubal sterilization
11. chip camera

PNEUMOFLATOR

The first requirement for laparoscopy is the provision of a safe pneumoperitoneum. The mechanically monitored pneumoflator is adequate for diagnostic laparoscopy and relatively simple operations. It allows continuous flow of carbon dioxide (CO_2) with automatic refilling of the abdomen which can be augmented by rapid refill at a rate of 3 l/min under direct visual control. The mechanical pneumoflator is not sufficiently responsive when performing complex surgery. It is unsafe for a surgeon to operate and at the same time check that the pneumoflator is being used properly. The intra-abdominal pressure and the volume of gas must be kept within safe limits.

An electronic CO_2 pneumoflator should be used when complex operations are being performed (**1.1**). This is fully automatic and simultaneously measures the intra-abdominal and insufflation pressures which can be preset to cut out at a selected level. The gas deficit is also electronically determined and can be replaced at a rate of 6 l/min. This is often necessary when aspirating smoke during laser surgery or when using copious amounts of fluid during pelvic lavage or hydrodissection in conventional laparoscopic surgery. When using this instrument the surgeon can be confident that the pneumoperitoneum is maintained safely while he concentrates on the operation.

When performing operative laparoscopy it is safer to use carbon dioxide (CO_2) than nitrous oxide (N_2O). Carbon dioxide is 20-fold more soluble in blood and body fluids than air or oxygen. However absorbtion at a rate of over 100 ml/min may lead to hypercarbia and cardiac arrythmia. This can be prevented by hyperventilation and controlled positive pressure respiration. In all cases where CO_2 is used, the patient's pulse rate and blood pressure and blood gases should be continuously recorded to detect the earliest signs of circulatory or biochemical changes. Carbon dioxide pneumoperitoneum may also cause postoperative pain as a result of formation of hydrocarbonic acid which is irritant to the peritoneum. Nitrous oxide is safer as regards circulatory changes but any advantage in this respect is offset by the fact that it can support combustion. Methane gas may leak into the peritoneal cavity if there has been inadvertent puncture of bowel by the Veress' needle or trocar. Methane in combination with N_2O produces a mixture of gas which is explosive when high frequency current is used. Several serious complications and deaths have been reported. The main advantage of N_2O is that it does not produce as much peritoneal pain as CO_2 and therefore it has met with some favor in diagnostic laparoscopy and in laparoscopy under local anesthesia.

The gas is introduced into the abdomen with a spring-loaded needle (**1.2**) originally designed by Veress' of Budapest in 1936 for the production of pneumothorax in the treatment of pulmonary tuberculosis. The Veress' needle is available in three different lengths. Normally the 7 cm needle should be used but longer ones up to 15 cm in length are available for obese patients or for introducing the pneumoperitoneum through the posterior vaginal fornix. The longer needle may also be used as a palpating probe. The sharp needle point is automatically withdrawn into its sheath by the spring which allows the needle to be used as a probe for lifting organs and palpating their consistency.

TROCARS AND CANNULAE

The choice of trocar is debatable. The pyramidal trocar is easier to insert but is more likely to perforate a blood vessel in the abdominal wall. The conical trocar, although safer in that respect,

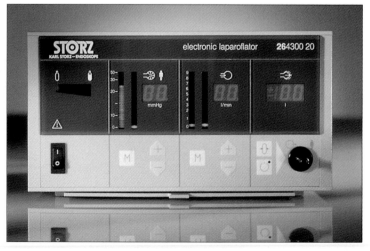

1.1 Electronic pneumoperitoneum apparatus.

requires a stronger thrust to insert it with consequent risk of accidentally perforating intra-abdominal organs. The primary trocar and cannula is always inserted blindly after production of the pneumoperitoneum. The secondary trocars and cannulae should always be introduced under direct visual control (**1.3**). The first trocar and cannula has an additional port for maintenance of the pneumoperitoneum.

As with all instruments, the trocars tend to become blunt with use. Disposable trocars have become popular in recent years because they are always sharp and so can be introduced with less force. However, they are expensive.

LAPAROSCOPES

The development of the rod lens in 1953 by Professor Hopkins of Reading has improved the performance of laparoscopes giving a brighter image with better definition and a wider viewing angle (**1.4**). A 5 mm telescope may be satisfactory for standard diagnostic laparoscopy. The 10–11 mm instrument is preferable for video laparoscopy and for operative procedures. The majority of laparoscopists prefer to use a 0° instrument. The 30° laparoscope was designed to enable the surgeon to see aspects of organs which are hidden from direct view. Orientation is easier with a straight telescope and, if ancillary instruments are used for manipulation, a satisfactory view can always be obtained. The lens system of the laparoscope provides magnification of x2 but this can be increased a further twofold by the addition of an endo-loupe to permit laparoscopic 'microsurgery'. Further magnification may be obtained with the use of video monitoring which, with modern high resolution cameras, allows very accurate definition.

Some gynecologists prefer to use the operating laparoscope instead of the standard telescope. The disadvantage is that the lens system is narrower and therefore there is less light available. The advantage is that there is a channel for the introduction of operating instruments or laser fibers. The operating laparoscope may also be used to introduce a second telescope for salpingoscopy or for intra-ovarian surgery in the technique of 'double-optic laparoscopy' (Chapter 4). The eye-piece may be parallel to the telescope or at an angle of 30°, the choice is a matter of personal preference

The pediatric laparoscope is essential for safe examination of the pre-pubertal child in whom even a 5 mm laparoscope is too large. This is becoming more important as laparoscopy is used more frequently by general surgeons both for diagnosis and to gain access to the abdomen for operations such as appendicectomy.

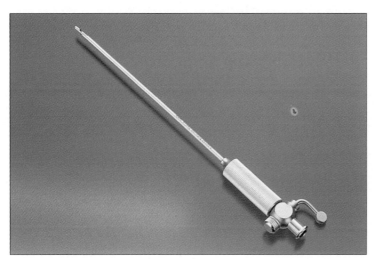

1.2 Veress needle.

1.3 Insertion of secondary trocar.

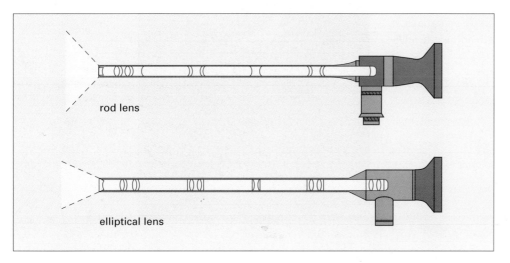

rod lens

elliptical lens

1.4 The rod lens gives a brighter image with a wider viewing angle.

LIGHT SOURCES

The standard light source with 150 watt power is satisfactory for diagnostic laparoscopy but, when performing operative laparoscopy or using closed circuit color television (CCTV), a cold light fountain with 250 watt halogen lamp is necessary. This maintains a constant color temperature and allows automatic variation of the light intensity by the camera (**1.5**). The modern laparoscopist should be trained in video laparoscopy which allows him to work while watching the image on a screen instead of through-the-lens viewing. This is especially important in procedures which may involve operating times in excess of an hour. Some surgical techniques may be uncomfortable or impossible because of difficulty in reaching the handles of the instruments while looking down the laparoscope. The modern chip camera (**1.6**) weighs as little as 130 g and has a zoom lens with automatic color setting and a high speed shutter to eliminate overexposure. Its development has been one of the major factors in the increased popularity and scope of laparoscopic surgery. It allows the operator to work in a comfortable position, the assistant to manipulate tissues more accurately and the trainee to be supervised more safely. The light source, video system including video recorder and the pneumoperitoneum apparatus can all be installed in a mobile cart.

FORCEPS

A variety of forceps are available for diagnostic and operative laparoscopy. The majority of forceps now have scissor grips instead of spring-loaded grips. These allow more accurate manipulation and have a stronger grasp. When using spring-loaded forceps the blades are withdrawn into the shaft of the instrument while they close so it is more difficult to apply them accurately. This may lead to tissue trauma especially during fine tubal surgery. Many modern forceps also have a mechanism to lock them firmly on to tissues. This allows the operator or assistant to exert constant traction during prolonged dissection of tissues. Two or three grasping forceps should be available. One or two should have atraumatic blades and another should have teeth for stronger traction (**1.7, 1.8**).

SCISSORS

Scissors should be fine enough to allow accurate dissection but strong enough not to be blunted by frequent use. This problem has recently been improved by the introduction of self-sharpening scissors but many of the instruments available still have a limited life span and must be replaced frequently. Some gynecologists prefer

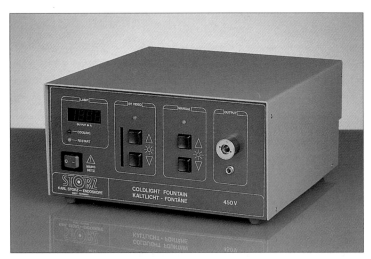

1.5 Video cold light fountain.

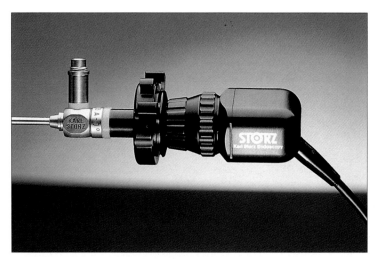

1.6 Chip camera with automatic exposure and zoom lens.

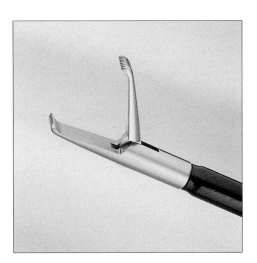

1.7 Non-toothed Forceps.

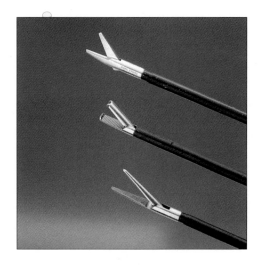

1.8 Atraumatic and toothed grasping forceps.

hook scissors (**1.9**) which are designed to pull the tissues into the blades and facilitate cutting but others prefer straight scissors which may be more accurate in use (**1.10**). It is important that one of the blades is fixed to allow the scissors to put tension on tissues before cutting them. This is more difficult if both blades move. Fine microscissors are available for performing delicate surgery when the standard ones would be too large (**1.11**).

Larger scissors introduced through a 11 mm diameter cannula may occasionally be necessary to divide strong pedicles. Similar forceps are used to grasp tough tissues (**1.12**). The 11 mm instruments can be introduced through the abdominal wall by enlarging the original incision with a dilating set which increases the diameter of the incision without further cutting.

ELECTRO- AND THERMOCOAGULATION

Safe and effective control of intraperitoneal bleeding is an essential prerequisite for any form of surgery and in laparoscopic surgery can be achieved in several ways. Bleeding may be prevented by careful recognition of the correct tissue plane and by taking care to cut only in an avascular area. Bleeding from minor vessels is also prevented by the raised intra-abdominal pressure produced by the pneumoperitoneum. When bleeding does occur from small vessels it may also be controlled by using lavage fluid at 40°C.

The mainstay of hemostasis, however, is electro- or thermocoagulation. The classic instrument for electrocoagulation was the forceps designed by Palmer for use with a monopolar current which he originally described for tubal electrocoagulation. Unfortunately the high frequency monopolar current was responsible for a number of complications resulting from accidental burns. First, excessive heat production can occur at the operation site and the heat may be directly transmitted to adjacent organs to cause thermal damage. Second, the current must return from the operation site to the return electrode on its way back to the generator. The pathway taken by the current is unpredictable but is usually along the surface of loops of bowel towards the pelvic side walls. The return plate should be large so that the power density of the current is low at the point of contact with the skin. Accidental injury to the bowel may result from contact with an active instrument or one with defective insulation. The burn may be outside the surgeon's visual field. However, while high frequency monopolar current should not be used for extensive coagulation, modern microdiathermy instruments provide a safe and effective method of cutting fine adhesions, performing neosalpingostomy or coagulating areas of endometriosis.

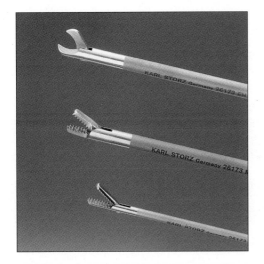

1.9 Hook scissors, needleholder and grasper.

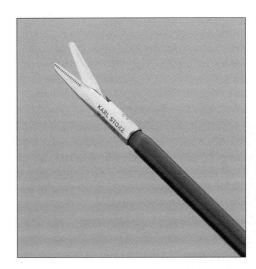

1.10 Straight scissors.

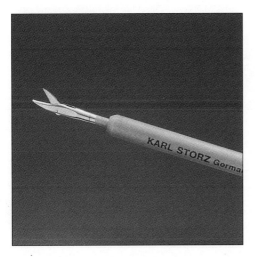

1.11 Microscissors (26169S).

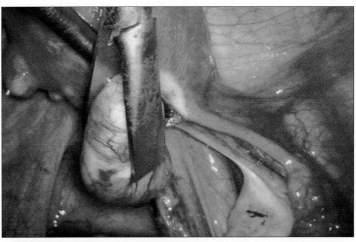

1.12 Grasping a fibroid at myomectomy.

The dangers of monopolar current in tubal sterilization were realized in the early 1970s when the operation became more popular throughout the world. In 1972 Frangenheim of Konstanz introduced bipolar electrocoagulation which is safer than monopolar current (**1.13, 1.14**). In this technique the current passes from one blade of the forceps to the other, coagulating the tissues between the blades (**1.15**). It is still possible for burns to be produced from direct transmission of heat to other tissues. Moreover, if two different electrical generators, one monopolar and the other bipolar, are connected simultaneously to the patient, it is possible for the current generated by the bipolar instrument to be attracted to the return plate of the monopolar generator and to cause inadvertent burns to organs distant from the operation site. It is imperative, therefore, that the monopolar generator is always switched off when bipolar current is being used.

The third type of energy used to secure hemostasis is thermocoagulation in which forceps are heated to 120–140°C for a preset time of 20–40 seconds (**1.16**). The proteins in the tissue between the forcep blades are coagulated. This is probably safer but the tissue response is slower than bipolar electrocoagulation. The thermocoagulator has a dial indicating the operating temperature and also an acoustic signal so that the surgeon is aware that the instrument is functioning without lifting his eye from the operation field.

LASER

Laser has become a popular surgical tool during the past 10 years. It allows precise tissue destruction with highly predictable results. The type, power and delivery system depend on the tissue reaction required, be it vaporization or coagulation. Both rigid and flexible systems are available for laparosopic surgery. An operating or standard laparosope may be used.

The commonest laser in use is the CO_2 laser which must be delivered via a rigid system of prisms and lenses. The articulated arm of the laser is connected to the laparoscope via the laser coupler which has a joystick for adjusting the direction of the laser beam, a quick-release attachment for the laparoscope and an interchangable lens housing. Alternatively the laser may be connected to a second-puncture probe which may include a smoke evacuating channel. When CO_2 laser is being used it is necessary to have a back-stop to prevent damage to tissues beyond the target organ.

The other lasers in current use, argon, neodymium:yttrium-aluminum-garnet (Nd:YAG) and potassium-titanyl-phosphate (KTP) laser may all be delivered along flexible fiberoptic cables increasing their versatility but requiring directional devices on the introducing channel of the laparoscope.

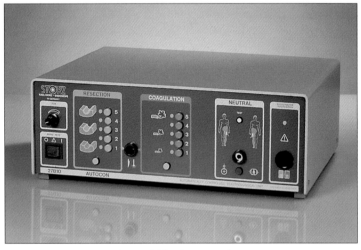

1.13 Combined unipolar and bipolar coagulator.

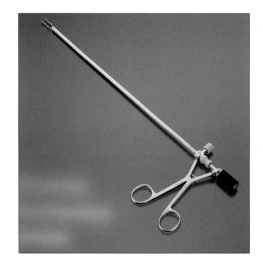

1.14 Bipolar forceps.

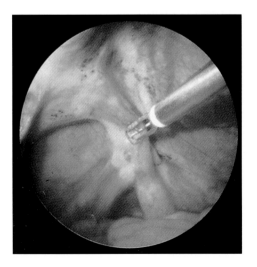

1.15 Coagulation of the uterosacral ligaments with bipolar current.

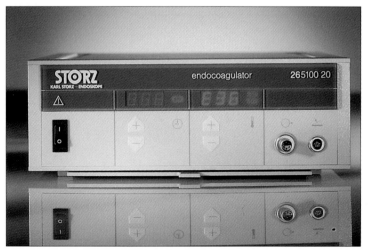

1.16 Thermocoagulator.

Safety for the theater staff as well as the patient is paramount when laser surgery is being performed. All staff must wear special goggles to prevent eye damage. Some of the risks to operating room staff may be minimized by using video cameras instead of having filters on the lenses. Warning notices must also be placed on all entrances to the operating room and windows must have blinds to prevent eye damage to passers-by. The foot switch of the laser must always be kept separate from the switch for the electric generators. It is essential to have staff who are specifically trained in the management of laser apparatus and to have a laser safety officer who is responsible for supervising all aspects of safety.

CO_2 laser is valuable for incising tissues but is not an effective coagulant. It is always necessary to have available additional means of securing hemostasis such as thermo- or bipolar electrocoagulation.

SUTURES, CLIPS AND STAPLES

Hemostasis and tissue apposition may be achieved in laparoscopic surgery by using sutures, clips or fibrin glue. The value of sutures is limited by the difficulty in performing fine surgery when the working distance between the surgeon's hands and the tissue is 35 cm or more. The needle must be strong enough to be held with the laparoscopic needle holder but the finest suture material available for endoscopic surgery is 6/0. It is, therefore, impossible to emulate microsurgical suturing in laparoscopic surgery despite the advantages of magnification and the excellent vision obtained with modern endoscopes. Nevertheless suturing is necessary in some operations although its use in others is debatable. This is because sutures may produce tiny areas of tissue ischemia which may predispose to the formation of adhesions.

Ligatures are of value when it is unsafe to use thermal energy. In this case an endoscopic ligature may be applied round the pedicle and the knot tightened by pushing down the tip of the applicator (**1.17**, **1.18**). Sutures may be tied intracorporeally or extracorporeally. The latter knots are simply tightened with a knot pusher.

Hemostatic clips may be applied to control bleeding or to ligate vessels before dividing them (**1.19**, **1.20**). Their development has contributed much to the techniques of advanced laparoscopic surgery which have been popularized in the late 1980s and early 1990s.

Staples have now been developed to occlude vessels and simultaneously divide tissues. These are applied with disposable

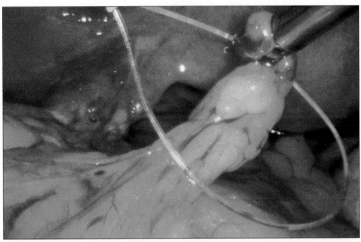

1.17 Endoloop being applied to a pedicle.

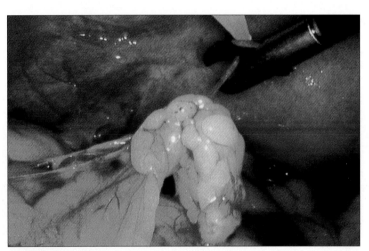

1.18 Suture being cut after pulling loop tight.

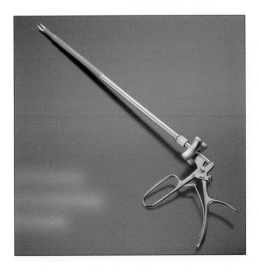

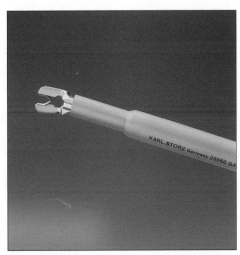

1.19–20 Clip applicator.

instruments which insert up to three rows of staples in two separate lines. A cutting blade in the applicator then divides the tissues between the rows of staples. This makes division of structures such as the broad ligament rapid and safe.

Tissue glue may be used to cover surfaces to prevent adhesion formation or to reperitonize areas where the peritoneum has been removed or destroyed by laser. Tissue glue may also be used to close defects in the ovary following ovariotomy.

PERITONEAL LAVAGE AND HYDRODISSECTION

It is essential to remove blood and wash away fibrin deposits to prevent adhesion formation. Heparinized Ringer lactate solution may be delivered under pressure via a two-way cannula powered by an Aquapurator pump (**1.21, 1.22**) which allows irrigation and aspiration of fluid and debris. The same instrument may be used to perform hydrodissection. In this technique an incision is made between two tissue planes and the force of the fluid used to dissect the tissues without danger of bleeding or perforation. The dissection may usually be completed bloodlessly by scissors when the adherent organs have been separated from one another. Hydrodissection also allows fluid to be injected deep to the peritoneum to provide a back-stop for laser and protect deeper structures.

CLIP AND RING APPLICATORS FOR TUBAL STERILIZATION

Female tubal sterilization is probably the commonest laparoscopic operation performed by most gynecologists. A variety of techniques are available including monopolar and bipolar electrocoagulation and thermocoagulation. Mechanical devices have increased in popularity in the past two decades because of the complications experienced in the 1970s from electrocoagulation, These devices include spring-loaded clips, locking clips made from titanium and silastic and silicone rings applied over a loop of tube. The applicators may be used through the channel of an operating laparoscope or through a second puncture according to the preference of the surgeon.

CONCLUSION

The basic instruments for diagnostic laparoscopy should be available in every gynecological operating room. Any diagnostic laparoscopic procedure may develop into an operative laparoscopic procedure if the surgeon has the skill and the instruments to treat the patient in this manner. The instruments should be acquired as the surgeon's training develops and his capability increases. Initially the surgeon should be able to carry out simple laparoscopic surgery and, after approrpriate training and experience, more complex procedures. When that stage is reached laparotomy for most gynecological conditions should become a rarity.

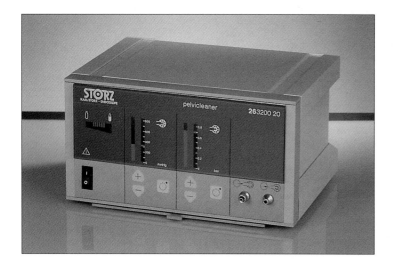

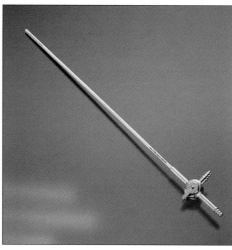

1.21–22 Aquapurator pump.

DIAGNOSTIC LAPAROSCOPY

2

Alan G Gordon

INTRODUCTION

Diagnostic laparoscopy is one of the commonest operations in modern gynecological practice. Direct visualization of the abdominal and pelvic organs allows a definitive diagnosis to be made in many conditions where clinical examination and less invasive techniques such as ultrasound fail to identify the problem. Every trainee should be taught the technique of laparoscopy. This should include the routine use of safety protocols during the introduction of instruments and the systematic examination of the abdomen and pelvis. Moreover every gynecologist should be capable of proceeding from diagnostic laparoscopy to perform a range of surgical procedures which will be discussed in subsequent chapters in this Atlas.

TECHNIQUE OF LAPAROSCOPY

POSITION OF THE PATIENT

The patient should be anesthetized using muscle relaxants, endotracheal intubation and intermittent positive pressure respiration as described in Chapter 1. The anesthetist should continuously monitor the patient's heart rate, blood pressure and blood gases. It is common practice to place the patient in a modified lithotomy position with the legs flexed to 45°. However, it is better to abduct the legs without flexion. This allows an assistant to manipulate the uterus and does not interfere with the use of ancillary instruments. There should be a 15° Trendelenburg tilt to allow the bowel to be lifted out of the pelvic cavity. The tilt may have to be steeper if more complex surgical procedures become necessary. It is prudent to ensure that the bowel is empty and can be easily lifted out of the pelvis. The patient's buttocks should protrude over the end of the operating table which should have a non-slip mattress to prevent her sliding cephalad on the table.

PREPARATION FOR LAPAROSCOPY

The operating room nurse should have available all the basic laparoscopy instruments and also those for operative laparoscopy and laparotomy. The surgeon should cleanse the abdomen with a suitable antiseptic solution, paying particular attention to the umbilicus. At the same time the assistant should cleanse the vulvar and vagina, catheterize the bladder and apply a tenaculum to the cervix to manipulate the uterus.

INSERTION OF PNEUMOPERITONEUM

The surgeon should first check the patency of the Veress' needle and ensure that the spring mechanism is functioning. A small incision should be made in the base of the umbilicus and the needle inserted while the abdominal wall is lifted with the other hand. This prevents damage to the underlying viscera and the major vessels (**2.1**). The needle should be held by the milled ring and should be heard to give two clicks as it passes through the fascia and then the peritoneum. The insertion should always be at 90° to the surface through the deepest part of the umbilicus. The abdominal wall is at its thinnest at that point and the peritoneum is firmly applied to it. It will not peel off with pressure from the needle and predispose to an extraperitoneal insufflation of gas. Insertion of the needle at another site may be necessary if there are adhesions beneath the umbilicus but it should be remembered that the abdominal wall at these sites may be thicker and the peritoneum more loosely applied.

The position of the tip of the Veress' needle should be checked by the aspiration test. A 20 ml syringe with normal saline is attached to the Veress' needle and aspirated to ensure that the needle is not in bowel or a major vessel. About 10 ml of saline should then be injected rapidly and aspirated again (**2.2, 2.3**). If the needle is correctly sited the saline will be distributed between loops of bowel and no fluid will be withdrawn. If the needle is in the abdominal wall or in an adhesion, clear fluid will be withdrawn; if it is in bowel or a blood vessel the aspirate will be stained brown or red. In this case the surgeon must decide whether or not to proceed to laparotomy. Alternatively the test may be performed by attaching an empty syringe to the Veress' needle, aspirating to make sure no feces or blood is withdrawn and then injecting 20 ml of air and repeating the aspiration. If the needle is sited correctly, nothing will be withdrawn but, if the needle is in the wrong position, gas or brown or red fluid will appear.

Transumbilical insertion of the needle may be difficult or dangerous if the patient is grossly obese or has scars on the abdominal

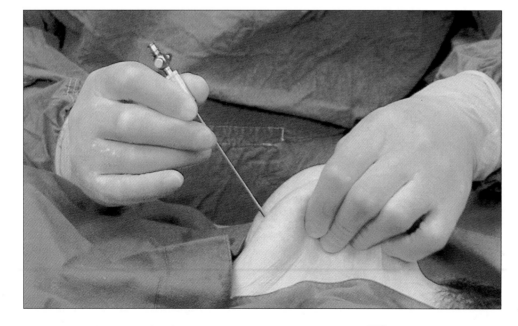

2.1 Insertion of Veress' needle.

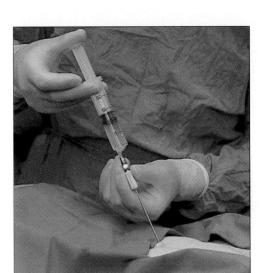

2.2 Aspiration test.

wall from previous operations. In this case the pneumoperitoneum may be introduced through the posterior vaginal fornix using a tenaculum to pull the cervix forwards which puts the uterosacral ligaments and the floor of the pouch of Douglas on tension (**2.4**). The needle may then be inserted using the same safety precautions as before to ensure that it is correctly sited before inducing the pneumoperitoneum.

The pneumoperitoneum is formed by introducing 1–2 liters of carbon dioxide (CO_2) at a rate of 1 l/min. Higher flow rates should only be used under direct vision after the laparoscope has been inserted. When the pneumoperitoneum is complete, the peritoneal cavity should be tested for adhesions using the sounding test. This is performed by attaching an intravenous needle to the 20 ml syringe which should now be half filled with saline. The pneumoperitoneum should be explored below the umbilicus at several points. The presence of space is confirmed by the ability to aspirate gas bubbles and its depth may be estimated by the length to which the needle can be inserted and gas aspirated (**2.5, 2.6**). Only then should the primary trocar and cannula be inserted.

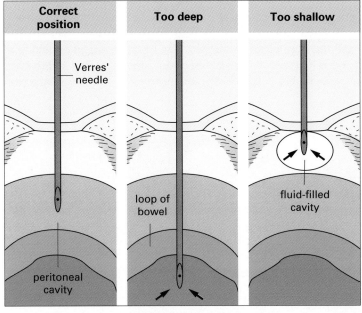

2.3 Position of the Verres' needle during aspiration.

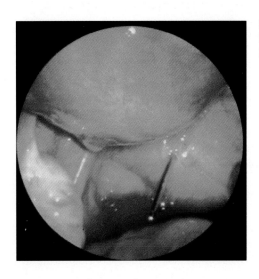

2.4 Veress' needle inserted through posterior fornix.

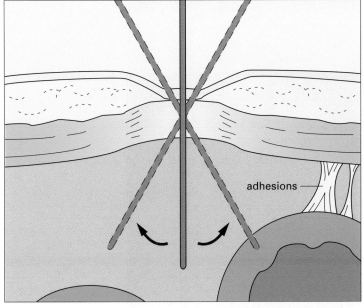

2.5 Sounding test.

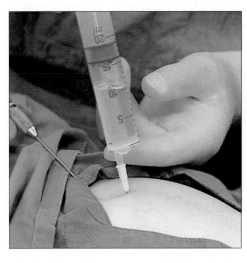

2.6 Sounding test.

INSERTION OF THE LAPAROSCOPE

During insertion of the primary trocar and cannula the upper abdominal wall should be compressed by the free hand to make the lower abdominal wall tense. The trocar and cannula may then be safely inserted along a zig-zag path using the extended fore finger to prevent sudden and deep penetration. If the line of insertion is straight there may be risk of herniation of omentum or bowel through the incision.

When the trocar and cannula have been inserted correctly gas may escape. This indicates the tip is in the peritoneal cavity. The trocar should be removed and a warmed laparoscope introduced. It is always necessary to use secondary portals of entry through which ancillary instruments can be introduced to allow organs to be retracted or lifted so that all their aspects may be examined. The ancillary instrument may be a long Veress' needle, a probe or a pair of forceps. The secondary trocar and cannula must always be inserted under direct vision. They may be introduced within the 'safety triangle' whose base is formed by the bladder and whose apex is the umbilicus while the obliterated umbilical arteries form its lateral walls. Alternatively they may be inserted lateral to the artery which should always be identified by direct vision through the laparoscope or by transilluminating the abdominal wall.

INSPECTION OF THE ABDOMINAL ORGANS

Inspection of the abdominal organs must always be performed in a systematic manner. The inspection should start with cecum and appendix (**2.7**) and proceed upwards on the right side to the ascending colon until the hepatic flexure is reached. The right lobe of the liver and gall bladder should now be inspected (**2.8**). It may be necessary to reverse the Trendelenburg tilt to allow gas to flow to the upper abdomen to obtain a clear view of the liver. The telescope should then be withdrawn a little to allow it to pass the ligamentum falciparum and reach the left lobe of the liver. The anterior aspect of the stomach should be inspected but the spleen cannot normally be seen without retracting the stomach which is rarely indicated. Finally, the descending colon should be inspected as far as the sigmoid colon. It should be remembered that there are normally adhesions between the descending colon and the pelvic side wall and, sometimes, also to the left round ligament. These are physiologic and need not be disturbed unless better access to the left

adnexa is needed. The diagnosis of diverticular disease may be confirmed by palpating the consistency of the bowel with the probe or forceps. The altered consistency of the bowel is often obvious.

INSPECTION OF THE PELVIC ORGANS

The pelvic organs may be examined when inspection of the upper abdomen is complete. Detailed inspection is only possible by manipulating the uterus to bring all its aspects into view and by using an ancillary probe or forceps to aid the full examination of the fallopian tubes and ovaries. It is impossible to perform a complete examination of the pelvic organs using a single puncture technique. The examination must be systematic. It is usual to commence with the uterus and proceed in a clockwise direction.

The uterus should first be examined starting with the fundus followed by the anterior and posterior walls (**2.9**). The size and shape of the uterus should be noted as should the presence of intramural or subserous fibroids and adhesions which may limit uterine mobility.

The anterior cul de sac should next be explored. The bladder peritoneum is a frequent site of peritoneal endometriosis (**2.10**) and occasionally adhesion of the bladder to the uterus may be seen resulting from previous surgery. The round ligament should next be seen followed by inspection of the tube in its full length from cornu to fimbriae. It is nearly always necessary to lift the tube with

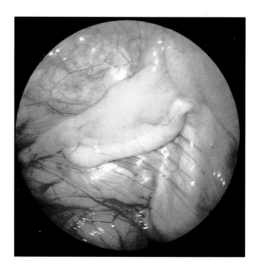

2.7 Inspection of appendix.

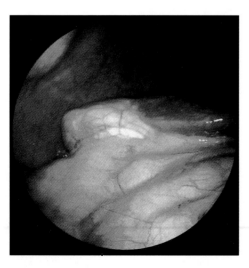

2.8 Normal liver and gall bladder.

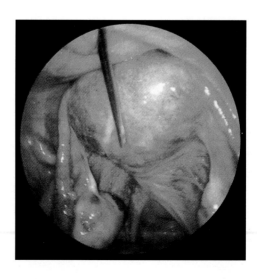

2.9 Inspection of uterus.

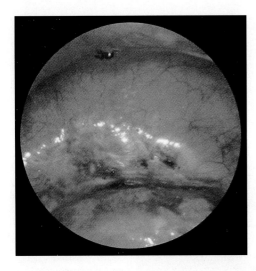

2.10 Endometriosis on surface of bladder.

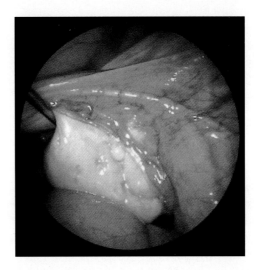

2.11 Lifting ovary with probe under the ovarian ligament.

a probe or forceps to see the fimbriae. This should always be done as there may be adhesions or phimosis even if the tube is patent. Peritubal adhesions and adhesions between the tube and ovary must be looked for as they may interfere with its motility and result in infertility. They may also be the only visible sign of endometriosis. Mild adhesions may be lysed with electrosurgery, scissors or laser. If there are more extensive adhesions it may be necessary

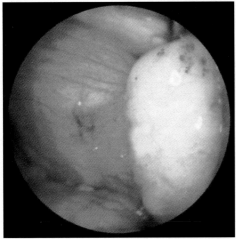
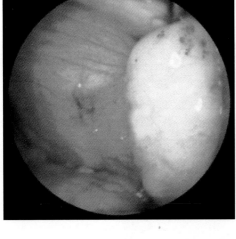

2.12 Adhesions on medial surface of ovary.

to investigate tubal morphology further by salpingoscopy (Chapter 4) to decide on the optimum form of treatment.

When the tube has been inspected, attention should turn to the ovary. This can only be examined with the help of a retractor to enable both aspects to be seen (2.11) without which fine adhesions could be missed (2.12). The ovary may be lifted by a second instrument placed under the round ligament of the ovary or, less commonly, under the infundibulo-pelvic ligament. Detailed inspection of the ovary should also include seeking evidence of its function as well as signs of disease such as endometriosis.

The broad ligament may be the site of endometriosis as may the uterosacral ligaments or the floor of the pouch of Douglas. The laparoscopist should be capable of treating such lesions by electrosurgery or laser (2.13).

The examination should now continue in a clockwise direction to inspect the left side of the pelvis and will be complete when the anterior cul de sac has been reached again. Failure to use a systematic approach such as this is a common cause of significant pathology being missed.

INDICATIONS FOR DIAGNOSTIC LAPAROSCOPY

NON-ACUTE CONDITIONS

Diagnostic laparoscopy is indicated in a number of non-acute conditions which are listed in 2.14.

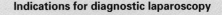

2.13 Laser to endometriosis in rectovaginal septum.

Indications for diagnostic laparoscopy
Non-acute conditions
Infertility Chronic pelvic pain Suspected endometriosis Suspected chronic pelvic inflammmatory disease Evaluation of uterine anomaly Prior to tubal reconstructive surgery

2.14 Indications for laparoscopy.

Infertility

The investigation of infertility is one of the commonest indications for diagnostic laparoscopy. Following inspection of the uterus for fibroids and developomental abnormalities and the anterior cul de sac for endometriosis, attention should be focused on the fallopian tubes which must be inspected from cornua to fimbriae. An oval thickening of the proximal isthmus may suggest salpingitis isthmica nodosa (**2.15**). In this case one may see blue blebs of sub-peritoneal methylene blue in the diverticulae after chromopertubation. A more irregular swelling of the proximal tube is suggestive of isthmic endometriosis (**2.16**).

The ampulla should next be examined and its diameter and mobility assessed. Adhesions between the tube and ovary may interfere with tubal transport. These may be mild as in **2.17** where they are undergoing laser adhesiolysis or severe as in **2.18** where they interfere with both tubal mobility and ovum pick-up. Adhesiolysis by electrosurgery, scissor dissection or laser may restore fertility in mild or moderate adhesive disease. The degree of distension of the ampulla resulting from distal tubal obstruction should be noted. A thin-walled hydrosalpinx with little distension (**2.19**) carries a better prognosis for reconstructive tubal surgery than a distended thick-walled hydrosalpinx (**2.20**). In patients with infertility and an apparently normal tube, patency should be demonstrated by chromopertubation with dilute methylene blue. Initially bubbles appear

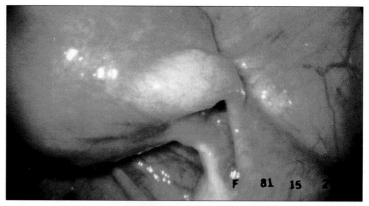

2.15 Salpingitis isthmica nodosa.

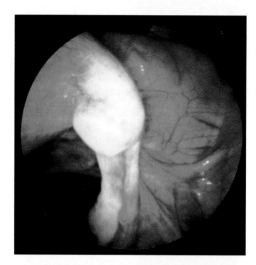

2.16 Isthmic endometriosis.

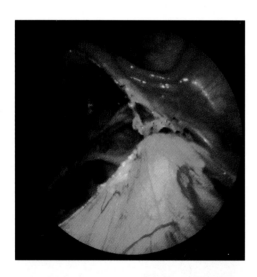

2.17 Mild peritubal adhesions treated with laser.

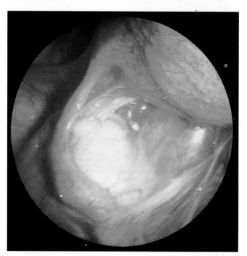

2.18 Severe peritubal adhesions.

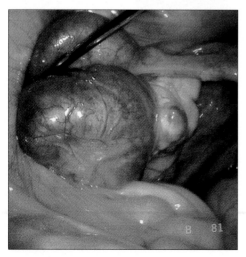

2.19 Thin-walled hydrosalpinx.

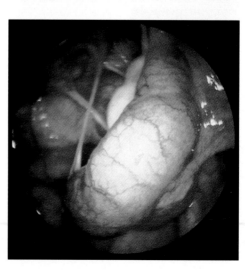

2.20 Thick-walled hydrosalpinx.

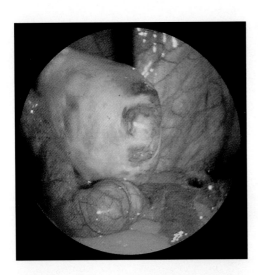

2.21 Gas bubbles coming from tube.

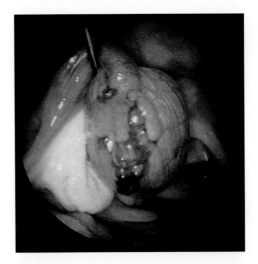

2.22 Methylene blue spilling from tube.

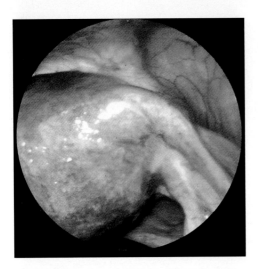

2.23 Proximal tubal block with intravasation of methylene blue.

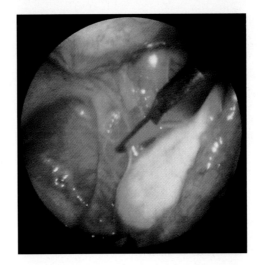

2.24 Peri-ovarian adhesions.

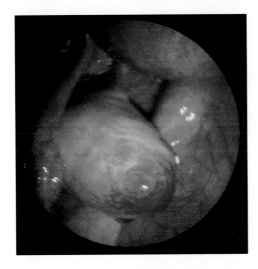

2.25 Follicular cyst.

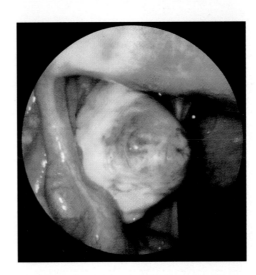

2.26 Stigma – double ovulation has occured.

at the fimbrial opening (**2.21**) followed by spillage of dye (**2.22**). If there is proximal tubal blockage no dye will be seen in the tube. Sometimes dye may be seen in the uterine veins due to intravasation of fluid under pressure (**2.23**). The presence of peritubal adhesions or distal blockage may be an indication for more detailed investigation of tubal mucosal morphology by salpingoscopy.

When the inspection of the tube has been completed, attention should turn to the ovary, which must be examined with the help of a probe or forceps to enable both aspects to be seen (**2.24**). Examination of the ovary should include evidence of its function. The presence of a follicular cyst (**2.25**) or the stigma following ovulation (**2.26**) are proof of ovarian activity. Other conditions such as polycystic ovarian disease may be diagnosed (**2.27**), as may congenital failure of ovarian function such as streak ovary (**2.28**) or an ovotestis (**2.29**). It should be remembered that the ovary is a common site of endometriosis.

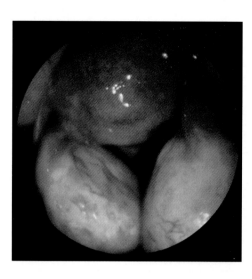

2.27 Polycystic ovary.

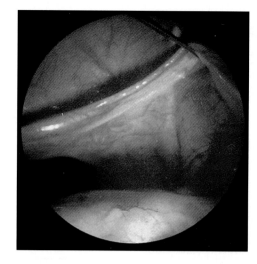

2.28 Streak ovary.

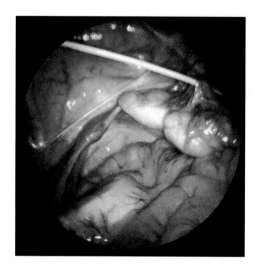

2.29 Ovotestis.

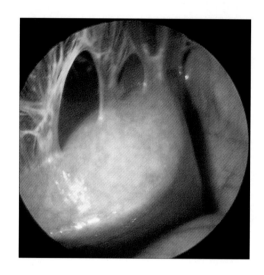

2.30 Fitz-Hugh–Curtis syndrome.

2.31 Omental adhesions.

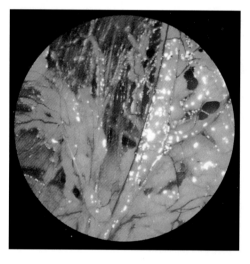

Chronic Pelvic Pain

Laparoscopy is often indicated in the investigation of chronic pelvic pain. The examination should be systematic and include evaluation of the whole abdominal cavity. Sometimes the only evidence of a chlamydial infection is the presence of subdiaphragmatic adhesions which constitute the Fitz-Hugh–Curtis syndrome (**2.30**). Omental adhesions or adhesions between the large bowel and abdominal wall (**2.31**) may cause pain by traction on the bowel. Peri-appendicular adhesions or irregularity in its outline may suggest endometriosis of the appendix which can be removed laparoscopically.

Suspected Endometriosis

Ovarian or pelvic peritoneal endometriosis may be diagnosed and treated by laparoscopic surgery. It is important to recognize the earliest signs of endometriosis which may present as slight alteration of the vascular pattern of the parietal peritoneum before progressing to red or black plaques (**2.32**). The sequelae of extensive adhesions may cause pain and be an indication for both diagnostic and operative laparoscopy (**2.33**).

Suspected Chronic Pelvic Inflammatory Disease

The diagnosis of the sequelae of chronic pelvic inflammatory disease (PID) and its differentiation from endometriosis can only be made by direct visualization of the lesions. There is frequently no significant history of a preceeding illness and the patient may present with chronic pain or infertility. Laparoscopy may reveal subdiaphragmatic adhesions. pelvic adhesions (**2.34**) or evidence of tubal damage.

Uterine Anomalies

It is important to recognize congenital uterine anomalies in the investigation of recurrent pregnancy loss. A broad fundus or a dimple in the fundus may suggest a septate or bicornuate uterus (**2.35**). In uterus bicornis there is a greater degree of failure of fusion of the Müllerian ducts (**2.36**). Laparoscopy is necessary to determine the precise status of the uterus, plan treatment and on occasion, monitor operative hysteroscopy during excision of a uterine septum. Other defects of development of the Müllerian ducts such as a unicornuate uterus (**2.37**) may influence the patient's obstetric performance.

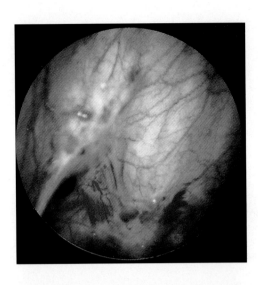

2.32 Peritoneal endometriosis.

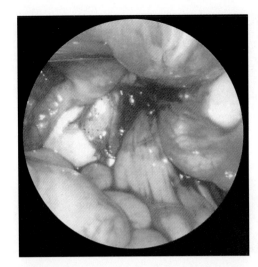

2.33 Extensive endometriotic adhesions.

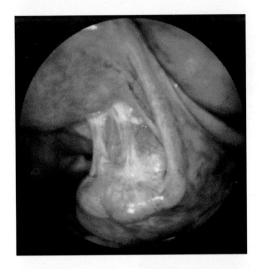

2.34 Post-inflammatory pelvic adhesions.

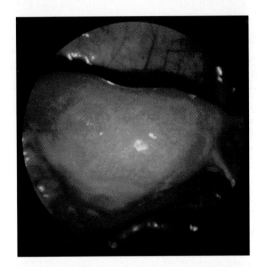

2.35 Septate uterus.

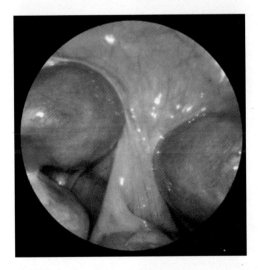

2.36 Bicornuate uterus.

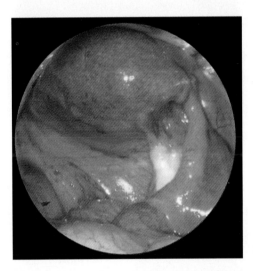

2.37 Unicornuate uterus.

Laparoscopy is sometimes of benefit to assess uterine fibroids which may be large and multiple (**2.38**) or in a position which may be difficult to treat such as the pouch of Douglas (**2.39**). However, modern high resolution ultrasound often obviates the need for such invasive procedures and should be used for assessment prior to endoscopic surgery.

Prior to Tubal Surgery

All patients with tubal disease require laparoscopy with, if appropriate, salpingoscopy to decide whether to offer reconstructive surgery or *in vitro* fertilization. It is only justifiable to offer tubal surgery if there is a reasonable prospect of success and this may only be assessed by direct visualization of the tube.

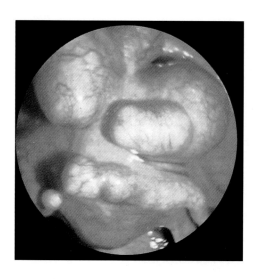

2.38 Multiple fibroids.

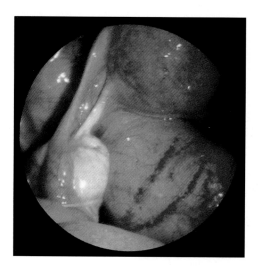

2.39 Fibroid in pouch of Douglas.

ACUTE CONDITIONS

Laparoscopy is indicated in a number of acute conditions (**2.40**). A full clinical history and careful examination together with appropriate haematological and sonar examination is always necessary In many cases the laparoscope is not only a diagnostic tool but may be used as a means of access to perform surgical procedures in preference to laparotomy. These will be discussed in the following chapters but it is appropriate to illustrate briefly the conditions which may be found in the acute abdomen. Even when laparoscopic surgery is not feasible, laparoscopy will frequently help to plan the correct incision and make unnecessary the large incision so often employed in exploratory laparotomies.

Acute Abdominal Pain

Acute abdominal pain may be caused by inflammatory processes but also by leakage of irritant material from a viscus. Rupture of an endometriotic cyst or perforation of a viscus may produce a confusing clinical picture which may impossible to resolve without laparoscopy.

Indications for diagnostic laparoscopy
Acute conditions
Acute abdominal pain Suspected ectopic pregnancy Acute pelvic inflammatory disease Torsion of adnexa

2.40 Indications for laparoscopy.

Acute Pelvic Inflammatory Disease

Acute pain may be caused by tubal infection with or without abscess formation (**2.41**) or by appendicitis. The latter may closely mimic salpingitis and differentiation may only be possible by direct inspection (**2.42**). In some cases of mild salpingitis the tubes may look normal and culture of the peritoneal fluid may be unrewarding. In these cases it is preferable to take intraluminal swabs from the fallopian tubes. The presence of subdiaphragmatic adhesions should always be sought.

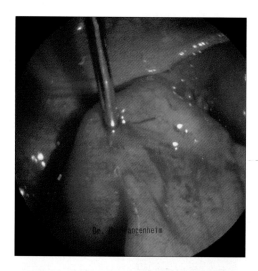

2.41 Acute salpingitis.

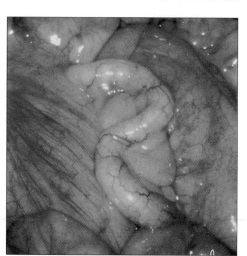

2.42 The appendix is in close proximity to the tube. Which is causing pain?

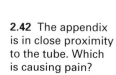

2.43 Unruptured ectopic pregnancy with leakage of blood.

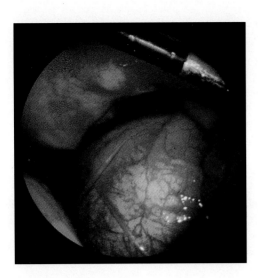

2.44 Torsion of ovary.

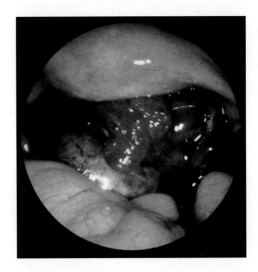

2.45 Infarcted torsion of ovary.

Ectopic Pregnancy

Ectopic pregnancy may be suspected clinically and confirmed with reasonable certainty by ultrasound and estimation of the level of human chorionic gonadotrophin in blood or urine. However, the final diagnosis often rests with laparoscopy when the distended tube with leakage of blood provides the final proof (**2.43**). Laparoscopy now provides the means of access to treat an ectopic pregnancy radically or conservatively.

Torsion of a Viscus

Torsion of a viscus such as the fallopian tube or ovary (**2.44**) is not common but presents as an emergency which can be diagnosed and treated by laparoscopic surgery. If the condition is recognised early enough and the organ is still viable, the torsion may be corrected laparoscopically. Recurrence of ovarian torsion may be prevented by shortening the ovarian ligament with a suture or clip. However, the venous return may be obstructed and the ovary become infarcted (**2.45**). In this case laparoscopic oophorectomy may be necessary if resection of the cyst is impractical.

CONTRA-INDICATIONS TO LAPAROSCOPY

The contra-indications to laparoscopy should be strictly observed (**2.46**).

ABSOLUTE CONTRA-INDICATIONS TO LAPAROSCOPY

Laparoscopy is dangerous in the presence of intestinal distension resulting from obstruction or ileus. Similarly a large abdominal mass such as a fibroid or ovarian cyst may be damaged. In any case this may be too large to consider laparoscopic surgery so laparotomy will be necessary. An irreducible external hernia contra-indicates laparoscopy because the raised intra-abdominal pressure may cause more bowel to enter the hernial sac and cause infarction. Hypovolemic shock is a contra-indication to any form of surgery and should always be corrected before operating. This applies especially to laparoscopy where the pneumoperitoneum may cause further cardiac embarrassment. Medical conditions such as cardiac or respiratory failure, severe obstructive airway disease or a recent myocardial infarct are also absolute contra-indications to laparoscopy.

RELATIVE CONTRA-INDICATIONS TO LAPAROSCOPY

Relative contra-indications will depend on the experience of the surgeon as well as the importance of the laparoscopy to the patient's health (**2.46**) Multiple abdominal incisions may make laparoscopy difficult but the problem may usually be overcome by modifying the technique or site of insertion of the instruments. Similarly gross obesity may require a transvaginal insertion of the Veress' needle and does not necessarily preclude successful laparoscopy. The instruments should not be inserted through an area of infected skin which should either be treated prior to laparoscopy or avoided by modifying the technique.

Contra-indications to laparoscopy
Absolute contra-indications

Mechanical and paralytic ileus
Large abdominal mass
Shock
Medical conditions precluding surgery:
  Cardio-respiratory failure or myocardial disease
  Severe obstructive airway disease
Irreducible external hernia

Relative contra-indications
Multiple abdominal incisions Abdominal wall sepsis Generalized peritonitis Gross obesity Blood dyscrasia and coagulopathy Hiatus hernia

2.46 Contra-indications to laparoscopy.

Generalized peritonitis is sometimes stated to be a contra-indication to laparoscopy. It has become one of the more important indications because it is often possible to treat the cause of the peritonitis by laparocopic surgery. Appendicectomy is commonly performed using the laparoscope. In peritonitis resulting from acute pelvic infection, repeated peritoneal lavage may prove to be an advantage.

Medical conditions such as ischaemic heart disease, endocrine disorders, blood dyscrasia and coagulopathy should be stabilized before any surgical procedure is contemplated. A hiatus hernia may be made worse by the pneumoperitoneum so the volume of gas should be limited and a steep Trendelenburg position should be avoided.

CONCLUSION

Diagnostic laparoscopy is now a basic skill which should be learnt by all gynecologists. It is indicated in an increasing number of conditions and must form an essential part of any gynecological service. In recent years the laparoscope has been used as a means of access to treat many conditions which hitherto demanded laparotomy. The modern gynecologist should be able to proceed from diagnostic to operative laparoscopy and, with proper training be able to perform most surgical procedures. The short hospital stay and postoperative recovery, the financial saving and the cosmetic incisions all make laparoscopic surgery an attractive option both to the patient and the providers of health care.

FURTHER READING

Gordon AG, Taylor PJ. Practical Laparoscopy. Blackwell Scientific Publications, Oxford, 1993

SALPINGOSCOPY

3

Ivo A Brosens

THE RATIONALE

The clinical value of tubal endoscopy is based upon the important role of the tubal mucosa in fertility. The intact fold structure of the mucosa with secretory and ciliated cells is essential for normal gamete transport and fertilization. Sterility and tubal pregnancy are frequently associated with underlying tubal pathology. The ampullary mucosa in infertility can show changes such as deciliation, flattening of the folds, inflammation, filmy or dense adhesions, fibrosis of the folds and wall and occlusive lesions. Some of these lesions such as deciliation and flattening of the folds have been shown in experimental and clinical hydrosalpinx to be reversible after restoring patency.

Scanning electron microscopy studies have shown that pregnancy can occur in the presence of deciliation and adhesions. However, the risk of ectopic pregnancy was increased to 50%. Pregnancy, either eutopic or ectopic, did not occur in patients when there was fibrosis of the ampullary segment (**3.1**).

At salpingoscopy a significant number of abnormalities are revealed which are not detectable by hysterosalpingography or laparoscopy. In hydrosalpinges the absence and presence of mucosal adhesions on hysterosalpingography were confirmed at salpingoscopy in respectively 48% and 57%, indicating that hysterosalpingography is inadequate to evaluate the tubal mucosa (**3.2**).

CLINICAL INDICATIONS

Salpingoscopy is indicated in patients with suspected tubal pathology.

PELVIC INFLAMMATORY DISEASE (PID)

Pelvic inflammatory disease is frequently associated with tubal mucosal lesions. Woodruff and Pauerstein believed that the extent of peritubal and periovarian adhesion was the primary determinant of tubal blockage and that intratubal damage was secondary. Mucosal lesions can occur as a result of hydrosalpinx formation and these changes are reversible. Experimental work has demonstrated that the mucosal damage resulting from mechanically induced hydrosalpinx such as deciliation, flattening of the folds and epithelial desquamation can recover following salpingostomy and that pregnancy can occur after the mucosa and the stretching of the myosalpinx have recovered.

There is poor correlation between peritoneal and tubal mucosal lesions. Mild pelvic adhesions with patent tubes can be associated with severe mucosal lesions. Differences in the severity of mucosal lesions between both fallopian tubes are common. At salpingoscopy it is important therefore that the full fold system of both ampullary segments are visualized in order to evaluate the extent and severity of adhesions or fibrosis.

In proximal tubal block transabdominal salpingoscopy is the only technique which allows accurate examination of the distal tubal segment. In the presence of a normal ampullary segment restoration of patency of the proximal segment yields an intrauterine pregnancy rate of 60%.

	n	IUP		TP		NP	
Deciliation	17	2	12%	2	12%	13	76%
Adhesions	29	4	14%	3	11%	24	78%
Fibrosis	12	0	0%	0	0%	12	100%

Tubal mucosal lesions at scanning electron microscopy and pregnancy outcome

IUP: intrauterine pregnancy
TP: tubal pregnancy
NP: non-pregnancy

3.1 Tubal mucosal lesions at scanning electron microscopy and pregnancy outcome.

HSG	Salpingoscopy		
	Normal	Abnormal	Conformity
Normal tube	11	12	48%
Abnormal tube	9	12	57%
No visualization	2	5	0%

Hysterosalpingography versus salpingoscopy in patients with hydrosalpinges

3.2 Hysterosalpingography versus salpingoscopy in patients with hydrosalpinges.

ENDOMETRIOSIS

Endometriosis can be associated with an extensive degree of pelvic adhesions and the tube is frequently involved in severe endometriosis. Hydrosalpinx can be present but the tubal occlusion is likely to be caused by compression or serosal stricture rather than by mucosal adhesions and occlusion. Salpingoscopy in these cases almost always reveals a normal ampullary mucosa. The tubal mucosa in endometriosis appears to be more resistant to the formation of adhesions than in pelvic inflammatory disease.

ECTOPIC PREGNANCY

There is now more evidence that after conservative surgery the recurrence of ectopic pregnancy depends on the underlying disease rather than on the operating technique or the damage at the site of implantation. This is no surprise as surgery and placentation usually affect only one or two folds in the ampullary segment. The other folds can remain unaffected and allow normal ovum transport.

Salpingoscopy can be useful in detecting early tubal pregnancy, recognizing tubal abortion, evaluating underlying tubal disease and the contralateral tube. Preliminary data suggest that salpingoscopy may be a useful tool for the prediction of the risk of recurrent ectopic pregnancy. Accurate detection of the presence and extent of underlying tubal disease allows a more rational approach in the selection of treatment and evaluation of the prognosis.

UNEXPLAINED INFERTILITY

Tubal mucosal adhesion can be detected at salpingoscopy in infertile patients with normal findings at laparoscopy. The incidence, however, appears to be about 3%. On the other hand salpingoscopy is recommended in patients with suspected tubal lesions such as mild fimbrial adhesions or with a history of tubal disease or ectopic pregnancy.

TECHNIQUE OF SALPINGOSCOPY

The rigid salpingoscope allows excellent visualization of the mucosa of the infundibulum and ampulla. The technique is based on distention of the tube by a saline infusion. The view is clear, bright and wide. Both the anatomical structure of the mucosa and the fine vascular network of the folds can be investigated. The instruments are the salpingoscope sheath with a connection for a saline drip, an obturator for assisting in cannulation of the tube, a 2.8 mm endoscope which is introduced through the channel of an operating laparoscope (**3.3a,b,c**). The tube is cannulated by the sheath with obturator and the tube is clamped with a round-ended atraumatic forceps at the level of the infundibulum (**3.4**). A saline drip connected to the sheath distends the fallopian tube. Air bubbles should be allowed to escape as they may create artifacts by compressing the folds giving the false impression of an abnormal tube. The obturator is then removed and the salpingoscope inserted into the sheath. The telescope is advanced into the tubal ampulla under visual control.

Complications rarely occur when the salpingoscope is maneuvered with care. Manipulation of the tube by the grasping forceps can produce some superficial serosal bleeding which usually stops after lavage with warm saline. Perforation of the tubal mucosa can occur if the telescope is advanced blindly. Excessive pressure of the saline drip can produce oedematous swelling of the mesosalpinx. However, edematous swelling of the mesosalpinx can also occur in diseased tubes probably when desquamation of the mucosa allows interstitial escape of the fluid.

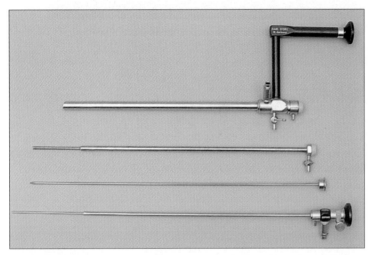

3.3a The operating laparoscope, the sheath, the obturator and the salpingoscope.

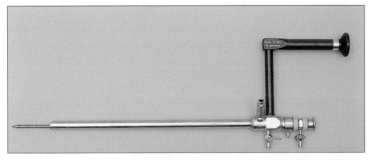

3.3b The sheath with the obturator protruding from the laparoscope.

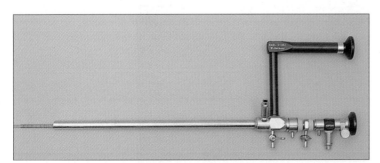

3.3c The assembled salpingoscope.

FINDINGS

NORMAL STRUCTURE

The infundibulum has a concentric structure of folds (**3.5**). In the ampulla there are four to five major longitudinal folds with several accessory folds arising from their sides (**3.6**). These major folds have a delicate structure with a fine vascular network (**3.7**).

Between the major folds there are four to five minor folds. At the level of the isthmoampullary junction the major folds level off to four or five small rounded folds which continue into the narrow, isthmic segment. The fluid in the ampullary segment may be turbid with flocculent material, particularly when salpingoscopy is performed around the time of menstruation or following hysteroscopy.

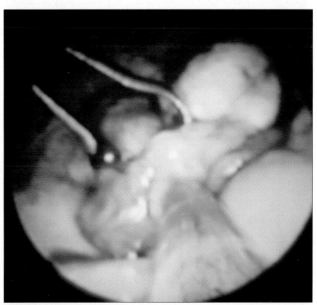

3.4 The salpingoscope is entering the tubal ostium.

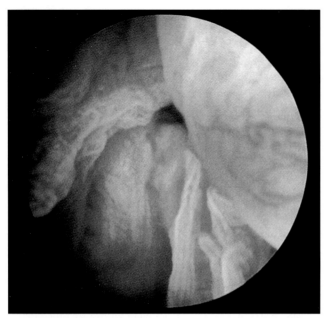

3.5 The tubal infundibulum showing the concentric arrangement of the folds.

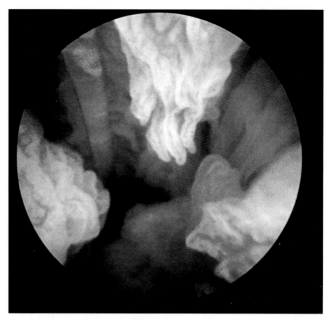

3.6 The tubal ampulla: three major folds can be seen with smaller folds between them.

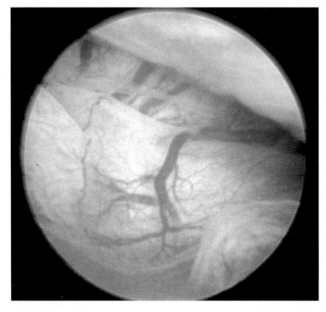

3.7 At x 20 magnification the vascular pattern of a major fold can be seen.

VASCULAR ABNORMALITIES

Cyclic vascular changes have recently been described. Vascular abnormalities of the small vessels can be seen in the folds. Their significance is not known. A marked vascularization with hemorrhagic spots are suggestive but not diagnostic of chronic inflammation.

LESIONS

Filmy adhesions between the ampullary folds are avascular and adhere between otherwise normal folds. These adhesions can occur focally or extensively in the ampulla. Severe adhesions are thick and vascularized and the fold structure is distorted. They usually extend over the entire length of the ampullary segment. Fibrosis produces partial or complete loss of the mucosal folds and makes the tube appear to be a rigid, hollow channel with some remnants of folds. **3.9** presents a classification of lesions in hydrosalpinges.

THE TORTUOUS TUBE

In the so-called convoluted or tortuous tube the lumen is very distensible, the folds are flattened and separated and the wall is extremely thin and transparent (**3.8**). Canulation of the ampulla can be difficult when the folds at the infundibulum are complex and tortuosity may prevent easy progress in the ampullary segment. The abnormality has been explained by herniation of the tubal mucosa in areas of aplasia of the myosalpinx. Segments or the entire ampulla can be involved. Hysterosalpingography or injection of methylene blue may create the impression of a hydrosalpinx due to the extensive dilation of the ampulla. The tortuous tube is, however, unlikely to be a cause of infertility, as it is found in parous patients.

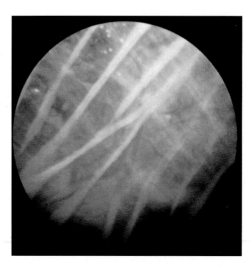

3.8 Tortuous tube: flattened and distended fold and segmental absence of myosalpinx.

Salpingoscopy: classification of ampullary fold lesions in hydrosalpinges	
Grade 1	Normal fold pattern
Grade 2	Separation and flattening of the major folds (3.10)
Grade 3	Peripheral filmy adhesions (3.11)
Grade 4	Adhesions across entire lumen (3.12)
Grade 5	Fibrosis of the fold system (3.13)

3.9 Salpingoscopy: classification of lesions of the ampullary folds in hydrosalpinges.

CONCLUSION

Transabdominal salpingoscopy is an extension of laparoscopy by a double optic technique. It allows detailed visualization of the mucosal pattern of the tubal ampulla as far as the isthmoampullary junction. With experience it takes only few minutes to perform on both sides. Transabdominal salpingoscopy at laparoscopy should be performed in all cases when tubal disease is suspected. Comparative studies have proved that the technique is superior to hysterosalpingography and provides additional information when tubal disease is suspected. In conditions like complete tubocornual block, transabdominal salpingoscopy is the only technique which provides information on the ampullary mucosa. Salpingoscopic inspection of a phimosis or a hydrosalpinx can be performed quite easily and the findings are important in the management and selection between surgical repair or *in vitro* fertilization. Salpingoscopy may also prove to be a useful tool in detecting underlying tubal disease in ectopic pregnancy.

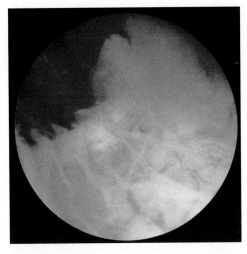

3.10 Hydrosalpinx (grade 2): distension and flattening of the major folds.

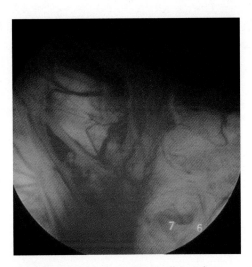

3.11 Hydrosalpinx (grade 3): distension and flattening of the major folds with filmy adhesions between them.

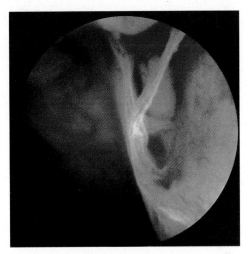

3.12 Hydrosalpinx (grade 4): fibrotic adhesions between distorded folds.

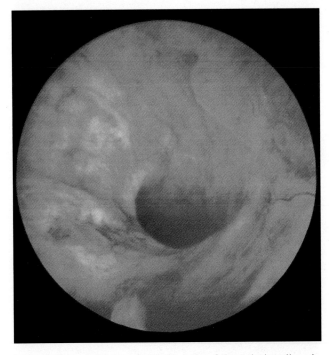

3.13 Hydrosalpinx (grade 5): fibrosis of the tubal wall and loss of fold pattern.

FURTHER READING

Brosens I, Gordon A. Tubal Infertility. Gower Medical Publishing 1990

Brosens I, Boeckx W, Delattin PH *et al*. Salpingoscopy: a new preoperative diagnostic tool in tubal infertility? *Br J Obstet Gynaecol* 1987;**94**:722–8

Cornier E. L'ampulloscopie per-coelioscopique. *J. Gynéc Obstét Biol Reprod* 1985;**14**:459–66

De Bruyne F, Puttemans P, Boeckx W *et al*. The clinical value of salpingoscopy in tubal infertility. *Fertil Steril* 1989; **51**:339–40

Henry-Suchet J, Loffredo V, Tesquier L *et al*. Endoscopy of the tube (= tuboscopy): its prognostic value for tubo-plastics. *Acta Eur Fertil* 1985;**16**:139–45

Karbowski B, Vasquez G, Boeckx W *et al*. An experimental study of tubo-ovarian function following restoration of patency in hydrosalpinges. *Euro J Obstet Gynaecol* 1988;**28**:305–15

Maguiness SD, Sjahanbakheh O. Salpingoscopic findings in women undergoing sterilization. *Human Reprod* 1992;**7**:269–73

Puttemans P, Brosens I, Delattin PH *et al*. Salpingoscopy versus hysterosalpingography in hydrosalpinges. *Hum Reprod* 1987;**2**:535–40

Vasquez G, Winston RML, Boeckx W *et al*. The epithelium of human hydrosalpinges: a light optical electron microscopic study. *Br J Obstet Gynaecol* 1983;**90**:764–70

FALLOPOSCOPY

4

Ian W Scudamore and Ian D Cooke

INTRODUCTION

The fallopian tube has long been known to provide a passage for the female germ cell to the uterus. In more recent years it has become recognized as having an important functional role in transporting and nurturing the ovum and early embryo. This function of the tube can be impaired after damage caused by infection which can result in permanent distortion of tubal anatomy and disturbance of function. There is frequently a tubal factor found in the diagnostic assessment of couples with infertility and this may influence the treatment and prognosis. The treatment options for the couple may include surgery or assisted reproduction techniques. Surgery using microsurgical principles either laparoscopically or at laparotomy, is directed toward restoring tubal anatomy which often means restoring tubal patency. It is becoming increasingly well documented that the results of such treatment are very dependant on the function of the tubal luminal mucosa at the time of the operation. Some assisted reproduction techniques such as gamete or zygote intra-fallopian transfer (GIFT or ZIFT) are also dependent on healthy tubal mucosa and should not be selected where there is significant intra-tubal pathology.

To assess the fallopian tube the standard modern techniques most used are hysterosalpingography (HSG) and laparoscopy. These techniques are directed mainly toward investigating the gross anatomical sequelae of tubal damage — tubal stenosis and occlusion, tubal restriction by adhesions and tubal dilatation. They provide an indirect assessment only of the lumen of the tube although a specific pattern of the epithelial rugae may be seen on HSG. In assessment of tubal obstruction they have a significant error rate and provide little qualitative assessment of an apparent proximal tubal obstruction or the epithelium in the isthmus or ampulla. Salpingoscopy, discussed in Chapter 3, has the great advantage of making a direct assessment of the tubal epithelium and allows staging of the degree of mucosal damage which seems to correlate well with pregnancy rates following tubal surgery. However, it requires general anesthesia and is unable to assess the proximal part of the tube due to the diameter of the rigid endoscope. Furthermore, access to the tubal lumen from the fimbrial end may be restricted by adhesions or require salpingostomy be performed first which prevents the technique being used to select good prognosis patients prior to surgery.

Falloposcopy is a technique first described by Kerin in 1990. Limitations of illumination and instrumentation had prevented trans-cervical cannulation and visualization of the tubal lumen until Kerin's group developed their coaxial technique and called it Falloposcopy (**4.1, 4.2**). The coaxial technique involves hysteroscopic guide-wire cannulation of the tube, passage of a Teflon catheter over the wire, replacement of the guide-wire with the falloposcope and retrograde imaging of the tube. Subsequently a technique of Falloposcopy using linear eversion technology has been developed. Linear Eversion Falloposcopy uses a pressurised tubular polyethylene 'balloon' which can be unrolled from within a plastic polymer cannula after having the falloposcope preloaded into its lumen (**4.3**). The 'balloon' carries the endoscope into and along the tube, protecting the tube and endoscope from damaging one another and negotiating curves and strictures without exerting shear forces on the tubal wall. The pre-loaded endoscope is used to identify the positioning of the catheter tip adjacent to the tubal ostium prior to everting the 'balloon' into the proximal tube. Hence the procedure does not need hysteroscopic guidance and can be performed without anaesthesia in outpatients. If resistance is felt during ever-

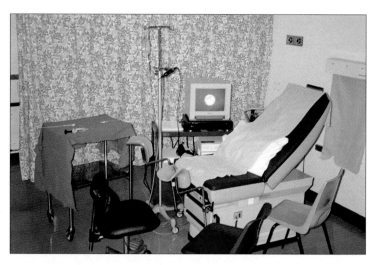

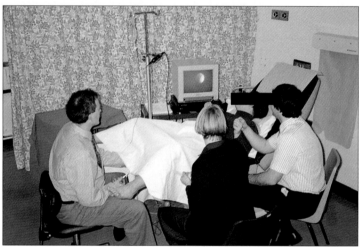

4.1, 4.2 Outpatient falloposcopy is performed in an environment dedicated to outpatient gynecological procedures (**4.1**). An adjustable gynecological examination couch is provided for the patient. The camera, light source and peristaltic pump are on the lower shelf of a mobile trolley with the video recorder and monitor on the upper shelf. A 1000 ml bag of sterile saline is suspended from an I.V. pole and the camera/endoscope coupling device is attached to the same pole with a screw clamp. The endoscope is attached to the coupling device and has been passed into the catheter through the portal at its rear end. The linear eversion catheter is on the draped trolley and is connected to the syringe pressure device (on the trolley beside the catheter) and to the saline flush through the peristaltic pump. **4.2** demonstrates the set-up during falloposcopy and the ability of the patient to follow the examination and observe the findings.

sion the endoscope can be advanced to the tip of the 'balloon' and the reason for the resistance investigated. Once the 'balloon' and endoscope are everted up to 10 cm into the tube (**4.4, 4.5**), imaging of the tubal lumen is carried out during withdrawal of the balloon, keeping the endoscope at the tip of the 'balloon' and flushing sterile isotonic crystalloid around the endoscope. The image obtained is displayed in real time on a video monitor and recorded simultaneously.

Being able to perform office falloposcopy has significant advantages. The patient can tell the surgeon when she has discomfort in one side which is quite characteristic of tubal cannulation or occlusion. If a tube is occluded she will not tolerate the saline flush, whereas if it is patent this is either painless or associated with pelvic peritoneal discomfort. She is able to participate in her investigation,

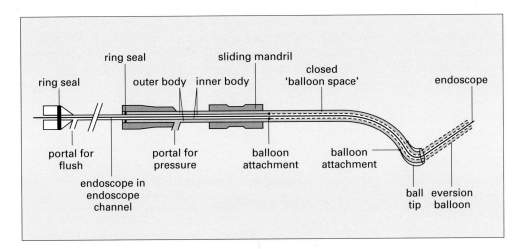

4.3 Design of the catheter. A schematic drawing of the linear eversion catheter illustrating the features of the catheter enabling atraumatic eversion of the balloon and endoscope into and along the fallopian tube.

ask questions and to see the video screeen confirming health or damage to her tube (**4.6–4.19**). These are things that often help couples to understand the choices they have and then to make rational decisions. The risk of anesthesia is avoided and there is no need for hospital admission, the patient going home at the end of the procedure. This makes it possible to assess the state of the endotubal epithelium before deciding if surgery or assisted conception are the preferred method of treatment minimizing the need for invasive investigation and the use of operating room facilities.

Initial comparisons have now been made of falloposcopy with HSG, laparoscopy and salpingoscopy in both proximal and distal tubal disease. Kerin described a classification and scoring system of endotubal disease in 1992 which seemed to correlate with subsequent pregnancy rates and also demonstrated endotubal isthmic plugs could be displaced with the technique, restoring tubal patency. Using the same scoring system, Venezia noted discrepancies between HSG and falloposcopic findings in 40% of cases. These

were mainly when HSG suggested proximal occlusion and the tube was patent or when HSG demonstrated patency but mild endotubal disease was present. In patients with unilateral or bilateral proximal occlusion on HSG and laparoscopy, Scudamore found in 1994 that bilateral occlusion was more likely to be associated with proximal pathology, some tubes with proximal and distal disease still had normal mucosal appearances and that unilateral occlusion was associated with contralateral abnormality in 40% of cases. The same group have made a comparison of outpatient falloposcopic scoring of tubal health with inpatient assessment by salpingoscopy at open microsurgery, and found a good correlation between falloposcopic and salpingoscopic scores.

These findings suggest that falloposcopy is a technique that can be used to compliment HSG, laparoscopy and salpingoscopy in the investigation of tubal disease. HSG can be considered a screen for possible tubal pathology and then falloposcopy to investigate any anomaly. After falloposcopy, those patients with apparently healthy

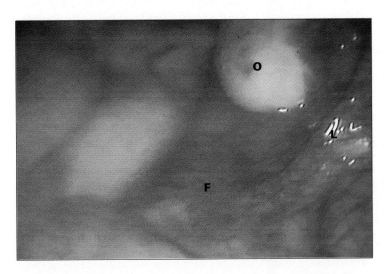

4.4 The endoscope and eversion balloon will follow the natural curve of the fallopian tube into the pelvis, around the ovary and into the vicinity of the ovarian fossa. In this image the light of the endoscope can be seen to be within 1–2 cm of the fimbrae of the tube in the ampullary segment. The ovary is anterior to the light and appendices apiploicae can be seen on the large bowel floating in the clear saline flush in the pelvis medial to the tube and ovary.The ovary is marked O, the light of the endoscope L and the fimbriae F.

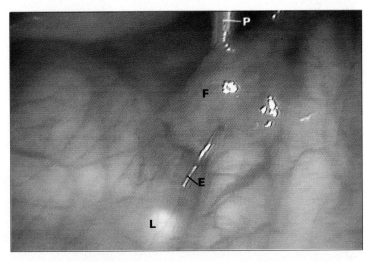

4.5 This image demonstrates the endoscope protruding beyond the fimbriae of the tube with the light from the endoscope clearly seen on the peritoneum. A laparoscopic palpiteur is seen in the 12 o'clock position in lifting the fimbriae from behind the bowel to facilitate laparoscopic visualization of the fimbriae and falloposcope. The light reflecting from the peritoneum is labelled L, the endoscope E, the fimbriae F and the palpiteur P.

tubal mucosa could proceed to laparoscopy. At this point, if surgical treatment is feasible it may be performed laparoscopically (with or without salpingoscopy) or an open microsurgical approach may be preferred. Those patients considered inappropriate for surgery due to the presence of endotubal disease at falloposcopy could proceed directly to assisted conception.

As the falloposcopic image is a real time video image obtained through a 0.5 mm diameter fiberoptic endoscope containing over 2000 imaging fibers it is best viewed as a moving image. The mobility of the tubal folds is an important part of the assessment and is not available on still images. Furthermore, comparison of still images with salpingoscopy is inappropriate as the rigid lens system and larger endoscope diameter give salpingoscopic images much better colour and definition. A still image recorded from the video loses a considerable amount of definition but can provide some idea of the image characteristics assessed at falloposcopy.

At office falloposcopy the assessment of the tube takes into account a number of factors:

- pain during eversion is generally worse in damaged tubes but allows lateralization of symptoms
- pain during flush is generally worse if the tube is occluded with generalised peritoneal pain if it is patent
- degree of dilation of the tubal lumen and ability of the tubal epithelium to 'close over' the endoscope when the flush ceases
- size, mobility and preservation of architecture of epithelial folds
- vascular pattern in folds and on the wall of a damaged tube
- degree of patency, stenosis or occlusion
- presence and characterization of adhesions

Using these criteria a score per segment of each tube can be given based on criteria suggested by Kerin (1991). This allows for objective recording of the findings and provides a means for testing the technique and grading the degree of damage as minimal/mild, moderate or severe.

The images reproduced on these pages attempt to illustrate important visual features in performing falloposcopy and assessing the tubal appearances within the limitations of still images obtained from original video material. These limitations must be emphasised as the visual quality of the moving image is much better and interpretation of still images is inappropriate in falloposcopy.

CONCLUSION

Falloposcopy is a technique which allows trans-cervical assessment of the luminal appearance of the fallopian tube. This can be performed as an office procedure. The fiberoptic image is most useful in 'real-time' with the tubal appearances being given a 'score' on a number of features to grade the tubal health. Much work needs to be done to correlate the appearances with tubal function and clinical outcome; however, the technique has promise in the investigation of tubal disease and the selection of appropriate treatment modalities. This chapter attempts to illustrate some principles of linear eversion falloposcopy and the images that are obtained within the limitations of still photographs taken from video material obtained using miniaturized fiberoptic technology.

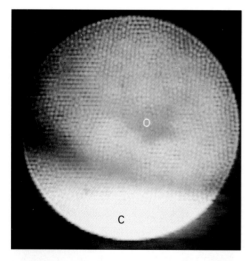
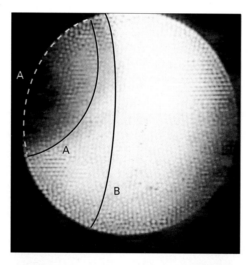

4.6, 4.7 Catheter tip and ostium. After the catheter tip is placed in the uterine cornu the endoscope is used to identify the ostium prior to eversion of the balloon. The ostium may be represented as an elliptical opening (O) adjacent to the gently curved white catheter tip (C) in the lower half of **4.6** from 4 o'clock to 8 o'clock. Sometimes it appears as the beginning of the tubular intra-mural segment. In **4.7** the tubular intra-mural segment is in the upper left quadrant (A) and the catheter tip vertical (B).

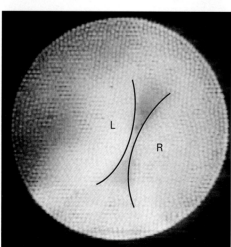
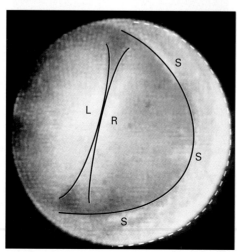

4.8, 4.9 Closed balloon from inside balloon lumen. With pressure in the balloon it closes in front of the endoscope with a characteristic two or three cusp appearance. In **4.8** the two cusp appearance can clearly be seen (the left cusp marked L, the right cusp R). In **4.9** the endoscope is just within the spring attachment of the balloon to the inner body which can also be seen. The balloon cusps are marked L and R again, and the spring S. This appearance is most likely when the balloon is fully everted and the endoscope is 1–2 cm behind the balloon tip.

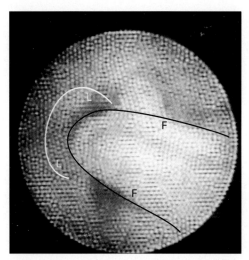
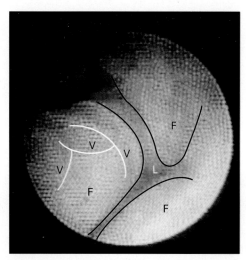
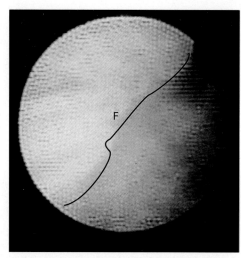

4.10–4.12 Ampullary folds. Normally these are freely mobile and contain discrete vascular channels. These channels may be in the center of the fold as in the finger-like fold F with its base at 4 o'clock in **4.10**. The appearance of an arcade of vessels (V) is present in the fold between 7 and 9 o'clock in **4.11**, albeit much clearer on real-time video. In both **4.10** and **4.11** the lumen of the tube is not dilated, the fold structure is well preserved with the folds 'falling' onto the endoscope when flush is ceased. In **4.12**, the folds are the projections with their bases between 8 o'clock and 1 o'clock (F) and the dark area on the right side of the image is representative of tubal dilation and hydrosalpinx. This tube is dilated with reasonable epithelial preservation.

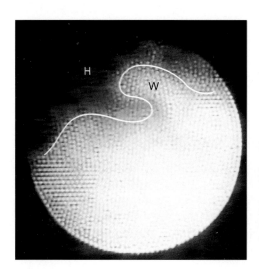
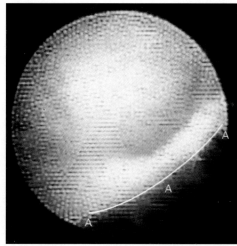

4.13, 4.14 Ampullary damage. Damage to the epithelial folds will result in a flattened appearance of the tubal wall with only remnants of the original folds present and in some cases discrete adhesions can be seen. In **4.13** the lumen of the hydrosalpinx is in the upper left of the image (H) and the flattened wall with fold remnants only (W) can be seen running across the image from 2 o'clock to 8 o'clock. In **4.14**, the lumen is in the lower right quadrant and there is a clear adhesion (A) on the wall from 3 o'clock to 7 o'clock.

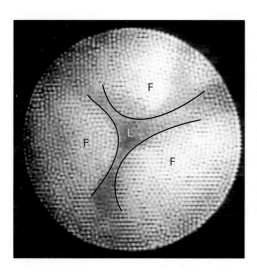
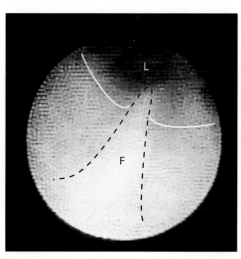

4.15, 4.16 Tubal isthmus. The healthy isthmus has 4–5 longitudinal folds which fill the lumen when no flush is being instilled. This appearance is illustrated in **4.15**. The impression of the longitudinal nature of the folds (F) and the visualization of the entire lumen (L) of narrower diameter is more clearly demonstrated on a moving image. These folds may be flattened and the tube somewhat dilated if a hydrosalpinx is present. In **4.16** a flattened longitudinal fold (F) is seen from 7 o'clock toward 1 o'clock and only 30–40% of the wall of the lumen (L) can be seen due to the degree of tubal dilation. On occasions irregular debris adherent to the wall can be seen on the real-time image.

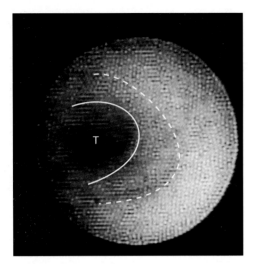 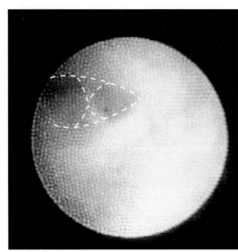 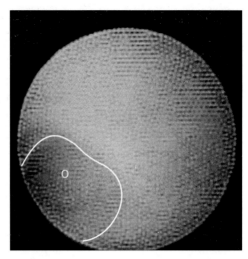

4.17–4.19 The proximal tube. The proximal segment of the tube is normally quite flat and the whole tubal lumen can be clearly seen. **4.17** demonstrates the characteristic appearance of a regular 'tunnel' in the upper left quadrant (T) with a circular lumen. Sometimes adhesions or a stenosis are encountered (eliptical dotted lines), as demonstrated at 11 o'clock in **4.18**. An adhesion can be seen crossing the stenotic lumen vertically. These stenoses may be amenable to treatment by tuboplasty using the linear eversion balloon to pass through them and dilate the lumen to 1.5–2mm. In the case of a complete proximal occlusion, eversion of the balloon will meet resistance and the endoscope can be used to visualize the cause of the resistance. In **4.19** the proximal tubal wall is irregular and there is an occlusion of the lumen in the lower left quadrant of the image (O).

FURTHER READING

Bauer O, Dietrich K, Bacich S *et al.* Transcervical access and intra-luminal imaging of the fallopian tubes in the non-anaesthetized patient; preliminary results using a new fallopian access technology. *Human Reprod* 1992;**7**(suppl. 1):7–11

Corfman RS. Falloposcopy: frontiers realized ... a fantastic voyage revisited [editorial]. *Fertil Steril* 1990;**54**:574–6

Grow DR, Coddington CC, and Flood JT. Proximal tubal occlusion by hysterosalpingogram: a role for falloposcopy. *Fertil Steril* 1993;**60**(1):170–4

Kerin J, Daykhovsky L, Segalowitz J *et al.* Falloposcopy: a microendoscopic technique for visual exploration of the human fallopian tube from the uterotubal ostium to the fimbria using a transvaginal approach. *Fertil Steril* 1990;**54**:390–400

Kerin JF, Williams DB, San Roman GA *et al.* Falloposcopic classification and treatment of fallopian tube lumen disease. *Fertil Steril* 1992;**57**:731–41

Kerin JF, Surrey ES, Williams DB *et al* Falloposcopic observations of endotubal isthmic plugs as a cause of reversible obstruction and their histological characterization. *J Laparoendoscopic Surg* 1991;**1**:103–10

Scudamore IW, Dunphy BC, and Cooke ID. Outpatient falloposcopy: intraluminal imaging of the fallopian tube by trans-uterine fibre-optic endoscopy as an outpatient procedure. *B J Obstet Gynaecol* 1992;**99**:829–35

Scudamore IW, Dunphy BC, and Cooke ID. Falloposcopic comparison of unilateral and bilateral proximal tubal occlusive disease. *Human Reprod* 1994;**9**:340–2

Venezia R, Zangara C, Knight C *et al.* Initial experience of a new linear everting falloposcopy system in comparison with hysterosalpingography. *Fertil Steril* 1993;**60**:771–5

PELVIC INFLAMMATORY DISEASE 5

Patricia E Munday and B Victor Lewis

INTRODUCTION

Pelvic inflammatory disease (PID) is defined as inflammation of the upper genital tract, and comprises endometritis, salpingitis, oophoritis, pelvic peritonitis, and tubo-ovarian abscess. The incidence of PID has increased significantly over the past few years, mirroring the increased incidence of sexually transmitted diseases (STD). This supports the view that PID is frequently a complication of STD. The true incidence and prevalence are difficult to ascertain because of the diagnostic difficulties and the wide variety of clinical pictures, from those who are seriously ill and require admission to hospital, to patients with no symptoms. Some patients may present with other problems such as deep dyspareunia, or infertility due to chronic disease. Furthermore patients may be seen by gynaecologists, genitourinary physicians and general practitioners, who have different approaches to diagnosis and management. The incidence of PID in the UK, based on hospital in-patient statistics, has doubled in the last two decades, and reached 16,000 admissions in 1985. In the two decades up to 1980, PID accounted for 200,000 admissions a year in the USA, but since then there has been a slight decline. The incidence of asymptomatic and mildly symptomatic infection is unknown, but serological studies of women presenting with tubal infertility suggest that asymptomatic chlamydial PID is at least twice as common as frank clinical disease. PID, like other STD, is most commonly found in young sexually active females, with a maximum incidence in the 20–24 year-old age group. The most vulnerable group are sexually active girls under 20 years old.

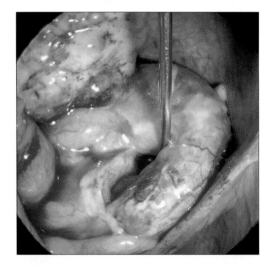

5.1 Acute appendicitis.

CLINICAL FEATURES

Acute salpingitis usually presents with lower abdominal pain, pyrexia and signs of peritonitis, with marked rebound tenderness. The differential diagnosis includes abortion, ectopic pregnancy, acute appendicitis, and possibly mesenteric lymphadenitis. However in many patients the disease may be mild, with little or no abdominal or pelvic pain, and no pelvic tenderness. If the condition is inadequately treated, chronic infection may ensue and the patient may present with chronic abdominal pain, dyspareunia or infertility.

PATHOGENESIS

Infectious micro-organisms may reach the fallopian tubes by direct spread following suppurative acute appendicitis (**5.1**) or inflammatory bowel disease. The tubes can also be affected by blood-borne spread, particularly in tuberculosis (**5.2**), although this is a rare condition in the UK. However, tuberculosis is more common in immigrants from the Indian Sub-Continent, and West Africa, so the incidence of tuberculous PID might increase. It will be interesting to see whether tuberculous pelvic peritonitis reappears in the community as HIV infection becomes more widespread, since infections with mycobacteria are common manifestations of HIV disease. The usual cause of PID is ascending infection following spontaneous or induced abortion, in the immediate puerperium following childbirth (particularly Caesarean section or operative delivery), and from lower genital tract infection (particularly caused by *Chlamydia trachomatis* and *Neisseria gonorrhoeae*). The intrauterine contraceptive device may also act as a focus for infection.

Once an infecting micro-organism has reached the fallopian tubes, acute infection ensues (**5.3**). Although infection may resolve spontaneously or with appropriate antibiotic therapy it may persist if treatment is delayed or inadequate. If infection does occur, the fimbriae close and the tube becomes filled with pus (**5.4**), forming a pyosalpinx which may rupture on laparoscopic exploration with release of pus into the pelvis. In response to generalized peritoneal infection a fibrinous exudate forms on the surface of the bowel and on the tube. Fine adhesions develop between bowel and adnexa, and the omentum may also become involved in the inflammatory process becoming adherent to the pelvic organs and interfering with access to the pelvis. If the acute infection fails to resolve fully, fibrous adhesions form between the tube and ovary and posterior surface of the uterus (**5.5–5.7**). The ovary

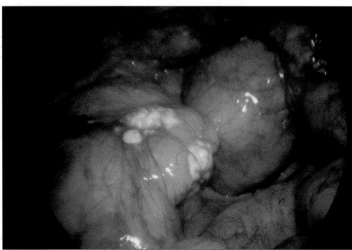

5.2 Pelvic tuberculosis with caseous deposits.

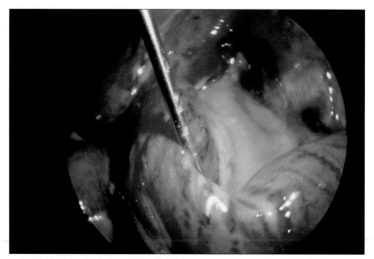

5.3 Acute suppurative salpingitis.

often becomes buried in dense adhesions and is firmly adherent to the broad ligament, so that ovum release is impossible. Loops of small intestine and sigmoid colon adhere to the uterus and adnexa, obliterating the pouch of Douglas. Hydrosalpinges may occur if there is incomplete resolution of the infection and the fimbrial ends of the tubes remain blocked (**5.8–5.10**). Some infections do not cause frank pus and a thin walled, fluid-filled cyst is often found. Some claim that this is characteristic of chlamydial infec-

tion (**5.11**). Furthermore, there are now some data to suggest that tubal damage may be immunologically mediated rather than a direct response to infection.

MICROBIOLOGY

For many years *N. gonorrhoeae* was thought to be the major cause of PID due to ascending infection although in many cases the organism could not be demonstrated in the genital tract. In 1976, *C. trachomatis* was first isolated from the fallopian tube of a patient with acute PID and since then it has become clear that this organism is responsible for many cases. Indeed, the majority of well designed studies indicate that *C. trachomatis* is the most important cause of PID in the western world, and perhaps also in the developing world. It is currently thought that at least 60–70% of cases are caused by *C. trachomatis* and *N. gonorrhoeae*, but in some, secondary infection with other organisms, particularly anaerobes, may obscure the picture and give the impression of polymicrobial infection. The proportion of cases due to *N. gonorrhoeae* is dependent on how well this infection is controlled; in Scandinavia gonococcal infection is now rare whereas studies from the USA suggest that gonorrhea is still the major cause of PID in some communities.

At one time it was believed that *Mycoplasma hominis* was a common cause of PID, but it is now thought to be the cause of only

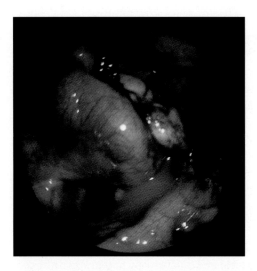

5.4 Ruptured pyosalpinx with pus.

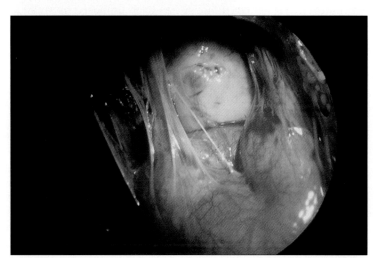

5.5 Chronic pelvic inflammatory disease with adhesions to large bowel.

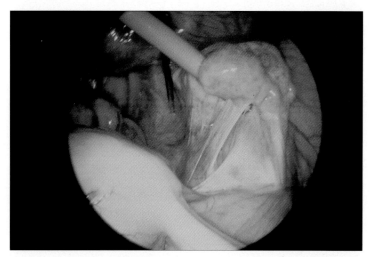

5.6 Chronic pelvic inflammatory disease — adhesions between ovary, tube and pelvic side wall.

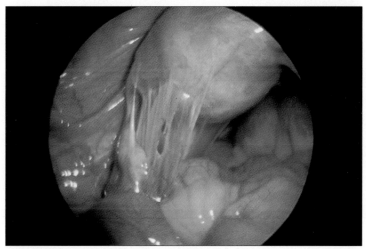

5.7 Chronic pelvic inflammatory disease.

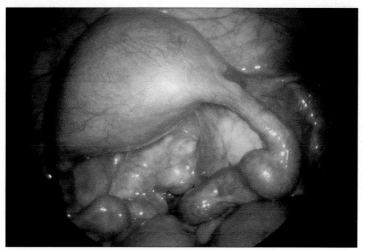

5.8 Bilateral hydrosalpinx distended with methylene blue.

occasional cases. *Mycoplasma genitalium* is difficult to culture, but serological data suggest it may be a cause of some cases of PID. Anaerobes, in particular *Bacteroides* spp. and peptostreptococci are commonly found in the peritoneal fluid in patients with severe PID, especially in septic abortion. *Actinomycosis israelii* is often found in association with intrauterine contraceptive devices, and may cause large inflammatory masses. Herpes simplex virus, and a variety of respiratory bacteria, e.g. *Haemophilus influenzae* have occasionally been isolated from the tubes, but their contribution to PID is small. The results of recent studies suggest that there may be an association between bacterial vaginosis (BV) and PID. It is not clear whether micro-organisms associated with BV are themselves etiological agents in PID or whether BV is a marker of infection with recognised pathogens.

In order to establish a microbiological cause for a particular case of PID it is necessary to take swabs from the affected site, namely the fallopian tubes, and this requires laparoscopy. Identifying organisms by taking swabs from the cervix, the urethra, the upper vagina, and the endocervical canal is important and may give the clinician some guidance, but the results of such tests do not always correlate with those from specimens taken directly from the tubes. Furthermore,

swab-taking from fallopian tubes at laparoscopy is technically difficult, and may yield negative results even in the presence of definite infection. Clinically normal tubes may also sometimes yield pathogenic micro-organsims, as *C. trachomatis* has been identified in this site in some women with pelvic pain and tubes which appear normal at laparoscopy.

Gonorrhea, chlamydial infection and actinomycosis are considered in greater detail below.

DIAGNOSIS

LABORATORY TESTS

In acute PID, laboratory tests may help to confirm the diagnosis. Such investigations include a raised white blood cell count, with excess of granulocytes, a raised erythrocyte sedimentation rate, and elevated C-reactive protein. CA125, the tumour marker, is raised in many cases of PID. None of these markers are specific for PID and the sensitivity is low as many women have normal results.

ENDOMETRIAL BIOPSY

In view of the diagnostic difficulty in mild cases of PID when the physical signs are equivocal and laparoscopy inappropriate or contra-indicated, endometrial biopsy has been proposed as an additional diagnostic tool. There is a strong association between plasma cell endometritis and salpingitis (**5.12**). However, it may be difficult to obtain an adequate endometrial biopsy in a patient with acute PID because of the discomfort.

PELVIC ULTRASOUND

Conventional ultrasound examination is only useful in identifying large inflammatory masses and excluding ectopic pregnancies. Although transvaginal ultrasound increases the sensitivity of the technique, it cannot identify early or mild disease.

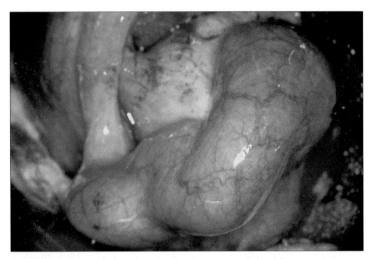

5.9 Early hydrosalpinx developing in acute salpingitis.

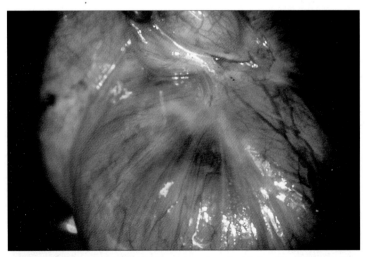

5.10 Fine adhesions closing fimbriated end of fallopian tube distended with methylene blue.

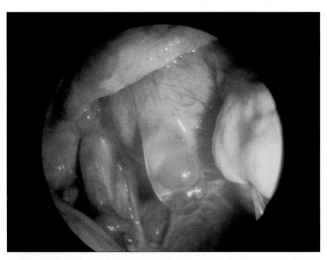

5.11 Chlamydial salpingitis with encysted fluid.

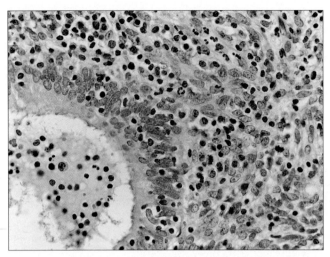

5.12 Chronic endometritis with increased cellularity of the stroma and an occasional plasma cell; the epithelium of the gland shows cellular infiltration (x560). By courtesy of Dr M C Anderson.

LAPAROSCOPY

In the late 1960s, Swedish investigators showed that the clinical diagnosis of PID was inaccurate in one third of those with typical clinical features. When women with less typical features are examined by laparoscopy the likelihood of an accurate diagnosis is even smaller, yet it is clear that many such women do have PID and may develop sequelae if the diagnosis is not considered. Laparoscopy is thus essential to establish the diagnosis, and in Scandinavia is generally incorporated into protocols for the management of all women with abdominal pain. It is a cost effective investigation, particularly if a definitive diagnosis can be established, because it prevents the unnecessary treatment of patients without PID with repeated courses of expensive antibiotics. Laparoscopy should always be performed by the double puncture technique, and Trendelenberg tilt may be necessary to visualize the pelvis clearly and mobilize the gut. In acute salpingitis the tubes are red and edematous with pus dripping from fimbriae. This can be aspirated for culture for *N. gonorrhoeae* and aerobic and anaerobic bacteria. However, since *C. trachomatis* is an intracellular organism, a speci-

men must include a cellular component and therefore the fimbrial end of the tube should be swabbed if possible. Since the tubes are normally sterile, any organisms identified should be regarded as pathogens. In chronic PID, laparoscopic diagnosis can be combined with surgery with division of adhesions and mobilization of the ovaries, this being preferable to laparotomy.

COMPLICATIONS

FITZ-HUGH–CURTIS SYNDROME

Fitz-Hugh and Curtis independently described peri-hepatitis (**5.13**) with "violin string adhesions" between the liver surface and the anterior abdominal wall, which they thought was caused by *N. gonorrhoeae*. More recently, *C. trachomatis* has been found to be an important cause. In one study a number of admissions to a surgical ward of women with right upper quadrant pain, initially attributed to acute cholecystitis, were found to be due to chlamydial peri-hepatitis. The upper abdomen should therefore always be carefully examined at the time of laparoscopy, because the detection of adhesions between the diaphragm and the superior surface of the liver may help to establish the diagnosis. It is unusual to identify either gonococcal or chlamydial infection by taking swabs but some patients do have very high titers of anti-chlamydial antibody.

TUBO-OVARIAN ABSCESS

The prevalence of tubo-ovarian abscess is variable, but may occur in up to a third of patients with PID. In most cases the infection is polymicrobial with a predominance of anaerobes. In over 50% of cases abscesses are bilateral. Acute symptoms will respond to medical management with high dose antibiotics, but surgery is required to confirm the diagnosis and to drain the abscess. When a pelvic abscess occurs (**5.14**), the tubes are often grossly distended with permanent damage to the mucosa. The prognosis for fertility is very poor, and only 14% of the patients reported in one series conceived subsequently. Laparoscopic surgery is rarely helpful following a large abscess or hydrosalpinx, and the patient is best advised to consider *in vitro* fertilization if infertility is an issue.

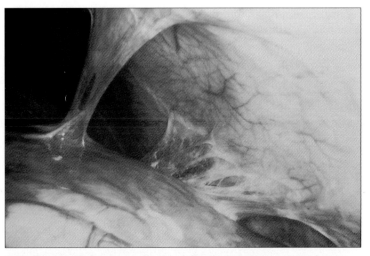

5.13 Fitz-Hugh–Curtis syndrome. Adhesions between superior surface of liver and inferior surface of diaphragm.

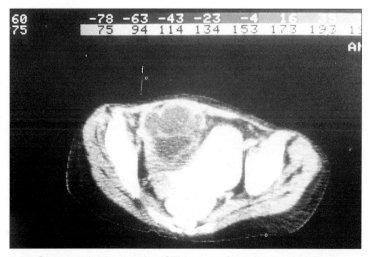

5.14 Computed tomography (CT) image of pelvic abscess. By courtesy of Dr J McGregor.

TUBAL INFERTILITY

Tubal infertility following PID depends on the severity of the initial attack, and the number and frequency of subsequent episodes of infection. Westrom found that 2% of women were infertile after one episode of mild salpingitis, compared with 29% after an episode of severe disease. After one infection 12.8% of patients were infertile, and after three attacks the incidence of infertility was 75%. The infecting organism may be important, and *N. gonorrhoeae* has been associated with blocked tubes. However, more recent studies have suggested that the outcome is worse after non-gonococcal than gonococcal PID which may be due to inappropriate treatment of the former. The tube is blocked less commonly at the cornual end (**5.15**) than the fimbrial end (**5.16**). In distal blockage, fluid and pus collect in the lumen of the tube, and cause pressure necrosis of the cilia, without which the tube cannot function. It is often easy to open a large hydrosalpinx, but the tube is unlikely to function adequately. Scanning electron microscopic examination of a biopsy of endosalpinx (**5.17**) may give a clue as to the future prognosis for fertility. If the endothelial cells and the cilia are destroyed, the prognosis is poor because the tube will not function in egg transport.

ECTOPIC PREGNANCY

Tubal damage which does not lead to complete obliteration of the lumen may nevertheless delay transportation of the fertilized ovum to the uterine cavity resulting in ectopic pregnancy. Women with ectopic pregnancies have a higher frequency of chlamydial antibodies than women with intrauterine pregnancies although many give no history of preceding PID.

CHRONIC PELVIC PAIN

Chronic pelvic pain and dyspareunia are well recognized sequelae of PID. Westrom reported 18% of women with laparoscopically proven disease still complained of pain after a mean of 9.5 years of follow-up. The pain in chronic PID can be severe, and may lead to marital stress and severe coital difficulties. In those cases with gross tubal damage and extensive adhesions, bilateral salpingectomy may be needed. Indeed, pelvic clearance with removal of both tubes and ovaries, and the uterus, may be the only option, particularly in women who have completed their families and are over the age of 40 years. Laparoscopic salpingectomy can be performed even in extensive PID, once the tubes have been mobilized using scissors, bipolar coagulation and endoloop ligatures. However, laparoscopically assisted vaginal hysterectomy may be difficult in these patients because of the very extensive disease process. It is important to remember that PID may occur in association with other causes of pelvic pain, particularly chronic appendicitis and endometriosis, and laparoscopy is the only method of establishing this diagnosis.

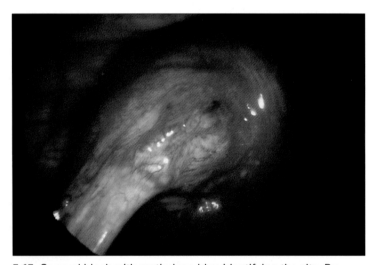

5.15 Cornual block with methylene blue identifying the site. By courtesy of Dr J McGregor.

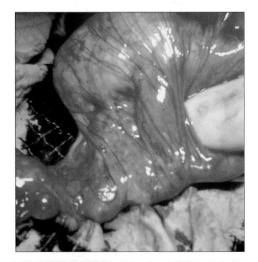

5.16 'Clubbed' fallopian tube with dense fimbrial adhesions.

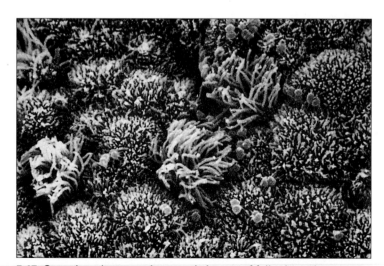

5.17 Scanning electron microscopic image of fallopian tube showing decilliation. By courtesy of Dr J McGregor.

TREATMENT OF PID

MEDICAL

Bed rest and avoidance of intercourse are important in the acute phase. Admission to hospital is required for diagnostic purposes and in patients who are sick enough to require parenteral therapy. Mild cases may be managed as out-patients if careful follow-up can be arranged. Antibiotic therapy should be selected to treat the presumptive pathogens, *N. gonorrhoeae, C. trachomatis* and anerobes. Local antibiotic sensitivities will determine the choice of anti- gonorrheal drug but the regimen should incorporate a tetracycline or erythromycin to treat chlamydial infection and metronidazole or its equivalent to treat anerobes. Newer antibiotics are currently under evaluation but assessment of clinical cure remains a problem and some investigators have used "second-look" laparoscopy to identify residual disease. If a sexually transmitted pathogen has been isolated at any site, notification of sexual partners is essential to prevent reinfection. It is sometimes easier to identify pathogens in men than in women and many experts now recommend that all partners of women with PID should be screened for infection and treated when necessary.

SURGICAL

When laparoscopy is used to confirm the diagnosis it is possible to extend the procedure to divide adhesions. Chronic PID is also often suitable for laparoscopic treatment. Adhesions should be divided under direct vision using scissors or a carbon dioxide laser. Avascular adhesions are easily divided, but if the adhesions contain blood vessels they should first be grasped with bipolar forceps before being divided (**5.18**). Thick vascular adhesions can be ligated, either with clips, endoloops, or intra-abdominal sutures, before being divided. The region of the ovary needs particular care. If the ovary is adherent to the pelvic side wall by dense adhesions, it must first be mobilized, because it may be adherent to the peritoneum overlying the ureter. If the carbon dioxide laser is used, an adequate smoke extractor system must be used to allow clear vision, and in some instances a back stop is required to prevent undue penetration of the laser beam and damage to underlying structures, particularly the ureter and large blood vessels. If fertility is desired every effort should be made to preserve the ovaries because of the possibility of *in vitro* fer-

tilization. A small hydrosalpinx can easily be opened through the operating laparoscope. The fimbrial end of the tube is held by grasping forceps, and opened with sharp scissors. The scissors are then inserted through the fimbriae and into the lumen of the tube, opened wide and withdrawn. The everted edge of the tube can either be sutured to the peritoneal surface or treated with a defocussed carbon dioxide laser, which causes the everted edges of the tubes to open. In the presence of a gross hydrosalpinx, opening the tube is easy, but it will not function, and the better option may be to perform a laparoscopic salpingectomy using either the endoloop or the bipolar electrocoagulation. In some instances a stapling instrument can be introduced through a 12 mm trochar to cut and staple the mesentery of the tube, so that it can easily be removed.

GONORRHEA

Gonorrhea is a sexually transmitted infection caused by a gram negative intracellular diplococcus, *Neisseria gonorrhoeae*. In the last decade there has been a decline in the number of cases of both lower genital tract infection (**5.19**) and gonococcal PID but it is still a disease of major importance in the developing world.

CLINICAL FEATURES

Most men develop symptoms within two or three days of acquiring the infection and seek treatment, but approximately 10% of men may be asymptomatic and thus be a reservoir of the disease. In contrast women are usually asymptomatic although some do have discharge or dysuria. The discharge may be purulent, but the appearance is not specific and the diagnosis is often made in women only when they are examined as the sexual contacts of men with symptoms. In women the endocervix, urethra and rectum are the primary sites of infection, but the throat may also be infected. Spread to the upper genital tract infection occurs in about 10% of cases and is most likely to occur during menstruation.

Incidence of gonorrhea and non-specific genital infection (NSGI) in women in England, 1979-1990/91		
	Lewis/Munday	
	Gonorrhea	NSGI*
1979	20061	21746
1980	20346	27410
1981	18746	29947
1982	19098	34214
1983	17929	36406
1984	17871	39855
1985	17555	46326
1986	16255	51501
1987	10377	44548
1988	7891	43583
1989	8415	44843
1990/91	7511	43698
*NSGI is a surrogate marker of chlamydial infection		

5.19 Statistics collected in English sexually-transmitted-disease clinics show a rapid decline in the number of cases of uncomplicated gonorrhea in women in the 1980s. This should be contrasted with the increase in number of cases of NSGI, which includes chlamydial infection. Chlamydial diagnostic tests were not widely available in the early part of this period.

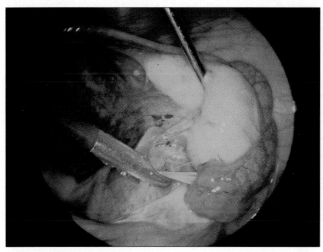

5.18 Adhesiolysis with scissors.

DIAGNOSIS

Accurate diagnosis is dependent on correct swab-taking and transportation of specimens to the laboratory, the use of selective media for culture and the performance of confirmatory tests. Since *N. gonorrhoeae* infects the cervix, urethra and rectum, swabs should be taken from all these sites. A high vaginal swab will miss the infection in up to 30% of cases. A positive swab is most likely from the cervix, but an additional 6% of cases have positive cultures only from the urethra, and 5% from the rectum. A swab should also be taken from the pharynx if there is a history of orogenital contact. The diagnostic success is increased by sampling more than one site, and on more than one occasion. Direct plating of specimens at the patient's bedside is optimum, but specimens may be sent to the laboratory in transport media. Gonococci require culture on selective media, e.g. Thayer–Martin, to suppress the growth of contaminating bacteria (**5.20**). Colonies have a characteristic appearance, but another identification test is essential to confirm the diagnosis. When facilities for direct microscopy are available, examination of a Gram stained smear of secretions (**5.21**) will lead to a rapid presumptive diagnosis of gonorrhea in 50% of cases in women with a high degree of specificity.

TREATMENT

Single-dose penicillin regimens have been in widespread use for the treatment of lower genital tract gonorrhea for more than 40 years, but the dose required to eradicate the organism is now high. Intramuscular regimes have largely been replaced by orally active penicillins with the addition of probenecid (1 g) which delays the renal excretion of the drug. In 1976 there were two independent reports of strains of *N. gonorrhoeae* which were totally resistant to penicillin because they contained a beta-lactamase- (penicillinase) producing plasmid, which inactivated antibiotics with a beta lactam ring structure. These strains, known as penicillinase producing *N. gonorrhoeae* (PPNG), spread rapidly from Africa and Asia, where they are now endemic. However, there has not been a major epidemic in

Western countries, where their prevalence is less than 5% of strains isolated). Some strains of *N. gonorrhoeae* show resistance to penicillin which is chromosomally mediated. A number of tetracycline-resistant strains have been described. Treatment of PPNG and other resistant strains is with an injectable cephalosporin e.g. cefotaxime 500 mg, or spectinomycin 2 g, or a quinolone derivative such as ciprofloxacin 500 mg orally. Multi-dose regimens are required to treat gonococcal PID. In order to identify treatment failure, all isolates should be tested for their antibiotic sensitivity. Re-infection is common if a partner remains untreated, and skilled contact tracing may be necessary to identify the source and secondary contacts. Follow-up tests are essential, and all infected sites should be swabbed on at least two occasions. Between 30 and 60% of women with gonorrhea have a concurrent chlamydial infection, so that a diagnostic test for *C. trachomatis* is essential. Trichomoniasis is also found commonly in association with gonorrhea.

Inadequately treated gonorrhea may lead to chronic PID, manifested by pain and dyspareunia as a result of a fixed retroverted uterus, and/or a pelvic abscess with hydro- or pyosalpinges (**5.22**). Infertility and sometimes ectopic pregnancy are the end results. A history of acute pelvic infection or lower genital tract infection should be sought in all patients with infertility. Laparoscopy is the only accurate method of determining whether there is permanent damage to the reproductive tract.

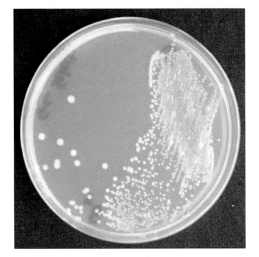

5.20 Culture plate showing characteristic colonies of N. gonorrhoeae on Thayer–Martin medium.

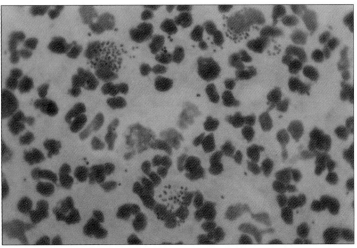

5.21 Gram-negative intracellular diplococci characteristic of N. gonorrhoeae.

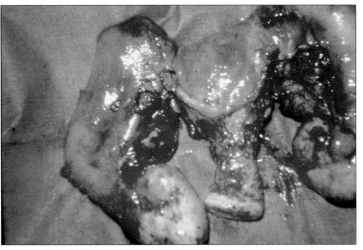

5.22 Operative specimen from patient with bilateral tubo-ovarian abscess secondary to gonorrhea. By courtesy of Dr J McGregor.

CHLAMYDIAL INFECTION

Chlamydia trachomatis is an obligate intracellular bacterium which causes genital and eye disease. It is transmitted sexually and is most commonly found in young adults. The infection may be asymptomatic in both men and women, and may be found in couples who have been in a stable relationship for months or years. There seems to have been a decline in prevalence of the infection, at least in women attending STD clinics from around 25% in the early 1970s to around 10% in the early 1990s. Nevertheless, data from various parts of the world now indicate that chlamydial infection is several times more common than gonorrhea.

SYMPTOMS AND SIGNS

C. trachomatis infects the cervix, urethra and rectum, but rarely if at all the pharynx. Although there may be symptoms of discharge or dysuria, these are often attributed to other causes. A mucopurulent cervicitis associated with hypertrophic ectopy is said to be characteristic of chlamydial cervicitis, and although this condition is commonly found in women with a chlamydial infection, the appearance is not very specific and many women with chlamydial infection have a clinically normal cervix. *C. trachomatis* is the commonest cause of non-gonococcal urethritis in men presenting with discharge or dysuria, which is less severe than in gonorrhea. However, a considerable proportion of men, perhaps up to 50%, are asymptomatic.

DIAGNOSIS

There are a number of techniques, including tissue culture, direct immunofluorescence and ELISA, which have advantages and disadvantages and may be appropriate in different situations. Tissue culture is regarded as the "gold standard" but is only available in a limited number of laboratories with special expertise. In experienced hands it is specific and sensitive. Specimen handling may be a problem as specimens must be taken into special transport medium and transported rapidly to the laboratory or frozen in liquid nitrogen. Direct immunofluorescence is simple to perform, but is labor intensive, and considerable experience is needed to recognise the characteristic appearances of fluorescent chlamydial particles (**5.23**). Some authorities believe that this test may be even more sensitive than culture. A swab is smeared over the well of a special slide and fixed with acetone. No special transport requirements are necessary. ELISA is a semi-automated test widely used in diagnostic laboratories. There are a number of kits with different sensitivities and specificities, and clinicians should be aware of the characteristics of the particular test kit used. Although the test is not as sensitive as direct immunofluorescence, large numbers of specimens can be tested together making it more cost effective. The test should not be used in medico-legal work as its accuracy could be challenged in court. Specimens should be collected into special media provided with the test kit, but no special precautions are required for transportation. New tests which are currently being evaluated are based on the use of DNA probes, and the amplification of chlamydial DNA using the polymerase chain reaction (PCR) or the ligase chain reaction (LCR). Their place in routine clinical practice is yet to be established. In the future, it may prove to be possible to use urine instead of genital tract swabs to identify chlamydial infection and thus open up the possibility of widespread non-invasive screening for this infection.

Serum antibody may be detected by a microimmunofluorescence test but the test should be used with caution because serum antibody may not be produced in superficial infections, and when it is, may persist for long periods. Some tests fail to distinguish between antibody to *C. trachomatis*, and *Chlamydia pneumoniae*, a common cause of pneumonia in young adults. Recently diagnostic tests for locally produced IgA have been developed as an alternative to culture and antigen detection techniques, but they lack sensitivity and specificity, especially in women. Serology therefore should be regarded as a tool to help epidemiologists understand the pattern of disease rather than as a diagnostic test in the individual patient.

TREATMENT

Tetracyclines are efficient in eradicating *C. trachomatis* from the lower genital tract, 1 g daily of oxytetracycline or the equivalent in divided doses for seven days producing a cure rate approaching 100%. Regimens with less frequent administration such as doxycycline, 100 mg twice daily, may improve patient compliance. If tetracyclines cannot be used, for example in pregnancy, erythromycin, 250 mg four times daily for ten days, is an acceptable alternative, but the cure rate is slightly lower. Some of the new quinolones, e.g. ofloxacin, have good anti-chlamydial activity, but are expensive. A new antibiotic, azithromycin, has produced promising results in chlamydial infection when administered as a single dose of 1 g. Tests of cure are not necessary unless poor compliance or re-infection is suspected.

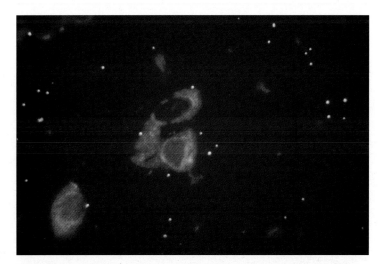

5.23 Chlamydial elementary bodies demonstrated by direct immunofluorescence (MicroTrak, Syva, UK). By courtesy of Syva UK Ltd.

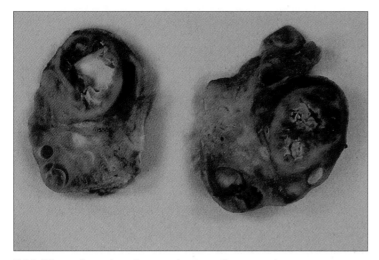

5.24 Bilateral ovarian abscess due to actinomycosis.

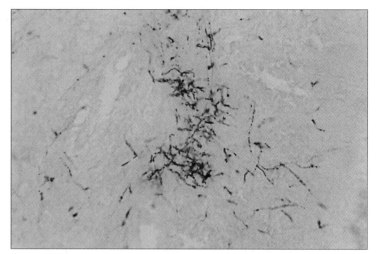

5.25 Branching filamentous actinomyces-like organism.

ACTINOMYCOSIS

Actinomycosis is usually caused by an organism, *Actinomyces israelii* which characteristically occurs in the presence of intrauterine contraceptive devices, especially inert devices. Although rare, actinomycetes infections can produce severe PID particularly with large abscess formation (**5.24**) and sterility, because of blocked tubes. The organism is most frequently identified on a Papanicolaou smear as culture is difficult and time-consuming (**5.25**). Penicillin is the antibiotic of choice, but treatment may have to be prolonged. However, chronic PID may result and then major surgery may be necessary to remove large inflammatory masses which may involve large and small intestine and omentum.

FURTHER READING

Jacobson L, Westrom L. Objectivized diagnosis of acute pelvic inflammatory disease, *Am J Obstet Gynecol* 1969; **105**:1088–98

Westrom L, Mardh PA. Acute Pelvic Inflammatory Disease (PID). In: *Sexually Transmitted Diseases*, 2e 1990. Eds: Holmes KK, Mardh PA, Sparling PF *et al.* McGraw Hill, New York, pp593–614

SUTURES, CLIPS, AND STAPLES 6

Michael P Diamond and Jaime M Vasquez

INTRODUCTION

The discipline of gynecological surgery was built on a combination of very basic principles. These included incision, dissection, traction and counter traction, achieving hemostasis and suturing. Good basic suturing skills are obviously essential to safe and effective surgery.

In the past decade laparoscopic surgery has advanced from simple procedures to complex operations. The laparoscopic surgeon is now able to treat effectively ectopic pregnancy, endometriosis, adnexal disease and extensive pelvic adhesions. The laparoscopic approach may also be used for hysterectomy and the excision of large pelvic tumors such as fibroids and ovarian cysts. The same basic principles, including suturing, which have evolved over the years in conventional surgery must now be adapted to allow the surgeon to work in a different environment. There are limitations to laparoscopic surgery. Normally only two or three secondary trocars and cannulae are inserted which limits access to the operation site. This reduces flexibility and adds to the technical difficulty of some of the more complex procedures. Nevertheless the surgeon can overcome these limitations by developing new skills.

The surgeon should master the techniques of suturing using preformed ligatures and the skill of tying knots both intra- and extra-corporeally. There are variety of suture materials and needles suitable for laparoscopic surgery and these will be discussed. There are a number of disposable staple applicators available with built-in knives which aid dissection and hemostasis. These may reduce tissue manipulation and trauma, decrease bleeding and edema and lead to a quicker postoperative recovery. Conversely these techniques have been criticized on the grounds of expense. There is no good clinical evidence available upon which to base these claims and counter claims. Whether the increased intraoperative costs can be justified by the early discharge from hospital, rapid postoperative recovery and decreased convalescence time remains to be demonstrated by controlled randomized studies.

SUTURES

Sutures are used to achieve hemostasis, approximate tissues, and promote healing. The quality of suture materials depends on several properties.

1 **Tensile strength.** Tensile strength is the amount of weight necessary to break a suture divided by its cross-sectional area. After placement of a suture into tissue, there is a marked variation in the retention of tensile strength.

2 **Good handling and knot tying properties.** Good handling and knot tying properties are related to the suture's memory, elasticity, plasticity, and physical configuration. Sutures which handle and tie better have less memory, more elasticity, less plasticity, and are usually multifilament.

3 **Infection risk**. The risk of infection is related to the suture's physical structure. Multifilament, twisted or braided sutures have a higher risk of infection, because they trap bacteria within their strands.

4 **Tissue trauma and inflammation.** Sutures are classified as absorbable and non-absorbable based on how rapidly their tensile strength is lost after placement into the tissue. An arbitrary definition of an absorbable suture is one which loses more than 95% of its tensile strength within approximately 60 days. Absorbable sutures are subdivided according to whether the material is natural or synthetic. Natural absorbable sutures produce an inflammatory response in tissues depending on their enzymatic degradation. Most sutures in use are synthetic, developed from polymerization techniques. Thus, in the following paragraphs, we will discuss absorbable synthetic sutures. Monofilament sutures cause less tissue reaction and trauma than multifilament sutures. Tissue response also depends on suture material and calibre. Synthetic sutures are less reactive than chromic catgut. Prolene 9-0 and 10-0 produce the smallest tissue response. Reaction persists longer with nylon and other non absorbable sutures. Also large sutures, regardless of type, incite greater tissue reaction than smaller calibre sutures.

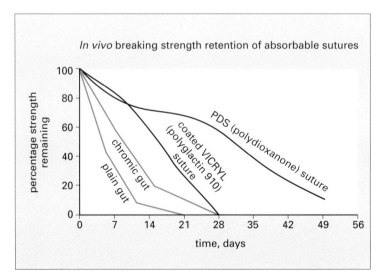

6.1 Absorption profile of different absorbable sutures (plain and chromic catgut, PDS and Vicryl). The percentage of suture area remaining at different times through the first 200 days after placement is shown.

6.2 *In vivo* breaking strength retention of absorbable sutures (plain and chromic catgut, PDS and Vicryl). The percentage of strength remaining at different times through the first 56 days after placement is shown.

SYNTHETIC ABSORBABLE SUTURES

Multifilament Sutures

Uncoated polyglycolic acid (Dexon) was introduced in the 1970s, followed by a less coarse version, Dexon-S. Dexon is a braided stiff suture, and handles easily. Because Dexon is degraded by hydrolysis, it provides prolonged and predictable loss of tensile strength. It can be coated (Dexon Plus) to help passage through tissue and knot tying.

Shortly after the development of Dexon, polyglactin 910 (Vicryl) was introduced. Vicryl is a copolymer that consists of nine parts glycolide to one part lactide. Vicryl is braided, a characteristic that leads to good handling and tying. Vicryl is also characterized by predictable loss of tensile strength and low tissue reaction. To improve the initial handling problems of poor knot rundown, high tissue drag and the cutting the surgeon's fingers, a coating was added to the Vicryl. However, this interfered with the reliability of the knots.

Monofilament Sutures

The synthetic absorbable monofilament sutures (unlike Dexon and Vicryl) available today include polydioxanone (PDS) and polyglycolic-3-methylene-carbonate (Maxon). PDS has the advantage of more gradual loss of tensile strength, less potential for infection, and easier passage through tissue. However, it is stiff, difficult to handle and difficult to tie. PDS has a slower rate of degradation than Maxon, but its stiffness and elasticity are greater and its coefficient of friction lower. These characteristics result in poor handling and knot performance, compared with Maxon. Other disadvantages include curling and pig tailing of the thread as the "out-of-the-package memory" is high. To overcome some of these drawbacks, a new generation polydioxanone (PDS-2) has been introduced. PDS-2 is easier to handle.

Maxon, the other monofilament copolymer, made by a combination of trimethylene carbonate and glycolide, is a suture with better handling properties. Fourteen days after placement, Dexon and Vicryl retain 50–60% of their tensile strength, while PDS and Maxon retain 75–85%. At four weeks, Dexon and Vicryl retain 5% of their tensile strength, while PDS and Maxon retain almost 60%. The superior knot performance of Maxon, compared with PDS, can be explained by the greater suppleness of Maxon. **6.1** and **6.2** give a relative comparison of the absorption patterns and the *in vivo* breaking strengths of absorbable sutures.

SUTURE REACTION

Uncoated Vicryl has been favored over Dexon-S in a comparison between the two sutures in rat uteri for inflammatory and tissue responses. **6.3** shows the minimal tissue reaction elicited in the rat with 4-0 Vicryl after 84 days of placement. Dexon and Vicryl are less likely to stimulate adhesion formation in the rabbit. Histological studies comparing polypropylene siliconized braided nylon (Prolene), Vicryl, and PDS, found nylon to be associated with fibrosis, whereas the histological response to Vicryl diminished with time. Nylon is associated with greater foreign body and inflammatory response than its absorbable counterparts Dexon-S and Vicryl. Maxon has better handling and tying characteristics and a comparable tissue reaction with Vicryl. An additional advantage of Maxon is its prolonged retention of tensile strength.

Current efforts to improve microsurgical techniques for infertility therapy have led to the exclusive use of absorbable microsutures in the female reproductive tract. This decision is based on research on histology in rats and rabbits.

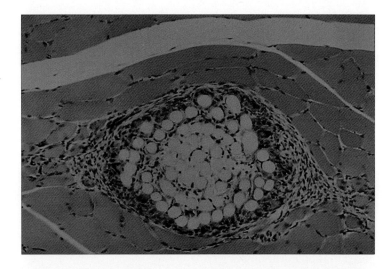

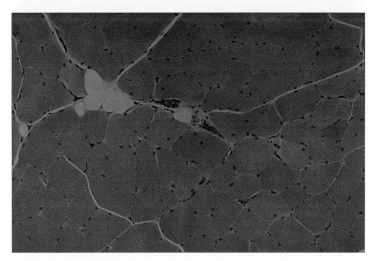

6.3a,b Vicryl (polyglactin 910) suture size 4-0 implanted in rat gluteal muscle. **6.3a** Seven days postimplantation — no absorption noted at this interval, slight foreign body reaction at the periphery of filaments. **6.3b** Vicryl suture implant site 84 days post-implantation — no identifiable filaments remain, a few mononuclear cells and fibrocytes are still present.

SUTURES AND ADHESION PREVENTION

Adhesion formation is the result of serosal injuries followed by repair. The fibrinolytic system plays a role in the formation and resolution of adhesions. Suture placement results in an inflammatory response. This inflammatory response leads to the formation of a fibrinous adhesive exudate. The resolution of this exudate is an oxygen dependent process, and ischemia produced by the sutures depresses the fibrinolytic system, resulting in the organization of fibrin matrices and adhesion formation.

Traditionally, the infertility surgeon faced with a tissue defect tried to reconstruct normal anatomy as accurately as possible. Although not proven, this approach theoretically gave the best postoperative reproductive function. Thus, defects in pelvic peritoneum, and raw surfaces following either ovarian cystectomy or adnexal surgery were sutured to achieve primary closure. However, recent studies suggest that this practice may promote postoperative adhesion formation. A possible explanation for the decrease in *de novo* adhesions noted by the Operative Laparoscopic Study Group (1991) was related, at least in part to the avoidance of sutures. Thus, these observations suggest that contrary to the previous general consensus, the less suturing the better. Confirmation of this hypothesis awaits appropriately controlled clinical trials. However, when structural integrity and anatomic relationships appear to be compromised or when there is a need to secure hemostasis, endoscopic suturing becomes the only acceptable option.

There has been controversy on whether absorbable or non-absorbable sutures are better for adnexal infertility surgery. When the ovaries are sutured following surgical incision adhesions were found in about 40% of Surgilon-closed ovaries and in 95% of Vicryl-closed ovaries. The adhesions were filmy in most of the patients in the Surgilon group but in few of the Vicryl patients. Dense and vascular adhesions were found in fewer of the Surgilon group compared with the Vicryl group. Subsequent conception rates were 68% in the Surgilon group and 33% in the Vicryl group. No difference was found in the quantity of postoperative adhesions or in postoperative reproductive outcome when nylon and Vicryl are compared in rabbit ovarian surgery.

Long- and short-term reactions of reproductive tract tissue to five microsurgical suture materials have been compared. The five materials were polyglactin 910 (Vicryl), polyglycolic acid (Dexon-S), polypropylene (Prolene), nylon (Ethilon and Dermalon) and chromic catgut. The calibres ranged from 6-0 to 10-0. The least tissue reaction was seen with 9-0 and 10-0 suture materials; Dexon-S caused a slightly greater reaction than did Vicryl. Prolene, 8-0 and 9-0, produced the smallest tissue response when compared with other sutures of similar size. Larger sutures incited greater tissue reactions. Vicryl had less late reaction as compared with the other sutures. Reactions persisted longer with non-absorbable sutures, and the tissue response depended on both the suture material and calibre. Vicryl, 8-0 to 10-0, incited the least short- and long-term tissue reaction. Thus, Vicryl 8-0 to 10-0 seem optimal for reconstructive tubal surgery using microsurgical techniques.

CHOICE OF SUTURES

The choice of a specific suture in specific surgical situations should be made on the basis of objective data regarding physical properties such as biocompatibility, tissue drag, stillness, elasticity and mechanical performance. Knot performance is the most important factor of a suture. Knot performance of a suture depends on the coefficient of friction, stiffness and the elasticity of the fiber. Knot security, however, is dependent only on the diameter of the suture.

Endoloop Sutures

The Roeder loop, which was devised for tonsillectomy in children, has been adapted for laparoscopy. This knot has become popular in laparoscopic surgery because it is pre-tied and locked *in situ* by a push-rod. However, this knot resists reverse slipping only when used with catgut. Thus, none of the available non-absorbable materials can be used safely as a slip knot in laparoscopic surgery. The slipping strength of the Roeder loop is decreased when applied to braided or monofilament suture. The performance of Roeder knots with polyglactin is inferior to those tied with gut and does not improve with hydration. The Duncan loop results in a knot that is less prone to slipping due to the better design of the knot. Alternatively, the slipping strength of both loops may be increased by adding a simple half hitch to the knot after the loop has been applied (**6.4**). Unfortunately, the commercially available loops have been trimmed to preclude the application of an additional half hitch. Today, available pre-tied endoloops include O Chromic, O Plain, Polyglactin 910 (coated Vicryl), PDS-2, and Prolene. Endoloops are pre-tied into loops using either a Roeder loop or a Duncan loop (**6.5**).

A new clinch knot can be used to replace the Roeder loop. This knot can be safely used with monofilament material such as polydioxanone. The clinch knot locks easily, it takes less time to tie, and it is not as bulky as other knots (**6.6**). It can be used to secure the endo-knot.

Extracorporeal Suturing

Extracorporeal suturing becomes essential, when it is technically impossible to use endoloops. The needle is swaged on a monofilament or braided suture. The suture is placed through the tissues, and then the needle is brought outside the abdomen and the knot is tied extra corporeally, forming a Duncan or Roeder loop (**6.7**). A suture applicator is then used to push the knot into the abdominal cavity. This technique is used to ligate vessels, reconstruct organs and approximate opposing tissue surfaces. An alternative technique utilizes the same suture bringing both ends through the trocar sleeve and a half hitch is thrown. A Clarke knot pusher advances the half hitch through the trocar sleeve into the tissue. The instrument is then removed and a second half hitch is placed and again pushed into the abdominal cavity in such a fashion that a square knot is formed. As many knots can be tied as appropriate, depending on the suture and surgical site.

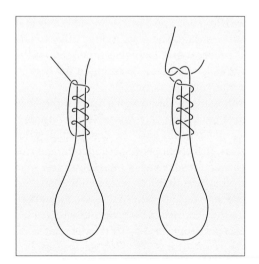

6.4 A half hitch adds security to the knot. The Duncan loop is seen prior and after adding this half hitch.

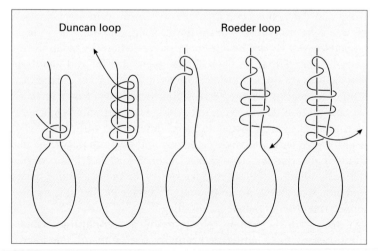

6.5 Duncan loop and Roeder loop.

Intracorporeal Suturing

lntracorporeal suturing is used to ligate bleeding vessels, reconstruct organs, approximate opposing tissue surfaces, and even suture anastomoses. Two methods have been used for this technique.

1 **Straight needle technique**. Most suture needles used laparoscopically are straight and are applied with a needle-holder with grooves designed to hold the needle at a right angle (straight needle technique). The straight swaged needle and suture are placed through a trapless trocar sleeve into the abdominal cavity, a simple instrument tie is used to place a surgeon's knot which is then trimmed. This technique is cumbersome, requiring great training and patience for efficiency (**6.8**).

2 **Fisherman's clinch knot**. The second method is the Fisherman's clinch knot, tied intracorporeally. This is a newer knotting technique derived from a common fishing knot. After suturing the tissue with a swaged needle attached to a long suture, a laparoscopic needle holder is used to grasp the needle. The needle holder is rotated several times, resulting in winding of the two strands of suture in the abdomen. A second needle holder through a separate cannula is used to grasp the needle. The first needle holder then grasps the short end of the suture and pulls it through the loops previously formed. Traction on both ends tightens the knot (**6.9**).

CLIPS

Clips preclude the need for time-consuming knotting techniques. Clips are mainly used to achieve hemostasis, either before or after transection. Clips should fulfil the following criteria for optimal performance:

• easy application;
• adequate performance in controlling bleeding;
• minimally reactive, regarding adhesion formation.

There are two general types, those with a latch mechanism and those without. The former sometimes requires a free pedicle although newer versions may be pushed through tissues. The latching clips require less memory and can be of absorbable material. Metal clips should be used if greater memory is required.

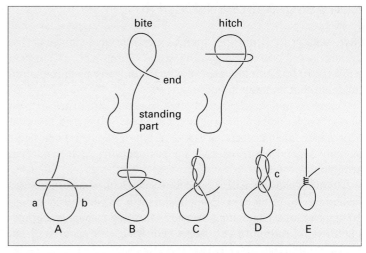

6.6 The clinch knot. A) After making a bite, a right-hand hitch is made around the standing part. B) The strand of the bite (b) is twisted over the strand (a). C) The end is passed over (b) and under (a). D) The end is passed over (c) to end up adjacent but running in the opposite direction to the standing part. E) The completed knot is tightened. The upper part of the diagram depicts knot-tying terms and displays a simple hitch.

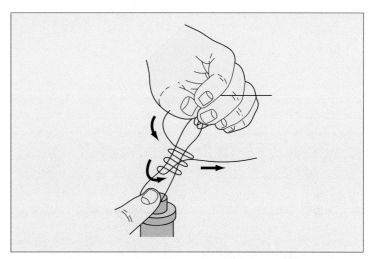

6.7 Extra-corporeal knotting – the completed suture. (From Gordon AG, Taylor PJ. Practical Laparoscopy. Oxford: Blackwell Scientific Publications, 1993, with permission).

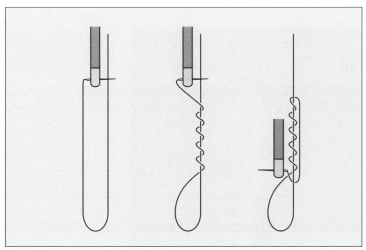

6.8 Intracorporeal knot tying with a straight swaged needle.

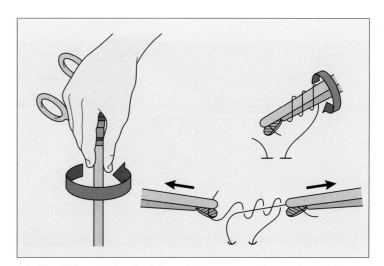

6.9 The Fisherman's clinch knot. Intracorporeal knot tying with a curved needle.

NON ABSORBABLE ENDOCLIPS

High-density surgical clips, such as metal, produce image degradation on computed tomography scans. Three types of surgical clips: tantalum, stainless steel, and titanium, have been compared in a phantom and animal model.

Tantalum and stainless steel produce severe streak artefacts on postoperative computed tomographic studies. In contrast, titanium clips lead to minimal artifacts. Thus, the type of clip to use may occasionally depend upon the need for postoperative high-resolution scanning.

Titanium clips were developed for hemostasis of moderate sized blood vessels. Automatic clip applicators can be introduced though 10 mm cannulae eliminating the need for a latch mechanism involving the tip of the clip. Thus, larger pedicles can be secured (**6.10, 6.11a,b**). Although, the clips are not absorbable, they are effective in providing hemostasis, are easily applied, and cause the same adhesion formation as do conventional sutures.

ABSORBABLE ENDOCLIPS

Biodegradable clips including polydioxanone and lactomer (copolymer of glycolic and lactic acids) are available. During the first two weeks after placement, inflammatory cells grow around these clips. Thus, the first phase of the inflammatory response is the proliferation of phagocytic cells. These inflammatory cells, including neutrophils, macrophages and mast cells, release high concentrations of proteases, collagenases, elastases, and cathepsins which may play a major role in the degradation of synthetic materials. However, after the second week, fibroblasts appear resulting in a collagenic fiber capsule. These fibrous capsules increase in thickness and might restrict the action of enzymes on the clips with a slowing in biodegradation.

PDS endoclips are available in 5 mm and 10 mm sizes. The PDS is hydrolyzed approximately 210 days after placement into tissue. The laparoscopic applicators used for clip placement crimp the clips into position, allowing a latch-like action to occur. The limitation of PDS clips is that latching is not possible with large pedicles.

STAPLES

Stapling as a substitute for suturing in surgery dates from 1908, when Dr Hultl, from Hungry, introduced a mechanical stapler. The first good quality staplers were later developed in the Soviet Union in the 1950s and gradually became popular in the USA. Today, staplers manufactured in the USA are much easier to use and have become popular in almost every surgical specialty, including obstetrics and gynecology.

Stapling is an accepted practice in abdominal and vaginal hysterectomy and in cesarean deliveries. Metal staplers were initially used for vaginal cuff closure, but need removal because of postoperative pain. Therefore, absorbable copolymer staples were developed to ensure softening and resorption over six months. Many surgeons believe that staples decrease operating time, tissue manipulation, blood loss, peritoneal contamination by vaginal flora and inspection. However, no prospective controlled, randomized study has documented these theoretical advantages. Furthermore, some investigators have suggested that there is no clinical advantage to surgical staples over traditional sutures for vaginal cuff closure in abdominal hysterectomy. The titanium stapler presently in use for vaginal cuff closure is shown in **6.12**.

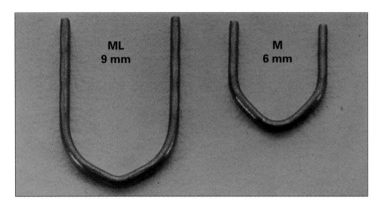

6.10 6 mm and 9 mm titanium clips used in pelviscopic surgery.

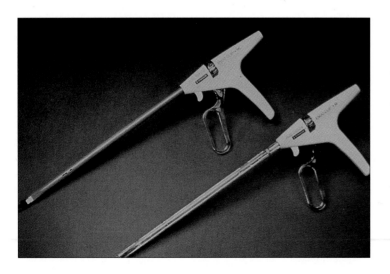

6.11a,b Clip applicators used in pelviscopic surgery.

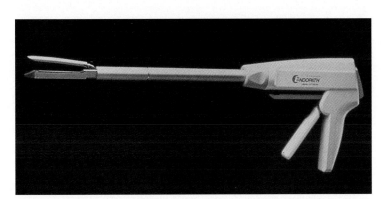

6.12 Hand-held titanium staple appliers used for vaginal cuff closure in abdominal hysterectomies.

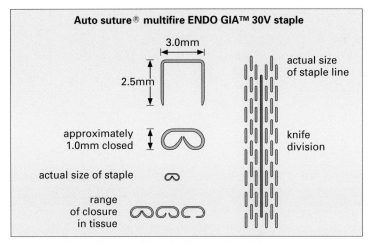

6.13 Rows of titanium staples and cutting line between staples.

Multifire staplers used for laparoscopically assisted vaginal hysterectomy consist of disposable handles and shafts, housing replaceable stapling cartridges. Staplers are available with vascular and standard staples. Staggered rows of titanium staples are placed across the pedicle with simultaneous cutting between the staple lines (**6.13**). For laparoscopic surgery, the staplers should be introduced though a 12 mm cannula (**6.14, 6.15**).

The fine titanium wire staples are driven against an anvil, closing it into a B-shaped configuration (**6.16**). Small vessels within the loop of the B are occluded. This has the advantage of securing hemostasis but the disadvantage of tissue damage. The length of the legs of the staple determines the diameter of the B-shaped loop and thus, the amount of the affected tissue within the loop.

In conclusion, the development of clips, and stapling and suturing instruments has produced enormous advantages in gynecological surgery. No instrument, however, can replace sound surgical judgment and technique.

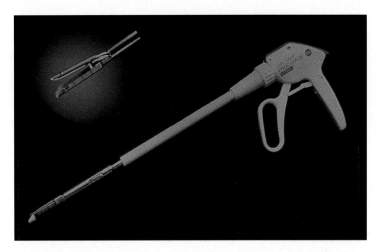

6.14 Disposable stapling device. Endo GIA™ (US Surgical).

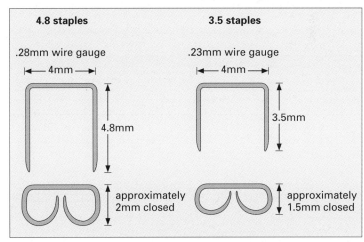

6.15 Disposable stapling device. Endopath™ (Ethicon Surgical).

6.16 Staple against anvil leading to a B-shape configuration.

FURTHER READING

Bruhat MA, Mage G, Chapron C *et al.* Present day endoscopic surgery in gynecology. *Eur J Obstet Gynecol Reprod Biol* 1991; **41**: 4–13

Gomel V. Operative laparoscopy: Time for acceptance. *Fertil Steril* 1989; **52**: 1–7

Grainger DA, Meyer WR, DeCherney AH *et al.* Laparoscopic clips. Evaluation of absorbable and titanium with regard to hemostasis and tissue reactivity. *J Reprod Med* 1991; **36**: 493–5

Martin DC, Diamond MP. Operative Laparoscopy: comparison of lasers with other techniques. *Curr Probl Obstet Gynecol Fertil* 1991; **9**: 563–77

McLaughlin DS, Diamond MP, Daniell JF *et al.* Laparoscopic assessment of ovarian healing following CO$_2$ laser microsurgery: Vicryl vs. Surgilon. *Microsurgery* 1987; **8**: 99–102

Semm K. Operative manual for endoscopic abdominal surgery. Chicago: Year Book 1987; **23**: 31–38

TUBAL STERILIZATION

7

Alan G Gordon

INTRODUCTION

Laparoscopic tubal sterilization is the most frequently performed endoscopic operation in current gynecological practice. The advantages of this approach to female sterilization over laparotomy or mini-laparotomy are that the incisions are small and can be cosmetically placed, the operating time is short and the procedure can be performed on a day care basis. Properly performed with modern techniques the complication rate should be extremely low. There is a small failure rate due either to incomplete occlusion or recanalization of the tube.

ELECTRICAL METHODS OF TUBAL OCCLUSION

The first suggestion that laparoscopic tubal occlusion might be possible was made in 1936 by Anderson in the USA. However, it is probable that the first actual sterilization operation using tubal fulgaration was performed by Power and Barnes in the USA in 1941. Laparoscopy became less popular in the USA during the following 20 years because of poor light sources and lens systems which made visualization difficult. During this time laparoscopic sterilization was popularized by Palmer in Paris and much of the credit for the early development of the procedure must go to him.

MONOPOLAR ELECTROCOAGULATION

In the classical method of monopolar electrocoagulation the current is conveyed from the electric generator to the tip of the forceps, and then to the target tissue. Heat is produced at the point of contact and localized tissue destruction takes place. The lateral spread of heat is dependent on the duration of application and the power of the current. The electric current must return from the point of application to the generator via the return plate which is usually applied to the patients leg. The return pathway is always along the path of least resistence and is usually over the surface of organs such as the bowel to the pelvic side wall and then to the return plate (**7.1**).

Laparoscopy is performed as described in Chapter 2. The patient is anesthetized with endotracheal intubation and positive pressure respiration. The legs should be flexed and supported in a modified lithotomy position to allow access to the vagina. The bladder is emptied and a cannula or probe is inserted in the uterus to facilitate manipulation. This allows better visualization of the tubes. The patient should be in a 15° Trendelenburg position to allow the bowel to fall out of the pelvis and avoid possible contact with the fallopian tubes or the laparoscopic instruments.

A standard 0° telesope should be introduced through an umbilical incision and the abdominal and pelvic organs inspected. The suitability of the tubes for coagulation should be assessed. Coagulation may be difficult if the tubes are distorted as a result of infection, endometriosis or previous surgery. There may be increased risk of thermal damage to other organs such as the ureter or bowel. Adhesions may also limit access to the tubes and may have to be divided before attempting coagulation. The tube must be inspected throughout its length to ensure recognition and to exclude distal tubal disease which may make sterilization unnecessary or undesirable.

The secondary trocar and cannula should be inserted in the midline 4 cm above the pubic symphysis. The isthmus of the tube should then be grasped, drawn gently away from contact with other organs and, when the tube is clearly seen, the generator should be activated. The tube will be seen to blanche before it bubbles and collapses. The process should be repeated in two or three places on the isthmus to ensure destruction of its full thickness. The tube may then be divided with scissors. This procedure results in loss of approximately half of the length of the tube which, while ensuring the success of the sterilization operation, makes re-anastomosis virtually impossible (**7.2**).

The tube may be divided either with scissors or by advancing the cutting sheath of the Palmer biopsy forceps which transects the tube with its serrated edge. The value of division of the tube is debatable. While it ensures that the continuity of the tubal lumen has been broken, it may produce a tubo-peritoneal fistula and thereby increase the risk of pregnancy.

The failure rate of monopolar tubal electrocoagulation is low but the complication rate is high. It fell into disrepute in the middle 1970s and is rarely performed in modern gynecological practice.

BIPOLAR ELECTROCOAGULATION

The dangers of monopolar electrocoagulation soon became evident and new instruments for bipolar electrocoagulation were developed by Frangenheim in Germany and Rioux in Canada in the early 1970s. In this procedure the current passes from the generator to one blade of a pair of forceps which acts as the positive electrode and through the intervening tisues to the second blade, the negative

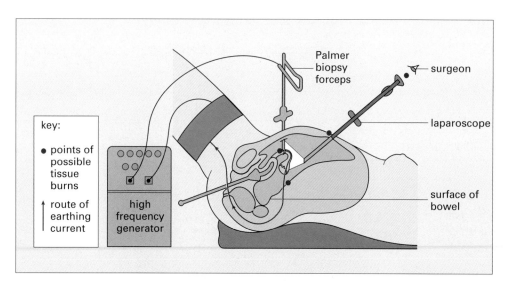

7.1 Electrical pathway in monopolar tubal coagulation.

electrode. Bipolar electrocoagulation is safer than monopolar coagulation because the current passes through only a small amount of the patient's body tissues.

However, there is still risk of inadvertent tissue damage by lateral spread of heat. Moreover, if a monopolar and bipolar system are in simultaneous use, the current may return from the bipolar forceps to the return plate and, in effect, act as a monopolar current with the risk of tissue damage on its return pathway. It is imperative, therefore, that the monopolar unit should always be switched off when the bipolar is in use.

Routine laparoscopy should be peformed and the secondary trocar and cannula inserted through a 5 mm incision above the pubic symphysis. The fallopian tube must be identified and care taken to ensure that it is not in contact with any other structure.

The tube should be grasped with the bipolar forceps (**7.3**) and the generator activated. Thermal destruction of the tube may be seen to spread from the forceps along the isthmus and into the mesosalpinx (**7.4**). The tube may then be divided with scissors (**7.5**). The cut ends should be coagulated again to ensure that they are sealed. This should prevent fistula formation. The risks of direct heat transmission are similar to monopolar coagulation but the risk of distant electric burns as the current returns to the return plate is eliminated.

THERMOCOAGULATION

The third technique, thermocoagulation, was developed by Semm in Kiel and involves the use of low voltage current to heat the resistance wires in the blades of a pair of forceps. The temperature and duration of effect are controlled by the endocoagulator. This has both visual and acoustic signals so that the surgeon is aware of its activity without lifting his eyes from the operation field. There is less risk of spread of heat to other structures and, because there is no electric current passing through the body tissues, the technique is safer than either mono- or bipolar electrocoagulation.

As in tubal electrocoagulation, routine laparoscopy is performed and the secondary trocar and cannula introduced. Crocodile forceps are inserted to coagulate the tubal isthmus. The coagulator is set to produce a temperature of 120–140°C for 20–40 seconds (**7.6, 7.7**). The surgeon recognizes when the instrument is activated by the increasing pitch of the acoustic signal as the tissue temperature rises. The signal is constant as the tissues boil and and the pitch descends when the current ceases to flow and the tissues cool. In this case also the tube may be divided with scissors (**7.8**).

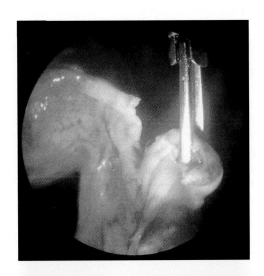

7.2 Coagulation and division of tube.

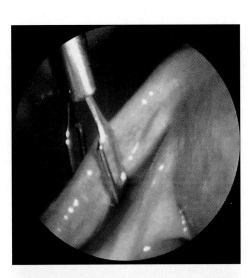

7.3 Tube grasped with bipolar forceps.

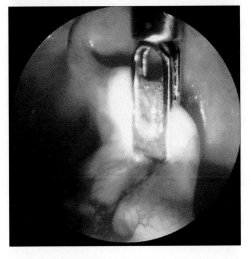

7.4 The coagulation effect involves the tube and mesosalpinx.

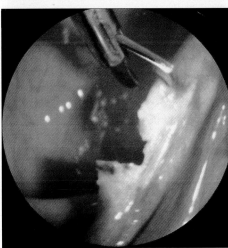

7.5 Tube divided with scissors.

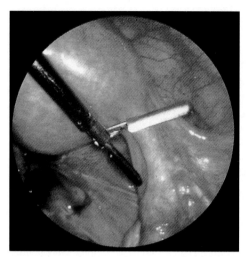

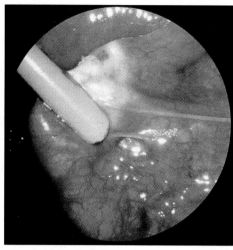

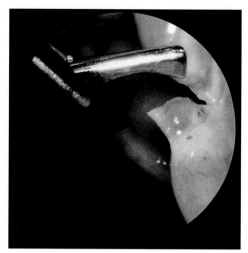

7.6 Crocodile forceps applied to tube.   **7.7** Coagulation of tube.   **7.8** Section of tube.

COMPLICATIONS

Monopolar Current

The use of high frequency monopolar current led to a number of serious complications in the 1970s including burns from direct spread of heat, burns to structures distant from the operation field, alteration in ovarian function, failure of tubal occlusion and difficulty in reversing the operation by reconstructive tubal surgery.

Burns

Direct spread of heat from the operation site may cause damage to nearby organs such as loops of bowel if they are in close contact with the fallopian tube or the forceps.

More commonly, electric burns to adjacent structures such as the small or large bowel, ureter and bladder may occur as the electric current returns to the dispersive plate. Burns to the bowel serosa may occur at the point of contact with the fallopian tube. If the area of contact is small, the power density of the current may be sufficient to cause a burn. It is possible for burns to occur outside the operator's visual field and fail to be recognized.

Bowel burns may be sufficiently severe to produce immediate blanching of the serosa or there may be an obvious fistula. Whether or not there is perforation, immediate laparotomy and oversewing of the damaged area of the bowel is mandatory. Less severe burns may lead to delayed avascular necrosis of the bowel wall. Symptoms may not develop for two to three days when their onset may be insidious with vague abdominal symptoms and variable fever. The diagnosis of fecal fistula may be difficult and delay in instituting treatment results in generalized peritonitis with drastic consequences to the patient.

Burns may also be produced to structures on the pelvic side walls such as the ureter or bladder. The peritoneum over the ureter may be damaged in the same way as the bowel serosa and, if the burn is deep, a ureteric fistula may be produced.

If the instruments have not been properly insulated and they come in contact with the patient's abdominal wall, there may also be burns of the patient's skin and even the surgeon may suffer burns to the hands or face.

Alteration in ovarian function

The application of mono- or bipolar electrocoagulation produces an extensive area of necrosis in the mesosalpinx which may damage the tubal artery as it runs along the mesenteric border of the tube. Since this also supplies some of the blood to the ovary, ovarian function may be disturbed and this probably accounts for some of the reports of menstrual disturbance following tubal sterilization.

Failure of sterilization

The failure rate of sterilization by electrocoagulation is small. In the author's series of 1100 procedures performed between 1969 and 1975 there were no intrauterine pregnancies but there were six ectopic pregnancies, none of which were life threatening but all requiring laparotomy.

Reversal of sterilization

Although the failure rate with tubal electrocoagulation was low, the extensive destruction mitigated against successful reversal which nearly always entailed a isthmo-ampullary anastomosis.

MECHANICAL METHODS OF TUBAL OCCLUSION

The problems resulting from the complications of the thermal methods of tubal occlusion led to the development of mechanical devices. These include several forms of clips, silastic rings and some little-used methods of tubal ligation through the laparoscope. Clips are usually applied using a double-puncture technique but many surgeons use an operating laparoscope to apply rings through a single incision. This makes the procedure quicker, especially if two rings are loaded on to the applicator at the same time.

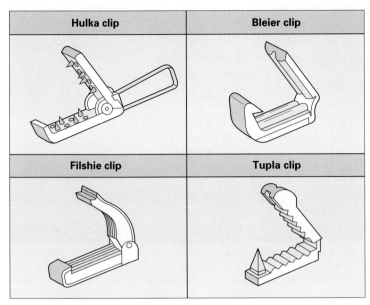

7.9 Types of clip.

TUBAL CLIPS

Four types of tubal clips were developed in Europe and North America in the 1970s but only two have survived the test of time (**7.9**). The Bleier and Tupla clips from Germany were both made of plastic and problems arose from weakness of the plastic hinges causing the clips to fracture The Hulka clip, originally developed in North Carolina and modified by Lieberman in London, was the first to gain wide acceptance. It was soon followed by the Filshie clip developed in Nottingham, England.

The Hulka clip is made of lexon and has teeth to prevent it slipping off the tube. It has a metal hinge. Compression of the tube is effected by the strength of a gold-plated stainless steel spring which slides forwards in the applicator when the clip is closed. It is usually applied by a double puncture technique. The secondary trocar and cannula should be inserted as above.

The applicator should, if possible, approach the tube in line with the mesosalpinx (**7.10**). The full thickness of the tube must be grasped by pushing the clip applicator firmly into the tissues to include part of the mesosalpinx with the tube. The tube is then pulled out to ensure the application is correct (**7.11**) before finally pushing the spring forwards to lock it on the clip. The tube may then be elevated with the applicator to check the application (**7.12**). The failure rate with the Hulka clip is low but, nevertheless, it is sufficient to encourage the use of two clips on each isthmus to try to reduce it. The peritoneum grows over the clip within a few days preventing it from being dislodged. Adhesion formation is rare.

The second clip in common use is the Filshie clip. This has two titanium leaves with a silastic lining. When the clip is closed on the tube the silastic gradually expands compressing the isthmus which undergoes avascular necrosis. After a few days the tube is transected and the two blind ends may become separated by a significant distance. The technique is similar to the application of the Hulka clip except that the instrument is easier to use with either hand and therefore a cosmetic suprapubic approach, is possible. **7.13–7.16** show the clip being applied to the isthmus of the fallopian tube and the final result.

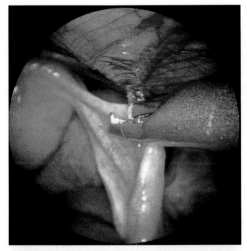

7.10 Application of Hulka clip.

7.11 Application of Hulka clip.

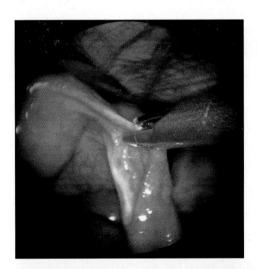

7.12 Hulka clip in situ.

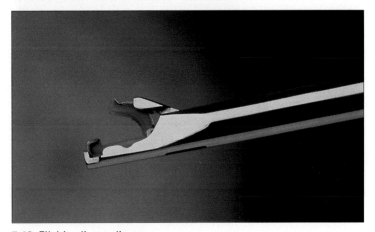

7.13 Filshie clip applicator.

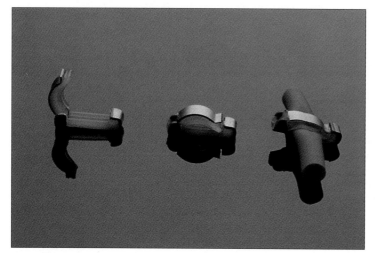

7.14 Filshie clip.

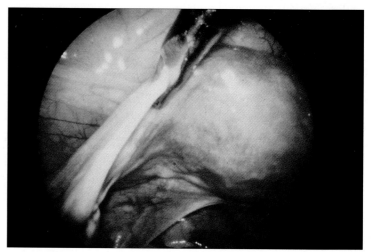

7.15 Application of Filshie clip.

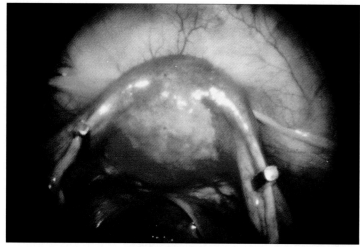

7.16 Application of Filshie clip.

FALLOPE RINGS

Yoon in Baltimore developed a silastic ring at the same time as Hulka was working on the spring-loaded clip in North Carolina. The operation can be performed with a single or double puncture technique. The advantage of the former is that it is easier to inspect the tube for correct application. The latter allows the operation to be performed through a single umbilical incision and, when two clips are loaded simultaneously, it can be performed very quickly without taking the laparoscope out of the abdomen. This has advantages when large series are being performed under local anesthesia.

As with the application of clips, standard laparoscopy is carried out and, when a double puncture technique is being used, the secondary incision is placed in the midline above the pubic symphysis. A small silastic ring is loaded onto an applicator using a cone-shaped instrument to effect initial dilation of the ring. A loop of tubal isthmus is formed by grasping the full thickness of the tube together with a small part of the of mesosalpinx (**7.17**). The loop of tube is then drawn into the lumen of the applicator by advancing the applicator towards the tube (**7.18**). If the tube is drawn into the lumen of the applicator by exerting traction on it, transection of the tube with resulting hemorrhage is likely. The ring is then pushed off the end of the applicator. When the tube is released from the chan-

nel of the applicator the fallope ring can be seen applied to the tube with a loop of isthmus completely occluded by the ring (**7.19**).

Failure of the sterilization may result from the tube being incompletely grasped by the forceps so that the loop does not contain the full thickness of the tube which, therefore, may not be fully occluded (**7.20**).

TUBAL LIGATION

A number of ingenious methods have been devised to occlude the tubes but they have not gained favor because of their complexity. It is possible to occlude the tube with an endoligature using a nonabsorbable material (**7.21, 7.22**). A similar operation has been devized using a wire loop and attaching a low-voltage electric generator to each end of the loop and passing a current through the loop to coagulate the tube. The only advantage of such techniques is that a loop of tube may be removed for histological examination for medico-legal purposes. The success of the other simpler and effective methods has prevented these techniques from general acceptance.

COMPLICATIONS

The complication rate of clip or ring sterilization is low and is related almost entirely to faulty techniques. The tube may be torn as it is drawn out to apply a clip or as it is pulled into the sheath of the applicator during ring application. This may cause bleeding. The main problems which arise with either clips or rings is when the tube is distorted by adhesions and is therefore difficult to mobilize. It may then be impossible to apply any kind of mechanical device and electric coagulation or laparoscopic salpingectomy may be necessary.

It is possible that application of a mechanical device may cause a mild infection to flare up and result in acute salpingitis (**7.23**) but this is rare.

Failed Sterilization
Pregnancies have been reported after all methods of sterilization including bilateral salpingectomy but the frequency is difficult to determine with accuracy.

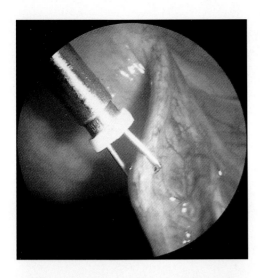

7.17 Application of fallope ring.

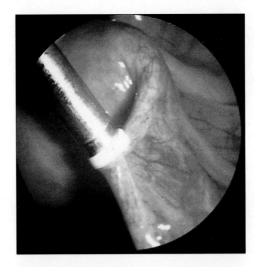

7.18 Application of fallope ring.

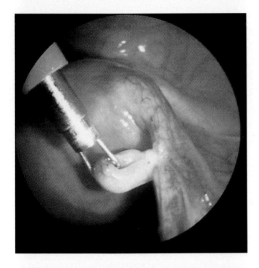

7.19 Application of fallope ring.

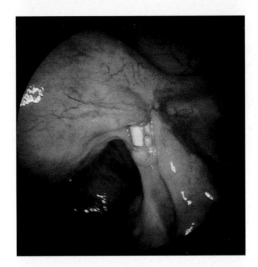

7.20 Incomplete application of ring.

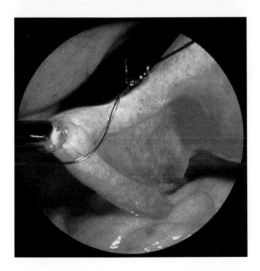

7.21 Tubal ligation.

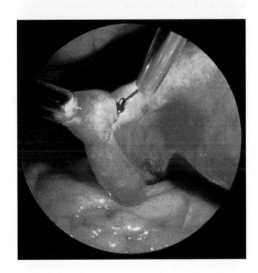

7.22 Tubal ligation.

The 1975 survey by the American Association of Gynecologic Laparoscopists (AAGL) showed that pregnancies can occur up to five years after electrocoagulation of the tube with a cumulative rate of 22.5/1000 cases. Even in skilled hands the pregnancy rate is 1–7/1000 individuals.

The pregnancy rate from the fallope ring is also 1–2/1000 patients although there have been no long-term studies. The Hulka clip had a failure rate in one series of 2–6/1000 patients. A study in England showed one pregnancy in 600 patients followed up for more than a year. All the information available therefore suggests

a small risk of failure with no difference between electrocoagulation or occlusion with fallope rings or Hulka clips.

7.24 shows the intrauterine and ectopic pregnancy rate from over 78,000 sterilizations reported by members of the AAGL in 1975.

A second large survey of over 77,000 sterilizations reported to the AAGL in 1976 confirmed that over a four or five year period 2–6 patients per 1000 became pregnant.

The most recent large scale survey by the AAGL was in 1988. It reviewed the data on almost 30,500 laparoscopic sterilizations and just under 10,000 postpartum Pomeroy procedures. The

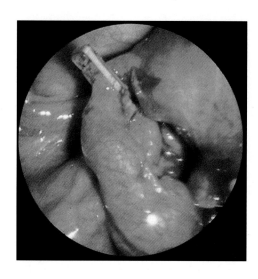

7.23 Acute salpingitis with clip.

	Pregnancy after sterilization	
	Intrauterine/1000	Ectopic/1000
Electric:		
Monopolar with division	2	0.5
Bipolar	1.6	0.2
Fallope ring	1.6	2.3
Hulka clip	7.3	0

7.24 Pregnancy rate after sterilization per 1000 individuals.

most significant finding was that 73% of monopolar coagulation failures were ectopic gestations compared to 16% of clip failures.

Pregnancy can occur after sterilization because of method or operator failure. Method failure undoubtedly occurs even when the operation is correctly performed. The tube can recanalize following electrocoagulation or below the closed jaws of a clip (**7.23**). A fistula can form if the tubes have been divided which may result in an eutopic or ectopic pregnancy. Operator failure may occur if the surgeon fails to adequately identify the tube and coagulates or clips the round ligament or the mesosalpinx. Sometimes the clip may fall off the tube if it has not been properly closed. In these cases legal action is likely to be successful even if the patient has signed a consent form with a disclaimer.

The best form of protection for the surgeon against legal action is clear pre-operative explanation, adequate training, precise documentation and, if possible, a video recording of the operation.

Luteal phase pregnancy is always a possibility if sterilization is performed in the second half of the menstrual cycle. Patients should be advised to practice contraception prior to admission. Uterine curettage may fail to disturb an early pregnancy and, at least in the UK, cannot legally be performed with the intention of terminating a pregnancy without preoperative documentation and consent.

CONCLUSION

Laparoscopic tubal occlusion presents an effective, safe and easy method of female sterilization. The hospital stay need not be more than a few hours and the return to normal duties should be within a few days. With the modern mechanical methods using clips or rings, the length of tubal destruction is such that microsurgical reconstructive tubal surgery carries a high chance of success.

LAPAROSCOPIC SURGERY
FOR INFERTILITY

8

Victor Gomel

INTRODUCTION

Laparoscopy was introduced into gynecological practice some three decades ago as a diagnostic technique. It was used primarily in the investigation of infertility. It allowed detailed inspection of the uterus, ovaries, fallopian tubes and pelvic peritoneum. Operative laparoscopy was originally confined to tubal sterilization. The concept of using the laparoscope as a means of access to perform other operations came later and was slow to gain general acceptance. Among the first procedures to be performed were those to promote fertility such as the treatment of periadnexal adhesions and distal tubal obstruction.

INVESTIGATION

The couple presenting with infertility should be offered a series of investigations. The complexity of these will depend on their age, previous obstetric performance, if any, and the duration of infertility. Initially all patients should have a detailed history and general and pelvic clinical examination. Other early investigations should include assessment of the the male partner's seminal fluid and determination of the female partner's ovulatory status. Hysterosalpingography (HSG) should be the initial investigation for the status of the uterine cavity and the fallopian tubes. This should always be performed by the clinician and not delegated to a radiologist who may or may not have a special interest in the technique. Too often a bolus of radiopaque dye is injected into the uterus followed by rapid inspection of the results on the screen. The dye must be injected slowly through a cannula which has been gently inserted into the cervical canal. Filling of the uterus and passage of dye along the fallopian tubes should be continuously observed. This causes no discomfort and produces valuable information. The physician may be able to identify uterine anomalies and intrauterine lesions, recognize cornual occlusion and diagnose non-occlusive proximal tubal disease, as well as distal occlusion. It is frequently possible to assess the status of the tubal mucosa. This information may then lead the physician to perform more detailed investigations including hysteroscopy, falloposcopy, laparoscopy and salpingoscopy. The prognosis for surgery for distal tubal disease is better in the presence of a relatively normal mucosal architecture. If prior HSG has demonstrated a normal uterine outline and tubal patency, the surgeon who discovers periadnexal adhesive disease will be encouraged to proceed with laparoscopic salpingo-ovariolysis. The information provided by the HSG will enable the surgeon to anticipate and schedule the appropriate operating room time for the procedure.

INSTRUMENTS

CUTTING INSTRUMENTS

Transection of tissues by laparoscopy may be accomplished with scissors, electrosurgery or laser.

Scissors

Laparoscopic scissors are used principally for mechanical division of tissues even though they may be provided with an electrosurgical capability. Scissors have been our preferred cutting instrument for salpingo-ovariolysis and other fertility promoting procedures on the tubes and ovaries. A number of different types of scissors are available.

Hook scissors have certain advantages. They allow the surgeon to lift an adhesion away from the surrounding tissues before sectioning it (**8.1**). However, the points of some hook scissors overlap which may be dangerous. The overlapping points present a sharp tip which may damage tissues when the scissors are used to retract or if they are left unattended within the peritoneal cavity. Straight or curved scissors are often preferable (**8.2**). If this type of scissors are used the surgeon should ensure that one blade is fixed and the other mobile as this allows tissues to be lifted and inspected before division.

Scissors must be able to cut effectively. Almost all scissors will become blunt with use. Maintenance and sharpening is difficult because of the disproportionate ratio between length and caliber which largely negates any advantage gained by sharpening. Disposable scissors provide one solution to the problem but are expensive for routine use. A new development is the provision of reusable scissors with replacable blades which combine the advantages of machine tooled instruments with the ability to replace/sharpen blades which have become blunt with use. These also have the advantage of being able to be rotated so that they can be aligned with the target tissue more easily.

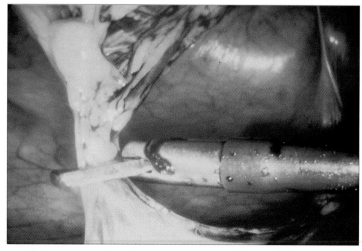

8.1 Omental adhesiolysis with hook scissors.

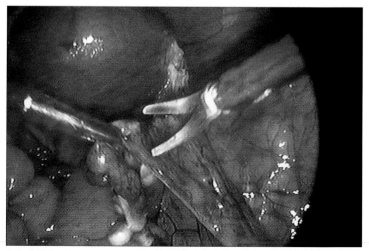

8.2 Salpingectomy with curved scissors.

ELECTROSURGICAL INSTRUMENTS

The general surgeon is often unaware of all the properties of the electric current he uses to cut or control bleeding. The laparoscopic surgeon must be aware of the physical characteristics of the form of energy used because the work is performed in a closed space. Knowledge of the bioeffects on the tissues, the pathways taken by electric current and the characteristics of the different forms of current is mandatory.

Effective cutting may be achieved with the use of a non-modulated monopolar current in the cutting mode. This is best applied with a retractable micro-needle. The coagulating mode may be used to achieve hemostasis. Alternatively, a blended current may be used which allows cutting but with some coagulating effect. A bipolar forceps may also be used to desiccate blood vessels. Electrosurgery is preferably used to prevent bleeding but is also essential to complete haemostasis at the end of the procedure.

Monopolar electrosurgery was considered dangerous in the 1970's because of the number of accidental burns to adjacent organs which occurred when high frequency current was used to occlude the fallopian tubes. Improved electrosurgical generators, properly employed monopolar techniques and a greater understanding of the principles of electrosurgery have made monopolar surgery safe with no greater risk of inadvertent damage than with other energy sources.

LASER

Four laser systems are in current use in gynecology: CO_2, KTP, Argon and Nd:YAG. The CO_2 is the most appropriate for laparoscopic fertility surgery because its depth of penetration makes it safe for use in proximity to vital structures and for working on the ovary. Its main disadvantage is that it cannot be effectively passed through a flexible fiber. Consequently the light beam must be guided into the peritoneal cavity along a straight hollow tube which may limit the direction of effective delivery.

The other three lasers may be propagated along a flexible quartz fibre which may be directed towards the target tissue. Some surgeons prefer to apply Nd:YAG in contact with the tissues using sapphire tips. These are expensive, may break off and cause greater thermal damage.

The Argon and KTP lasers require water cooling which necessitates installing new plumbing into the operating room. There is also greater adjacent thermal injury than with CO_2.

OTHER INSTRUMENTS

The other instruments commonly used in laparoscopic surgery include probes, grasping instruments, irrigation and suction cannulae and, occasionally needle holders. The latter are available in 3 mm and 5 mm diameters, the remainder are usually 5 mm diameter. Both atraumatic and toothed grasping forceps should be available. Heparinized Ringer lactate at 40°C is used for irrigation. The irrigation cannula also allows the surgeon to perform hydrodissection in adhesiolysis.

PRINCIPLES OF LAPAROSCOPIC SURGERY

The patient should be placed in a modified lithotomy position with her legs abducted, flexed to 5° and the knees bent to provent her sliding cephalad on the table. This gives access to the genital tract from below without interfering with the full range of movement of the laparoscopic instruments. An intrauterine cannula should be inserted which allows manipulation of the uterus as well as intra-operative chromopertubation. Manipulation of the uterus enhances pelvic exposure and allows the adnexae to be immobilized which, in turn, facilitates the procedure.

With proper positioning of the patient and adequate distension of the peritoneal cavity by the pneumoperitoneum, an excellent exposure of the pelvic organs can be achieved by laparoscopy. The ability to bring the laparoscope into close approximation with the target tissue allows the surgeon to obtain an even better view than by laparotomy. Additionally, the laparoscope magnifies 2x and further magnification is obtained by the use of the video screen.

A multiple puncture technique must always be used. A 7 mm to 10 mm laparoscope is introduced through the umbilicus. Secondary trocars and cannulae are inserted at McBurney's point and a similar position on the left side or in the midline suprapubically. The separation of the visual and operative axes provided by the technique allows better perception of depth, compensating for the loss of binocular vision inherent in laparoscopy. It is always necessary to use a high definition camera and a video screen which makes the stance of the surgeon comfortable and allows the other operating room personel to assist effectively. The video monitor should be placed at the caudal end of the operating table to enable all the staff to have a clear view of the screen.

There are limitations to laparoscopic surgery. The number of portals is limited so the variety of angles of approach to the target tissue is also limited. This disadvantage may be partially overcome by manipulation of the uterus by an intrauterine cannula and by using the uterus to steady the adnexa. This may be simply done by retroverting the uterus, lifting the adnexa and then anteverting the uterus again and displacing the fundus into the ovarian fossa. This manoeuvre brings the adnexa to lie on the anterior surface of the uterus which then becomes an "internal operatng table". Access may also be improved by traction on adhesions or organs with forceps to alter the alignment of the tissue. The introduction of rectal or vaginal probes and varying the horizontal and lateral tilt of the table may also improve access to a particular area.

An essential part of laparoscopic surgery is to carry out intra-operative irrigation and pelvic lavage to remove blood and other protein material which may promote adhesion formation. Prevention of desiccation of tissues is essential. The flushing cannula may also be used to perform hydrodissection. The irrigation fluid is introduced between tissue planes under pressure. The fluid always finds the pathway of least resistance and may be used to separate tissues without bleeding or risk of trauma.

Laparoscopic hemostasis is relatively crude in comparison to microsurgery. Although fine monopolar and bipolar forceps are available they are not as precise as those used in microsurgical procedures. Bleeding in laparoscopic surgery is limited by the pressure of the pneumoperitoneum and by the use of warm irrigation fluid. Troublesome oozing may be controlled by instillation of a very dilute solution of vasopressin. Specific bleeding vessels may be identified by examining the operation field under water. The pelvis is filled with irrigation fluid and the tip of the laparoscope immersed in the pool to visualize small bleeding vessels and desiccate them with micro-bipolar forceps under the surface of the fluid.

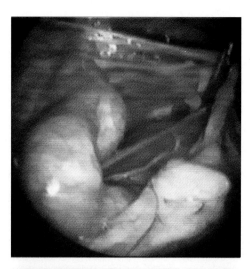

8.3 Extensive fine peritubal adhesions.

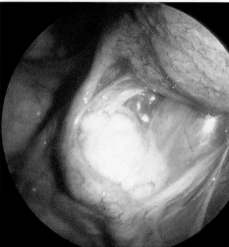

8.4 Periovarian adhesions secondary to chronic pelvic inflamatory disease.

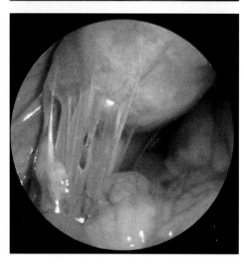

8.5 Fine adhesions resulting from infection involving both the tube and the ovary.

tle tissue handling and avoidance of drying. Peritoneal trauma caused by mechanical, thermal or chemical agents induces an inflammatory reaction. The inflammatory exudate contains fibrinogen which is transformed into fibrin. Fibrin deposition and fibroblastic proliferation are the basis of adhesion formation.

Laparoscopy is performed within a closed abdomen. This prevents the dessication of tissues which occurs at laparotomy. However, this advantage may be lost in operative laparoscopy when high volumes of CO_2 are insufflated.

Laparoscopic surgery, like microsurgery, requires the use of relatively few instruments. However, because of the length of the instruments it has not been possible as yet to design fine forceps and scissors as in microsurgical instruments. The force applied to the tissue is increased by the length of the instrument projecting from the cannula which acts as a fulcrum. This produces more tissue trauma than occurs with microsurgery.

A further limitation of laparoscopic surgery is related to the optical system. Perception of depth is significantly decreased by the monocular vision.

FERTILITY-PROMOTING PROCEDURES

Procedures which are of proven value in improving fertility include:
• Adhesiolysis
• Salpingo-ovariolysis
• Fimbrioplasty
• Salpingostomy

ADHESIOLYSIS

Pelvic adhesions are usually secondary to pelvic inflammatory disease (PID) (**8.3–8.5**) or the result of acute ruptured appendicitis. Postoperative adhesions are usually more cohesive and dense than those resulting from PID. The adhesions resulting from endometriosis are usually associated with the more extensive stages of the disease (**8.6, 8.7**).

Periadnexal adhesions are usually associated with other occlusive tubal disease. They may also be present without any evidence of tubal occlusion. In this case the adhesions envelop the fimbrial end of the fallopian tube and prevent the oocyte entering the tubal lumen. Adhesions may surround the ovary preventing oocyte release or they may cause distortion of the normal anatomical relationships between the tube and ovary and interfere with oocyte pick-up.

Adhesions are composed of connective tissue with a variable degree of vascularity. They may be filmy or thick. They may be avascular or contain a large number of blood vessels. There may be a variable amount of space between abnormally joined organs, some are cohesive and dense with virtually no space, others are loosely joined by relatively fine adhesions.

Patients with prior abdominal or pelvic surgery frequently have adhesions between the omentum and abdominal wall (**8.8**). Adhesiolysis should be carried out close to the parietal peritoneum where there is usually a relatively avascular attachment. Even the fatty and vascular omentum is usually attached to the peritoneum by a relatively filmy adhesion with few or no vessels in it. Traction with forceps will demonstrate the avascular area which can be easily divided with scissors. Occasionally there are large blood vessels. These should be coagulated with bipolar electrocoagulation prior to section.

The greatest problem in laparoscopic fertility surgery in comparison to microsurgery is the accurate alignment of tissue planes. Laparoscopic suturing is difficult and time-consuming despite the development of new needle holders. It is also difficult to use very fine suture material and needles. They tend to break or bend because of the large needle holders and the greater force necessary to insert the suture. The tendancy is to use fewer sutures with resultant failure of accurate apposition of tissue planes.

The "gold standard" of reconstructive surgery is microsurgery. The essential ingredients of microsurgery are the use of magnification and the avoidance of tissue trauma. Tissue trauma is minimized by gen-

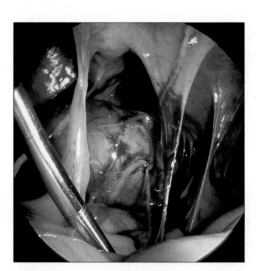

8.6 Adhesions secondary to endometriosis.

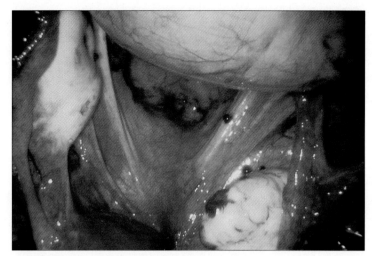

8.7 Adhesions resulting from endometriosis.

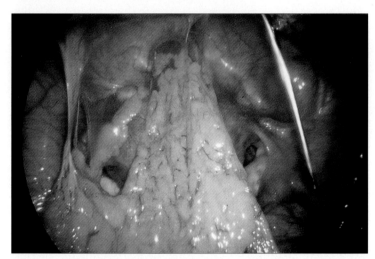

8.8 Adhesions resulting from previous myomectomy.

SALPINGO-OVARIOLYSIS

The first step in salpingo-ovariolysis is to evaluate the type and extent of the adhesive process and the structures involved. This is especially important if there is distortion of the anatomy when it is essential to define the correct relationships accurately. Failure to adhere to this rule may produce tissue trauma and increase the likelihood of complications. Adhesions should be divided at their attachment and not half way between the adherent organs. The line of section should be along the organ to be freed.

Adhesions usually have at least two layers which should be divided separately since they affix to different sites. Section should commence in a well exposed area. The sectioning instrument should approach the adhesion perpendicularly and divide the adhesion parallel to the surface of the organ avoiding damage to its serosal surface. Section with scissors may be performed close to the organ. When laser or electrosurgical energy are used, a small space should be left between the instrument and organ to avoid damage by lateral transmission of heat.

Effective and safe adhesiolysis requires the following considerations: 1) Recognition of the structures lying behind the adhesion. 2) Retraction of the adhesion with a probe or grasping forceps applied to the adhesion and not to the target organ. 3) A small initial incision in the adhesion revealing what structures lie behind it. The form of the adhesion will also be recognized and whether it is composed of one layer or two. 4) Short adhesions may be simply divided; longer, or more complex adhesions should be divided

at both attachments and the whole adhesion removed from the abdomen through a cannula.

Adhesions are best divided with scissors. Electrocoagulation should be used only when a significant vessel crosses the line of section. Adhesions secondary to PID are usually filmy and avascular. They are amenable to mechanical section or excision. Adhesions with little space between the organs such as when loops of bowel adhere to one another should be separated without the use of thermal energy. In this case a small incision should be made at one edge of the adhesion and the tissue planes separated by spreading the jaws of scissors or forceps or by hydrodissection.

Fatty adhesions are usually related to omentum or an appendicae epiploica. When such adhesions are put on stretch it is usually possible to see an avascular attachment where the omentum or appendix meets the serosa of the organ to which it is attached. Section with scissors is usually easy.

The procedure is completed with thorough pelvic lavage with Ringer's lactate solution at 40°C. This allows removal of blood and debris from the pelvis. The warm solution has a hemostatic effect but also allows recognition of persistent bleeders. These can be coagulated with a monopolar or bipolar instrument, the latter may be applied accurately under the surface of the irrigating fluid where the blood vessel is recognized by the little spiral of blood coming from it.

Finally it is prudent to leave 150 to 200 ml of Ringer's lactate solution containing 500 mg of hydrocortisone succinate in the pelvis. This probably prevents adhesion formation by allowing the pelvic organs to float in the fluid for a few hours and thus prevents dry non-motile surfaces sticking together.

FIMBRIOPLASTY

Salpingitis may cause varying degrees of tubal occlusion (**8.9**). Agglutination of the fimbriae may produce phimosis of the distal tubal opening. The tubal ostium may be covered with fibrous scar tissue. In other cases the distal tube may be completely occluded with formation of hydrosalpinx with a varying degree of tubal distension. Frequently peritubal and peri-ovarian adhesions are also present. The prognosis for tubal surgery in these cases will depend in large measure on the status of the tubal mucosa which may be ascertained by HSG and/or salpingoscopy.

Fimbrioplasty is the reconstruction of existent fimbriae in a partially or totally occluded fallopian tube. Periadnexal adhesions, when present, must be divided first. Stenosis or obstruction of the dis-

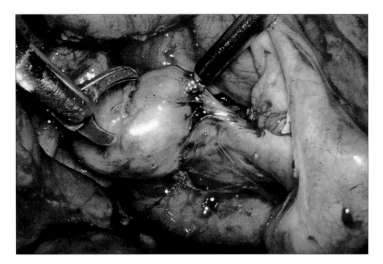

8.9 Hydrosalpinx.

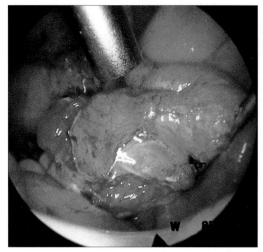

8.10 A low-power density mode of beam is aimed at the serosal surface of the tubes to cause surface coagulation.

tal end of the tube may be the result of agglutination of the fimbriae. In this case transcervical chromopertubation produces distension of the tube with delayed escape of dye into the peritoneal cavity. If the agglutinated fimbrial end is covered with a fibrous layer of tissue there will usually be complete occlusion of the tube. Less frequently there may be stenosis of the tubal ostium at the apex of the infundibulum (prefimbrial phimosis).

When the fimbrial end is covered by a layer of fibrous tissue, it will be necessary to divide this layer to expose the agglutinated fimbriae. This can be accomplished with microscissors, laser or a monopolar microneedle. The agglutinated fimbriae are separated by introducing a closed forcep into the tube through the phimosed opening. The jaws of the forceps are opened and the instrument is slowly withdrawn from the tube in the open position. This is repeated several times varying the direction of the jaws until satisfactory deagglutination is achieved. If the tissues are manipulated gently there should be no significant bleeding.

Prefimbrial phimosis is best corrected by making a longitudinal incision over the antimesosalpingeal border of the fallopian tube from the fimbriae to the ampulla proximal to the stricture. The tube should be immobilized by placing it on the "internal operating table" and, if possible, a teflon probe introduced through the fimbrial opening into the ampulla. The tube is then incised with a monopolar microneedle starting at the fimbriae and continuing towards the ampulla beyond the site of the stenosis. Bleeding from the cut edge should be controlled with a microelectrode or fine bipolar forceps. The procedure is completed with copious lavage and instillation of warm Ringer's lactate solution into the pelvis.

NEOSALPINGOSTOMY

Laparoscopic neosalpingostomy was reported from our unit in 1977. Although originally used only for repeat procedures, its success has gained acceptance as a primary approach in the treatment of hydrosalpinx. The results of surgery relate not only to the technique but to the status of the tubal mucosa which can be determined by HSG or salpingoscopy. If the tubal mucosa is abnormal then better results may be obtained by *in vitro* fertilization (IVF).

Any periadnexal adhesions are first divided. The distal fallopian tube and its relationship to the ovary must now be assessed. It is important to ascertain whether the distal tube is free in which case the tubo-ovarian ligament is clearly visible. Sometimes the dis-

tal end of the tube is adherent to the ovary in which case the ligament is not visible. It is then necessary to free the tube from the ovary before performing salpingostomy.

The technique of laparoscopic salpingostomy closely mimics that used in microsurgery (**8.10–8.13**). First the tube must be distended with fluid introduced through the uterus by a uterine cannula. This confirms proximal patency and helps to identify the cartwheel shaped scar at the site of block. The central dimple is opened with scissors, monopolar microneedle or laser. The initial incision runs from the central dimple towards the ovary to form a new fimbria ovarica. The tube should then be grasped at the edge of the incision, retracted and folded slightly backwards. This allows the surgeon to inspect the tube from within and recognize the avascular scars. Additional incisions may then be made along the circumference of the tube avoiding the vascular mucosal folds. It is essential to preserve the folds to maintain function of the fimbriae and infundibulum.

Once a satisfactory opening has been made, steps must be taken to achieve eversion. This may be done with 5-0 or 6-0 Vicryl sutures but there is no evidence that this improves the prognosis. Eversion may be effectively and simply achieved by desiccation of the serosa with bipolar current or a defocussed laser beam (**8.14, 8.15**).

Salpingoscopy can be performed, once the tube is entered at the central dimple, as described in Chapter 3 or by inserting a hysteroscope through one of the secondary cannulae and into the fimbrial opening. This will give the surgeon a reasonable estimate of the prospects of subsequent fertility. If the mucosa is normal or displays only flattening or mild to moderate adhesions, the prospects are good. If there are extensive adhesions, agglutination of the folds or loss of fold pattern with fibrosis it would be preferable to proceed to IVF sooner rather than later.

RESULTS

The data relating to the association of adhesions and pain and the efficacy of adhesiolysis for this indication are inadequate.

When considering the results of treatment for infertility associated with tubal disease, patency and total pregnancy rates are often taken as appropriate measures of outcome. However, patency does not equate with conception and many conceptions result in tubal pregnancy or with loss of an intrauterine pregnancy. The only acceptable measure of success is the "take-home baby rate".

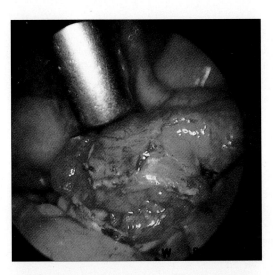

8.11 As coagulation begins, the edges begin to evert.

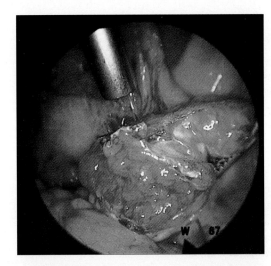

8.12 With continued coagulation, the edges continue to retract and the endosalpinx is seen.

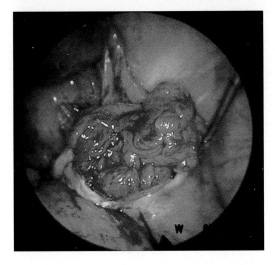

8.13 At the end of the procedure, the walls are held apart by the coagulated and contracted serosa. The eversion should be exaggerated as early cases were complicated by closure due to insufficient edge separation.

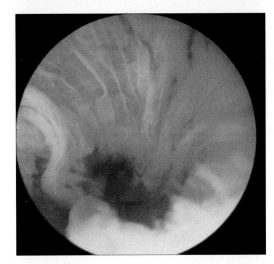

8.14 Hydro-salpinx with normal folds.

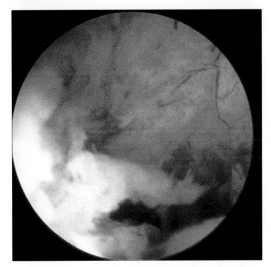

8.15 Hydro-salpinx showing damaged folds.

A successful outcome from tubal surgery can only be accepted if there has been total bilateral tubal blockage. Pregnancy may have been possible if there has been any degree of patency of either tube. Consequently studies of the value of tubal surgery on women with pre-existing tubal patency that do not have control groups may overestimate the results of the intervention.

SALPINGO-OVARIOLYSIS

In 1975 we described the results of laparoscopic salpingo-ovariolysis and fimbrioplasty. The intrauterine pregnancy rate in 24 patients followed up for a year or more was 59%. Eight years later we reported on a series of 92 patients, 79 of whom had severe peri-adnexal adhesions. After a follow-up period of at least nine months 62% had conceived, 59% with an intrauterine pregnancy. Half of these women conceived within six months of surgery. Other workers have reported relatively similar results.

FIMBRIOPLASTY

Fimbrioplasty is less frequently reported. Our series reported in 1983 showed that 47% of 40 patients had successful pregnancies and two had ectopics. Others have reported a 25–50% intrauterine pregnancy rate and up to 12% ectopic rate. It is, perhaps, surprising that some authors obtained fimbrioplasty results that are inferior to those of salpingostomy.

SALPINGOSTOMY

The first reports from our centre in 1977 showed that four out of nine patients had successful pregnancies after laparoscopic salpingostomy. In eight of the patients the laparoscopic procedure was preceded by an unsuccessful operation. Others have subsequently reported a success rate of 18–29% for laparoscopic salpingostomy.

CONCLUSION

Pelvic and periadnexal adhesions arise as a result of an inflammatory process secondary to infection, endometriosis or physical or chemical trauma. They are frequently associated with pain or infertility. With appropriate planning, instruments and technique these conditions may be treated effectively by laparoscopic surgery. The results of laparoscopic surgery of salpingolysis and fimbrioplasty approach or equal those obtained by microsurgery. The advantages to the patient of therapy at the time of the initial diagnosis, a shorter hospital stay and recovery period are self-evident.

The results of laparoscopic salpingostomy appear to be somewhat lower than those of microsurgery. However, the main factor in determining the results appears not to be the technique but the status of the fallopian tube. The factors which determine the result are the diameter of the tube, the thickness of the tubal wall, the nature of the tubal ampullary mucosa and the extent and type of adhesions. Full evaluation of the status of the tube at diagnostic laparoscopy should include assessment of all these factors by detailed examination and salpingoscopy. This can then be followed in appropriate cases by laparoscopic neosalpingostomy. The others will benefit more by referral for IVF.

FURTHER READING

Brosens I, Gordon A. The treatment of tubal infertility. In *Tubal infertility*, 1990. Lippincott/Gower, London, pp5.1–5.35

Bruhat MA, Mage G, Manhes H *et al.* Laparoscopy procedures to promote fertility: ovariolysis and salpingolysis results of 93 selected cases. *Acta Europa Fertilitatis* 1983; **14**: 476–9

Canis M, Mage G, Pouly JL *et al.* Laparoscopic distal tuboplasty: report of 87 cases and a 4-year experience. *Fertil Steril* 1991; **56**: 616–21

Daniell JF, Herbert CM. Laparoscopic salpingostomy using the CO_2 laser. *Fertil Steril* 1984; **41**: 558–63

Donnez J, Nisolle M, Casanas–Roux F. CO_2 laser laparoscopy in infertile women with adnexal adhesions and women with tubal occlusion. *J Gynecol Surg* 1989; **5**: 47

Dubuisson JB, Borquet de Jolinière J *et al.* Terminal tuboplasties by laparoscopy: 65 consective cases. *Fertil Steril* 1990; **54**: 410–3

Fayez JA. An assessment of the role of operative laparoscopy in tuboplasty. *Fertil Steril* 1983; **39**: 476–9

Gomel V. Laparoscopic tubal surgery in infertility. *Obstet Gynecol* 1975; **46**: 47

Gomel V. Salpingostomy by laparoscopy. *J Repro Med* 1977; **18**: 265–7.

Gomel V. Reconstructive surgery of the oviduct. *J Reprod Med* 1977; **18**: 181–90

Gomel V. Salpingo-ovariolysis by laparoscopy in infertility. *Fertil Steril* 1983; **340**: 607–11

Gomel V. Microsurgery in female infertility. Little Brown & Co., Boston, 1983

Gomel V. Distal tubal occlusion. *Ferrtil Steril* 1988; **49**: 946–8.

Gomel V, Taylor PJ. In vitro fertilization versus reconstructive tubal surgery. *JARGE* 1992; **9**:306–9

McComb P, Paleologou A. The intussesception salpingostomy technique for the therapy of distal oviduct occlusion at laparoscopy. *Obstet Gynecol* 1991; **78**:443–7

Tulandi T, Collins JA, Burrows E, *et al.* Treatment-dependent and treatment independent pregnancy among women with periadnexal adhesions. *Am J Obstet Gynecol* 1990; **162**: 354–7

LAPAROSCOPIC USE OF LASERS

9

James F Daniell

Lasers have been used laparoscopically in gynecology for over a decade. The use of the CO_2 laser at laparoscopy began independently in France, Israel, and North America and investigators have subsequently reported use of argon, Nd:YAG, and KTP lasers for laparoscopic laser surgery. All of these surgical lasers are now widely available and have been used clinically for many laparoscopic procedures. This chapter will review the laparoscopic use of both infrared and visible laser light energy from these four energy sources.

THE DEVELOPMENT OF LASERS FOR LAPAROSCOPY

The CO_2 laser was first used for laparoscopic surgery in France by Bruhat with independent development in Israel and the USA. After clinical trials for delivery of the CO_2 beam via laparoscopy, Eder Instrument Company (Chicago, Illinois) marketed the first system for laparoscopic use in 1982. In 1983, both the argon and the Nd:YAG laser were used in laparoscopic surgery using flexible fiberoptic delivery systems.

In the autumn of 1985, the KTP laser (Laserscope, San Jose, California) became available for clinical investigations in gynecology in North America. Initial evaluations were carried out in rabbits for treating endometriosis and other disease. The first KTP laser produced 16 W and was water cooled. Subsequent dual wavelength models producing 60 W Nd:YAG laser power were air cooled (**9.1**).

Synthetic sapphire tips have been attached to the fibre to focus and thus better control Nd:YAG laser energy. These tips are expensive, become hot, can fracture, and can only be used in direct contact with tissue. In practice, the use of sapphire tips with the Nd:YAG laser produces simple thermal tissue damage and not laser vaporization. Thus, this becomes a very expensive form of microscopic endocoagulation. Many laparoscopists still use sapphire-tipped Nd:YAG lasers, but the cost of the system has led physicians to discard them for simpler, safer, less expensive alternatives.

ADVANTAGES AND DISADVANTAGES OF FIBEROPTIC LASERS FOR LAPAROSCOPY

Having worked over a decade with the CO_2 and over five years with fiberoptic lasers, we have found they have distinct advantages in laparoscopy (**9.2**). The main advantage of fiberoptic lasers is the tremendous ease with which the laser energy can be delivered to tissue compared with the more cumbersome coupling devices needed with the CO_2 laser. The fiber is simply delivered through the operating channel of the laparoscope or through a secondary cannula into the abdomen and placed on or close to the impact site. No cumbersome alignment procedures are needed to apply the laser energy. Since the laser energy passes through clear fluids in the pelvis, the amount of smoke generated is reduced when performing operative procedures at laparoscopy, compared with the CO_2 laser. This simpler delivery system combined with less smoke generation means that operations can usually be performed more quickly than with the CO_2 laser. Another advantage of visible light (argon and KTP) lasers is the ability to either incise, vaporize, or photocoagulate rapidly by merely pulling the fiber tip back from the tissue slightly. We also feel there is less potential for bleeding, since Nd:YAG, KTP and argon lasers have greater hemostatic effects than the CO_2 laser.

As with all technology, there are some disadvantages of fiberoptic lasers. An eye safety filter must be placed over the laparoscope

before firing. This filter slightly alters the tissue color and adds an extra encumbrance to the eyepiece of the laparoscope, plus an extra cord running out from the operating field. A new small video insert filter that fits over the optics of the laparoscope has eliminated some of these problems. Another disadvantage of the KTP/YAG or argon lasers is that they cost more than CO_2 lasers or electrosurgical systems.

In spite of the above disadvantages we feel that the ease and simplicity of performing some procedures with these lasers, combined with reduced operative time, outweigh the disadvantages. This has led us to discard the CO_2 laser for laparoscopic surgery except when training physicians.

Since laser energy from fiberoptic lasers can be delivered through flexible fibers, it becomes simple to insert the fiber into the peritoneal cavity for laparoscopic surgery. The method used, when a minimum amount of laser firing is necessary, is to thread the fiber down the operating channel of a laparoscope. The advantages of this system are that it requires only one extra puncture and it gives the operator a good angle for operating in the pelvis by passing the fibre coaxially with the laparoscope. The disadvantage of this method is that it reduces the available light. In addition, the operator's depth perception is reduced because the fiber is passing down the axis of vision.

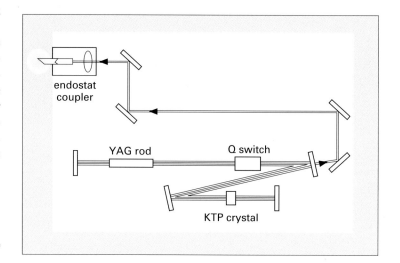

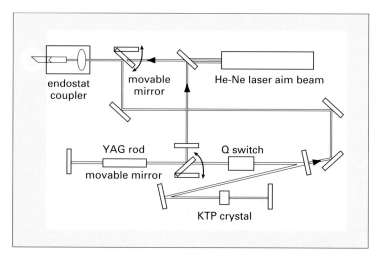

9.1a,b KTP/532 laser with Nd:YAG module. These two schematic drawings demonstrate how the KTP energy can be diverted to allow direct use of the primary 50 watt Nd:YAG laser present in each KTP machine. The lower panel shows the beam pathway with the Nd:YAG and associated helium–neon aiming laser, while the upper panel demonstrates the original KTP beam pathway.

The alternate method of use is to deliver fibers through secondary cannulae using a standard diagnostic laparoscope. A special steerable 5 mm probe (Marlow Medical, Willoughby, Ohio) has been designed which allows passage of the fiber as well as suction and irrigation. The probe tip can be rotated, from 180° to 90°, with the fiber thus being directed at the best angle (**9.3**). This probe is especially useful for treating the lateral surface of the ovary. Alternatively, the probe can be used as a backstop for the fiber or to accomplish traction on tissues in the pelvis. We have found this probe to be particularly helpful in advanced laparoscopic procedures such as salpingostomy, enterolysis, or treatment of advanced stages of endometriosis.

Since advanced operative laparoscopy demands the placement of extra trocars and cannulae, it is important to carefully select the incision sites. We normally place our first extra trocar and cannula in the midline suprapubically and use this with 5 mm instruments for retraction and dissection as necessary. If inspection of the pelvis reveals a need for a third cannula, we usually place it 5–6 cm lateral to the umbilicus at that same level and on the side opposite from the major site of disease. If a fourth cannula is needed, we place it on the opposite side. On occasion, three cannulae can be placed in the midline, but this often leads to problems with clashing of the instruments during manipulation. Care must be taken to avoid the inferior epigastric vessels when placing lateral incisions. Vascular complications can be reduced by transilluminating the abdominal wall and identifying the vessels in a briefly darkened operating room.

A plethora of ancillary instruments have been developed for laparoscopy. We feel that the minimum necessary are three 5 mm trocars and cannulae with scissors, atraumatic grasping forceps, and both unipolar and bipolar forceps. Any gynecologist who plans to undertake extensive operative laser laparoscopy should be experienced with multiple punctures and with the use of both unipolar and bipolar electrocoagulation at laparoscopy.

The use of video is essential for all operative laparoscopy. There are many advantages of video, some of which are listed in **9.4**. Since multiple punctures and extensive operative procedures require more than two hands, it is mandatory to have a coordinated, knowledgeable assistant. The only way that the assistant can be effective is by being able to visualize what is occurring, to anticipate the actions necessary to obtain optimum results. Video-controlled surgery can be with a direct coupler, which requires the operator to work while looking directly at the video monitor, or with a beam splitter, which retains the option of looking directly through the laparoscope or at the monitor.

Advantages of fiberoptic lasers for laparoscopy
Simple fiberoptic delivery
No backstop necessary
Effective under fluid
Minimal smoke formation
Excellent hemostasis
Both vapourization and coagulation possible
Short operating time

9.2 Advantages of fiberoptic lasers for laparoscopy.

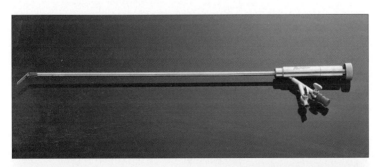

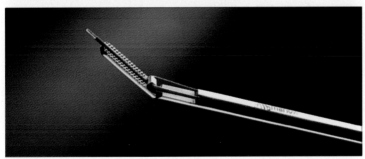

9.3a,b A steerable probe that allows simultaneous suction of smoke and irrigation. This multiple purpose probe also can be used for traction, manipulations in the pelvis, as a backstop, or to allow bending of the fiber to target hard-to-reach areas in the pelvis.

SPECIFIC PROCEDURES PERFORMED LAPAROSCOPICALLY

Every laparoscopic procedure that has ever been done has now been performed using various lasers for parts of the procedure. Our personal list includes:

1. Correction of hydrosalpinx
2. Treatment of polycystic ovaries
3. Conservative treatment of ectopic pregnancy
4. Adhesiolysis
5. Treatment of endometriosis
6. Enterolysis
7. Myomectomy
8. Adnexectomy
9. Laparoscopically assisted hysterectomy
10. Uterosacral ligament transection
11. Presacral neurectomy
12. Pelvic lymphadenectomy
13. Appendectomy

Advantages of video use for gynaecologic endoscopy
Allows assistant to help
Allows residents to be trained
Permits greater involvement by the operating room team
Educational tapes can be produced
Increases patient information
Makes possible accurate retrospective review of techniques

9.4 Advantages of video use during gynecologic endoscopy.

NEOSALPINGOSTOMY

In the past, the treatment of a hydrosalpinx had poor results, with the best surgeons reporting approximately 30% pregnancy rates with long-term follow-up in controlled series.

Laparoscopic treatment of hydrosalpinges has been attempted since the late 1970s, with early reports by Gomel and others. Following the reports of Bruhat on using the CO_2 laser for repair of hydrosalpinges at laparotomy, we began investigating the use of CO_2 laser energy through the laparoscope for neosalpingostomy and reported our initial results in 1983. We have switched to the KTP laser for this and have obtained better results by being more selective in our attempts at salpingostomy and by refining our laparoscopic techniques. When using the CO_2 laser, bleeding often occurred that required electrocoagulation of the edges of the tubes. Also, in some tubes we could not successfully evert the fimbriae. We find it easier and quicker to do laparoscopic salpingostomy using the 400 μm KTP fiber with four punctures.

An incision is made in the distal end of the tube and either one or two radial cuts performed. After the tube is opened, the 5 mm steerable probe is placed into the tube and used both as a backstop and for traction, so that the thinnest tubal portion can be identified for the next incision. After the tube is opened, the fiber is then held 2 cm from the lateral edges of the peritoneum of the open fimbriae, and 5 W of defocussed KTP laser energy is used to contract the peritoneum. (The Nd:YAG laser should never be used on the delicate fimbria.) This causes the tubes to evert outward like the petals of a flower. This laparoscopic "Bruhat technique" is much easier to accomplish using a fiber than with the CO_2 laser, with less risk of bleeding and less smoke production (**9.5a,b**).

Our recent results in patients in which the primary treatment of their tubal blockage was carried out using the KTP laser with a minimum of 18 months follow-up are given in **9.6**. A 31% pregnancy rate has been obtained, with an acceptable level of ectopic pregnancies in these patients. Most pregnancies in these patients do not occur until 9 to 16 months after surgery.

It is my opinion that in this age of out-patient ultrasound *in vitro* fertilization (IVF) with pregnancy rates of 30% per E.T., laparotomy for hydrosalpinges should be reserved for those patients who cannot afford or do not desire IVF and in whom the fallopian tubes can-

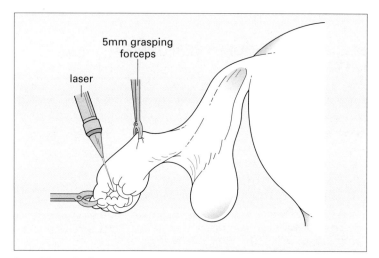

9.5a The tube is grasped with two atraumatic grasping forceps and held so that the laser beam can be aimed at right angles to the end of the tube. With this combination of traction and countertraction, the laser is fired from above, downward across the end of the tube, in the area where fiberoptic distal tubal occlusion has occurred. The laser is used to continue opening the end of the tube in a Y- or X-type incision.

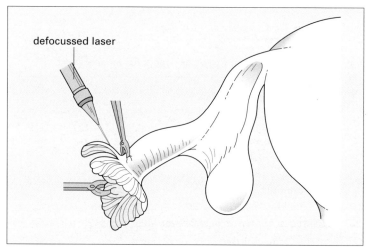

9.5b After completion of the desired number of radial incisions, the laser is defocussed by pulling the fiber back several centimeters from the tissue surface. Using this low power setting, with a defocussed beam, the surgeon is able to constrict and dessicate the peritoneum on the serosa of the tube. When fired behind the incised edges of the tube, the constriction of the peritoneum causes the edges to evert, making the tube flare open.

9.6 Results of CO_2 and KTP laser neosalpingostomy (eighteen-month follow-up).

Results of laparoscopic neosalpingostomy with lasers							
Type laser	Years	Total patients	Open tubes at 6 weeks HSG*	Attempting pregnancy	Pregnancy results		
					IUP*	Abort	Ectopic
CO_2	1982 – 1985	104[1]	58/71 (82%)	88	22(25%)	11(13%)	11(13%)
KTP	1985 – 1987	36 [2]	24/28 (86%)	32	10(31%)	3(9%)	5(16%)
Totals		140	82/99 (83%)	120	33(28%)	14(12%)	16(13%)

*HSG, hysterosalpingogram: IUP, intrauterine pregnancy
[1]Sixty procedures were in recurrent hydrosalpinges with at least 2-year follow-up
[2]Only three procedures were recurrent hydrosalpinges

not be repaired by a laparoscopic approach. The advantages to the patient from a laparoscopy include reduced discomfort, minimum recuperation, and reduction of cost and time off from work. Although further work and evaluation by other authors are needed, in the hands of experienced laparoscopic surgeons it appears that laparoscopic treatment of hydrosalpinges using laser energy is a reasonable alternative to laparotomy.

TREATMENT OF POLYCYSTIC OVARIES

Following reports of the successful use of laparoscopic ovarian electrocoagulation and ovarian biopsy to treat polycystic ovaries, we began investigating the use of laser energy to treat this condition. First, we used the CO_2 laser, with satisfactory results. However, the volume of tissue vaporized produced a tremendous amount of smoke, requiring a fairly long operating time. In 1986, we began to investigate the KTP laser for laparoscopic treatment of polycystic

ovaries. We have been able to reduce our operating time while still selectively destroying satisfactory portions of the ovarian stroma. Of 85 postoperative patients, 71% have spontaneously ovulated, with successful pregnancies in 56% (**9.7**).

Our present technique for treating polycystic ovaries involves laparoscopy with a three-puncture technique. A 5 mm grasping forceps is used to fix the ovary and the 600 μm fibre is introduced through a 5 mm cannula. The KTP laser at 20 W is used to vaporize multiple sites symmetrically over each ovary. Multiple subcapsular cysts are opened as the fiber is slowly pushed into the ovarian stroma. Small craters up to 2 cm deep are thus developed into the ovary with KTP laser energy. The bilateral procedure can usually be accomplished in less than 30 minutes, and the majority of the patients are discharged within eight hours. We feel that this is an excellent treatment for patients who desire a pregnancy and who have failed to respond to clomiphene in maximum doses. It gives these patients a "window of opportunity" during which they might conceive without the need for expensive ovulation induction therapy or open wedge resection. The effect is transient, as almost all patients failing to conceive revert back to an anovulatory state within six months to one year. In over 120 cases, we have had no complications in this procedure and recommend it to all our patients with polycystic ovarian disease who fail to respond to clomiphene or otherwise need a laparoscopy. Nd:YAG laser energy from a bare fiber should not be used because of the risk of excessive ovarian damage and potential ischemic ovarian failure. Switching from the CO_2 laser to the KTP laser has made this an easier, safer, and quicker procedure via laparoscopy. This is of particular advantage in patients who are obese. The advantages to these patients are obvious compared with the risks and discomfort of laparotomy, the expense of ovulation induction, and the known risks of hyperstimulation and multiple pregnancies.

		No CC		CC given	
Presurgery	Patients	Ovulated	Pregnant	Ovulated	Pregnant
Ovulation on CC	47	40	20	7	2
No ovulation on CC	38	20	15	17[1]	10
Total	85	60 (71%)	35	24	12

Table title: **Pregnancy after laparoscopic treatment or polycystic ovarian disease**

*Total conception = 48 (56%) – spontaneous, clomiphene citrate (CC), or human menopausal gonadotrophins (hMG)
[1]One patient was anovulatory with CC and required hMG for ovulation and conception

9. 7 Pregnancy after laparoscopic treatment or polycystic ovarian disease.

TREATMENT OF TUBAL PREGNANCY USING LASER ENERGY

There have been many reports of successful treatment of ectopic pregnancy using laparoscopic electrocoagulation and the CO_2 laser. However, we feel the techniques that we have used with the KTP/YAG laser have some advantages (**9.8**). In our experience, the risk of tubal bleeding is less when applying KTP laser energy through the 400 μm fiber than when using the CO_2 laser. In addition, trauma to the tube appears to be less with the small laser fiber than when using the needle electrodes available for laparoscopic electrosurgery. **9.9** lists our early results using KTP laser energy for laparoscopic ectopics. We agree with others that laparoscopic treatment of ectopic pregnancy is well tolerated by patients and cost effective.

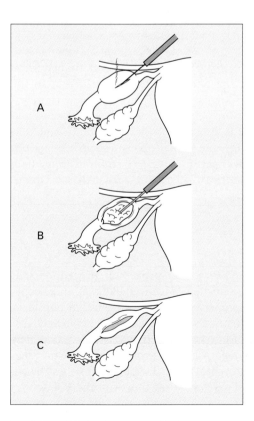

9.8 Linear salpingostomy for an ampullary ectopic pregnancy is performed with the use of the laser beam. (A) The laser is first used to make a linear salpingostomy. (B) It is followed by grasping and removing the products of conception. (C) The incision is allowed to heal without primary closure.

Laparoscopic treatment of ectopics January 1986 to January 1988	
Total patients	36
Ruptured tubes	2
Salpingectomy	6
Salpingostomy	30
Laparotomies done	0

Tubal patency on hysterosalpingogram:
19 out of 20 tested – 90% postoperatively
Repeated ectopic: 2 out of 2 attempting
pregnancy – 10%
Intrauterine pregnancy: 8 of 20 – 40%

9.9 Results of laparoscopic laser surgery for ectopic pregnancy.

TREATMENT OF ENDOMETRIOSIS AND ADHESIONS

Pelvic endometriosis is an ideal condition to be treated laparoscopically. It is usually multifocal and often associated with adhesions that cannot be successfully treated with drugs. The ability to perform laparoscopic surgery combines the patient's diagnosis and therapy into one event. Laparoscopy can confirm the diagnosis and establish the stage of the disease. Then using a laser, the experienced operator can treat the patient and perform successful adhesiolysis and destruction or reduction of disease. Endometriomas can be opened, drained, excised, and/or vaporized and other associated pathology corrected at the same time. The need for adjunctive postoperative drug therapy will then depend on the amount of disease remaining and the patient's desires and symptoms. Patients who wish to become pregnant can begin attempts at conceiving in the next menstrual cycle without the delays associated with drug therapy or recovery from major surgery. In addition, the likelihood of postoperative adhesions forming in the pelvis is probably less following laparoscopy as compared with the same techniques performed at laparotomy.

The techniques for treating endometriosis depend on the location and amount of disease present. Surface implants can usually be photocoagulated using a 600 µm fiber held close to the tissue. If vaporization is desired, the tip touches the tissue. An alternate method is to use accessory forceps for traction on the implants of endometriosis and then to dissect out the lesion using the tip of the laser fiber. It is important to remember that endometriosis will often burrow into the extraperitoneal space, and active disease that is not visible may be located in the margins of visible implants. Thus we treat each implant as we do viral lesions on the perineum, using an "airbrush" technique around the visible portions of the lesion in the center.

Endometriomas need to be carefully dissected from their attachments to the lateral pelvic sidewall. In our experience, it has usually been the sidewall that bleeds and not the ovary itself, so putting gentle traction on the ovary and using laser energy to vaporize the ovary free from the pelvis seems to be more effective than bluntly dissecting the ovary. Care must be taken to identify the ureter and to avoid major vessels lateral to the ovary. Once the ovary is freed from the adhesions to the sidewall, the endometrioma can be opened and the chocolate contents aspirated. Our method of handling an endometrioma depends on whether the capsule can be stripped from the ovarian stroma or not. If it is possible to tease the capsule free, it can be grasped and usually removed from the ovary by gentle traction. If the capsule remains adherent to the ovarian stroma, we use the 600 mm laser fiber at 20 W to vapourize the capsule by holding the fiber close to the surface of the inside of the endometrioma and passing it over the entire surface. The endometrioma bed will usually constrict and reduce the size of the opening in the ovary. Occasionally, laparoscopic sutures or clips can be placed to close large defects. Endometriomas larger than 10 cm are probably still best handled by laparotomy because of the large open ovarian surface areas that result from opening the cyst.

Adhesions associated with endometriomas are handled in the same way as other adhesions. The advantage of the KTP/YAG laser fiber is that the energy dissipates from the tip rapidly, so that structures more than 2 cm beyond the tip will not be affected by the laser beam. This means that it is not necessary to use a backstop behind adhesions which are not close to vital structures. However, when working close to the bowel, bladder, or the fimbriae, it is necessary to use a backstop because of the potential for damage distal to the target tissue. The easiest instrument for providing this extra safety is the 5 mm steerable probe, which can be placed through a 5 mm secondary cannula and manipulated as needed to provide both a backstop and traction behind the adhesion while firing the laser. Gentle traction on the adhesion is usually necessary so that it can be easily vapourized. We feel the KTP laser is particularly advantageous for adhesiolysis because of the speed with which the adhesions can be lysed with minimal risk of bleeding or smoke production.

Although some have reported the treatment of bowel endometriosis using laser energy through the laparoscope, we have minimal experience with this. Since bowel implants are usually invaginated, we feel that the risk of late bowel perforation is greater than the potential for successful destruction of the entire lesion. For this reason, we limit laparoscopic treatment of bowel endometriosis to those lesions that are exophytic or on epiploic fat or on the tip of the appendix. We will perform an appendectomy through the laparoscope if the appendix is affected with endometriosis. However, lasers play no role in laparoscopic appendectomy in our practice, as we use either pre-tied loop ligatures or automatic stapling devices for this operation.

ENTEROLYSIS

Laparoscopic bowel adhesiolysis, following surgery or pelvic inflammatory disease, can also be successfully accomplished in many cases using laser energy. We have reported our results in patients who have been referred for laparoscopic adhesiolysis after multiple abdominal operations. Many of these patients had previous bowel obstruction and are at high risk of complications at laparoscopic surgery. We counsel these patients concerning the risks of bowel injury and the possible need for immediate laparotomy and/or diverting colostomy. We prepare the bowel and always have a general surgeon standing by to repair bowel injuries that occur during enterolysis. We try to accomplish pneumoperitoneum in a standard fashion, and then introduce a 5 mm laparoscope for initial inspection. After confirming that we are in the peritoneal cavity and noting the proper site for placement of the 10 mm laparoscopic trocar and cannula, the larger laparoscope is inserted. The laser fiber placement is based on the location of abdominal wall adhesions. Many of these patients can be helped, although some have such extensive adhesions with bowel so adherent to the abdominal wall that it is impossible to lyse them safely. However, patients who have significant pain from postsurgical adhesions and who undergo successful laparoscopic lysis report improvement in two-thirds of cases. We have not yet had any late complications and have only had one bowel perforation that required immediate laparotomy in our initial series of 42 patients with extensive laparoscopic bowel adhesiolysis.

MYOMECTOMY

Laparoscopic myomectomy is a controversial procedure that requires proper patient selection, advanced skills at endoscopy, expert assistance, and proper equipment. We feel that non-laser techniques are less expensive and more effective for hemostatic dissection of large myomas from the myometrium. Thus, we have now switched from lasers to laparoscopic use of the argon beam coagulator (ABC) for our laparoscopic myomectomies. We lose less blood, produce less smoke, and save operating time with the ABC.

REMOVAL OF ADNEXAL MASSES

Our experience with the use of endoloop sutures, bipolar coagulation, and scissors transection or automatic stapling devices for oophorectomy, salpingectomy, or removal of periadnexal structures has been good. In these cases, the technique is mainly non-laser. However, we will occasionally use a laser to dissect the ovary from the pelvic sidewall or bowel, or to vaporize the pedicle after the bulk of tissue has been removed.

LAPAROSCOPIC ASSISTED VAGINAL HYSTERECTOMY

There is much interest at present in "laparoscopic" hysterectomy by both gynecologists and patients. Since 1989, we have explored various laparoscopic methods to "assist" hysterectomy vaginally. We feel the proper term for the procedure is laparoscopic assisted vaginal hysterectomy (LAVH). We use two basic techniques: either automatic stapling devices, or bipolar electrocoagulation and scissor transection. Although some laparoscopists are promoting lasers to assist LAVH, we feel they are unnecessary. In our opinion, lasers prolong anesthesia time and needlessly increase the cost of the procedure while adding no benefits to LAVH. Lasers play no role in either vaginal or total abdominal hysterectomy; thus, why try to use them for LAVH?

UTEROSACRAL LIGAMENT ABLATION

One of the more common operations we perform is laparoscopic uterine nerve ablation by transection of the uterosacral ligaments using laparoscopic laser energy (LUNA). We offer this procedure to all patients with dysmenorrhoea and who are planning laparoscopy. In 1955 Doyle reported relief from dysmenorrhoea by separating the uterosacral ligaments via colpotomy. More recent reports suggest laser transection through the laparoscope to be a successful treatment for dysmenorrhoea, either with or without endometriosis. We initially used the CO_2 laser for this, but encountered several cases of bleeding that required electrosurgery. There have been two deaths so far in North America from bleeding from uterosacral ligaments that occurred when these were transected with CO_2 laser energy. We feel that the hemostatic properties of the KTP/YAG laser add some degree of safety when the uterosacral ligaments are being transected. Our technique is to identify the ligaments, trace them out to the pelvic brim, trace the ureters, and note the area of insertion of the uterine artery into the lateral cervix. We then take a 5 mm probe and push against the posterior cervix to tent up the uterosacral ligaments. The laser fiber is then used to transect the ligaments at right angles just at the insertion of the ligaments into the posterior cervix (**9.10**). Sometimes the ligaments will be attenuated and difficult to identify. In these cases, we may refrain from cutting if we feel it is unsafe or the landmarks cannot be identified. Occasionally, rectosigmoid obliteration of the cul-de-sac in cases of endometriosis will preclude the ability to cut the uterosacral ligaments.

The majority of our patients have a reduction in their menstrual pain (**9.11**). In the initial postoperative period, most patients report pain, which probably reflects tissue swelling in the healing phase. We have not noted any effects on bowel or bladder function in these patients, and no patients have reported any reduction in ability to enjoy intercourse or obtain orgasm. It is important to counsel these patients preoperatively and make certain that they are aware that success is not guaranteed in all cases.

PRESACRAL NEURECTOMY

Laparoscopic presacral neurectomy (LPSN) is one of the newer operations being performed by laparoscopic surgeons. Our technique differs from that first described by Perez. We employ a transverse incision over the sacral promontory just out of the true pelvis. Because of the potential for bleeding with excess dissection in the retroperitoneal space, we merely transect the nerves and do not excise a specimen for pathology. Laser energy can be effectively used for incision of the peritoneum and to coagulate small vessels in this space. In a small initial series of 16 patients, we have had good results (**9.12**). However, we had one case of injury to the common iliac vein that required immediate laparotomy to control bleeding. We continue to perform LPSN in carefully evaluated and counselled patients with intractable midline pelvic pain. We believe, however, that this operation should only be attempted by gynecologists who are highly skilled at operative laparoscopy and who are willing to work in this risky retroperitoneal space.

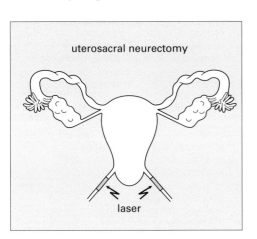

9.10 Vaporization of the uterosacral ligaments. A segment 1–2 cm long and 1 cm in depth is vaporized over the initial portion of the ligament. The ureter is identified laterally in all cases.

LUNA results wuth KTP laser (6-month follow-up)			
1988 – 1990	Worse	Same	Improved
Endometriosis 80 patients	3 (4%)	17 (21%)	60 (75%)
Primary dysmenorrhea 20 patients	2 (10%)	6 (30%)	12 (60%)
Totals 100 patients	5 (5%)	3 (23%)	72 (72%)

9.11 Results of LUNA.

Laparoscopic presacral neurectomy results*			
January 1991 – December 1991	Subjective results		
	Improved	Same	Worse
16 patients	13	1	2
* Minimum 6-months follow-up with pain questionnaire			

9.12 Results of pre-sacral neurectomy.

SAFETY

To undertake any sort of extensive operative laparoscopy without proper safety precautions, training, equipment, and assistance can result in unnecessary complications and their tragic sequelae. It behoves all of us who are interested in operative laser laparoscopy to be selective in the techniques we undertake. This will protect us, our hospitals, and our patients.

The safe use of lasers at laparoscopy includes the proper use of eye filters and protection for both the patient, the surgeon, and the assistants in the operating room. Since the laser energy of the argon or KTP is visible, it is less likely that the operator's eyes will be damaged. Inadvertent firing of the laser without eye filters will be immediately recognized because of the bright green color that is seen. This improves the safety of use of visible light lasers compared to the Nd:YAG, which is infrared and therefore not visible when fired. When working in a closed abdominal cavity, we do not require people in the operating room to wear safety glasses. The fiber itself is coated, which protects leakage of energy except from the tip of the fiber.

The operator is the only person at risk when the beam is being fired intraperitoneally through the laparoscope, and his or her eyes are protected by the eye filter that is placed over the eyepiece of the laparoscope. The laser cannot be fired if the eye filter is not working properly. If an attempt is made to override the eye filter with the KTP (this can be done, for instance, by placing the eye filter on another laparoscope that might be on the table), the operator will immediately be aware of this problem because of the intense brightness that is see when the laser is fired without the filter. This is not true with the Nd:YAG, which is invisible and thus requires constant awareness of unfiltered laser light when the instrument is fired.

Because of the potential of harm on those breathing the plume, we vent the smoke off through a specially designed disposable suction-irrigation system (PumpVac Plus, Marlow Medical, Willoughby, Ohio) which is also used for aspirating fluid and for hydrodissection (**9.13**). By using in-line filters, we protect the hospital filter system from being plugged by particulate matter that might be in the plume.

Other safety precautions are those that one would undertake with any sort of operative laparoscopy, such as gentle tissue handling, use of the proper instruments in the correct situation, and judicious use of both bipolar and unipolar electrosurgery. With proper attention to safety, the careful, trained endoscopist can perform extensive operative laparoscopic procedures with good results in the majority of cases, with minimal complications.

CONCLUSION

I strongly agree with Dr Alan DeCherney, who said in his prophetic editorial in *Fertility and Sterility* entitled "The Leader of the Band is Tired" that the obituary for laparotomy for infertility surgery has been written but not yet published. Today, many gynecologists are becoming interested in doing more advanced operative laparoscopic surgery. Procedures that in the past required open laparotomy can now be performed with combinations of hysteroscopy and/or laparoscopy. **9.14** lists the so-called old methods of treatment for some of these diseases compared with the new techniques that are giving good results in the hands of experienced operators.

In this time of cost containment in medicine, it will benefit physicians to reduce costs without cutting corners or compromising patient care. Careful, selective use of laser and non-laser laparoscopic techniques in gynecology can help cost containment by giving comparable results while avoiding major surgery with its increased expense, risks, morbidity, and discomfort. All gynecologists should investigate the potential for using advanced operative laparoscopic laser surgery in their practices.

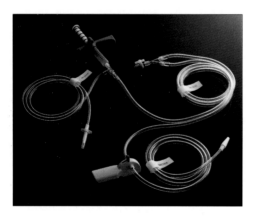

9.13 Disposable suction irrigation system.

Shifting trends in gynecologic surgery		
	Old therapy	New therapy
Dysmenorrhea	Laparotomy, presacral neurectomy	Laparoscopic presacral neurectomy
Menorrhagia	Hysterectomy	Endometrial ablation
Severe endometriosis	Laparotomy	Laparoscopy
Uterine septum	Abdominal metroplasty	Hysteroscopic resection
Uterine fibroids	Laparotomy	Laparoscopy or hysteroscopy
Cornual blockage	Cornual re-anastomosis	Hysteroscopic probing and dilation
Hydrosalpinx	Laparotomy	Laparoscopy
Ectopic gestation	Laparotomy	Laparoscopy
Ovarian pathology requiring removal	Laparotomy, oophorectomy	Laparoscopic surgery
Uterine pathology	Total abdominal hysterectomy	LAVH

9.14 Shifting trends in gynecological surgery.

FURTHER READING

Brumsted J, Gibson C, Gibson M, *et al*. A comparison of laparoscopy and laparotomy for the treatment of ectopic pregnancy. *Obstet Gynecol* 1988; **71**:889–93

Daniell JF. Surgical management of polycystic ovarian disease. In: *Ovulation Induction*, 1991. Ed: Collins RL, Springer-Verlag, New York, 145–60

Daniell JF. Laparoscopic evaluation of the KTP/532 laser for treating endometriosis — initial report: *Fertil Steril* 1986; **46**:373–7

Daniell JF, Kurtz BR, Gurley LD. Laser laparoscopic management of large endometriomas. *Fertil Steril* 1991; **55**: 692–6

Davis GD, Brooks RA. Excision of pelvic endometriosis with the carbon dioxide laser laparoscope. *Obstet Gynecol* 1988;.**72**:.816

Fayez JA. An assessment of the role of operative laparoscopy in tuboplasty. *Fertil Steril* 1983; **39**: 476–79

Feste JR. CO_2 laser neurectomy for dysmenorrhea. *Lasers Surg Med* 1984; **3**: 327–31

LAPAROSCOPIC MANAGEMENT OF OVARIAN CYSTS

10

Alain JM Audebert

INTRODUCTION

Ovarian cyst surgery is very common in gynecologic practice. There have been several published series providing data on techniques, complications and results of laparoscopic management. Nevertheless, the use of laparoscopy to treat ovarian cysts remains controversial because of the difficulty of recognizing a borderline or malignant cyst preoperatively and the risk of treating it incorrectly.

Laparoscopic surgery is the preferred treatment if the cyst is benign. Borderline and frankly malignant tumors should have laparotomy and complete excision (**10.1**). Functional ovarian cysts do not require surgery provided that the diagnosis can be made with confidence as a result of careful clinical and sonar examination (**10.2**). Detailed clinical and sonar assessment combined with appropriate laboratory investigations such as tumor markers should enable the clinician to recognize the nature of most tumors and indicate correct management.

It is not possible to exclude malignancy completely even when all the preoperative investigations are negative. Careful laparoscopic assessment is always necessary (**10.3, 10.4**). If immediate adequate histological confirmation of the diagnosis is not available or there is doubt about the nature of the lesion, laparotomy should be carried out. Alternatively it may be acceptable to remove the cyst laparoscopically and proceed to secondary laparotomy if histological examination suggests the presence of malignant change in the tumor.

Laparoscopic management of ovarian tumors is acceptable if these criteria are met. The clinician can then offer the patient the best treatment with the known advantages of laparoscopic surgery without compromising the cure rate in cases of malignancy.

CLINICAL PRESENTATION

There are no specific symptoms of simple ovarian cysts. Chronic pain, menstrual disturbances or infertility may all be associated with an ovarian tumor. Acute pain may occur if the cyst undergoes torsion or, less commonly, if there is bleeding into it. Early malignant change may be difficult to recognize. Advanced malignancy usually presents with the classical picture of a mass accompanied by ascites.

Ovarian cysts may be asymptomatic and be discovered at a routine clinical examination. However, clinical examination only detects 70% of tumors when they are less than 5 cm in diameter. Asymptomatic tumors may be discovered by ultrasound or plain X-ray of the

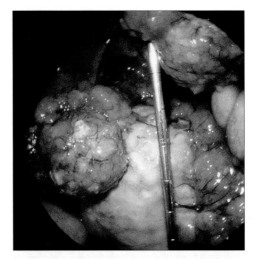

10.1 Bilateral ovarian carcinoma.

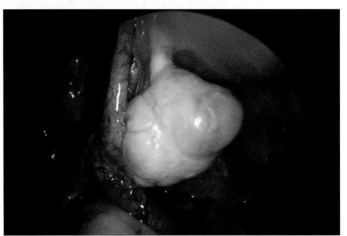

10.2 Mature Graafian follicle.

abdomen or during laparoscopy for another indication such as infertility. The prevalence of asymptomatic ovarian cysts in women of over 44 years in a series published from the UK was 1.25% for functional cysts, 1.3% for benign epithelial cysts and 0.05% for borderline or malignant tumors.

Some statistical points should be considered when deciding on treatment: 1) Ovarian epithelial neoplasms occur in 10 out of 100,000 women in North America and Northern Europe. 2) The prevalence of malignancy is related to age. In women under 35 years old, the risk of an apparently simple cyst being malignant is 4.5 per 100,000. 3) If the cyst is unilocular and less than

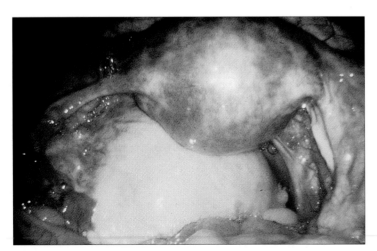

10.3 Benign unilocular serous cyst.

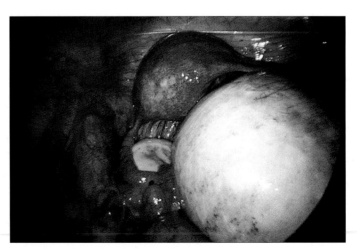

10.4 Benign unilocular serous cyst.

10cm in diameter the risk is very low. 4) Borderline tumors are more common and represent 9–16% of epithelial ovarian cysts. 5) The risk of recurrence of Stages 1a and 1b is about 10% after ovarian cystectomy. 6) The frequency of microscopic malignant change in a grossly normal looking contralateral ovary varies from 5–10%. The known risk factors for ovarian malignancy are listed in **10.5**.

PREOPERATIVE ASSESSMENT

The preoperative assessment of an ovarian mass is of vital importance. The whole treatment strategy depends on the assessment, which should include diagnostic imaging, tumor markings and should take into account the patient's age, the known risk factors for malignancy and the desire to preserve fertility.

Pelvic Ultrasound

Transvaginal ultrasound with color doppler has increased the sensivity of the preoperative assesssment of ovarian tumors.

Malignant change may be suggested by a number of features on ultrasound imaging. These include the presence of thick septa, solid parts or papillae, indefinite margins, bilateral tumors and ascites. A ultrasonographer trained in gynecologic imaging should be able to predict a benign tumor with 96% accuracy. The possibility of an echogenically clear unilocular cyst being benign is 90–95% (**10.6, 10.7**). No case of malignancy was detected in a series of 152 women over the age of 50 years with clear cystic lesions of less than 5 cm in diameter. Similar accurate predictions have also been reported in postmenopausal women. In other words, the risk of malignancy in a postmenopausal woman with an apparently simple cyst is about 6%. Our investigations involving pooling the data from several series suggests that the risk of malignancy in unilocular cysts is 2.3% for premenopausal women and 3% if they are postmenopausal.

Thus ultrasound is reasonably accurate in excluding malignancy but it appears to be less reliable in detecting malignancy in cysts which do not exhibit the accepted features of malignancy.

It is possible with ultrasound to distinguish between a pathological and a functional cyst. An uncomplicated functional cyst does not require surgical intervention and will usually undergo complete resolution. Experience has shown that when a persistent cyst is removed laparoscopically, some 16–43% are found to be functional and the surgery was unnecessary. This illustrates the value of careful preoperative assessment in reducing the frequency of such unproductive surgery.

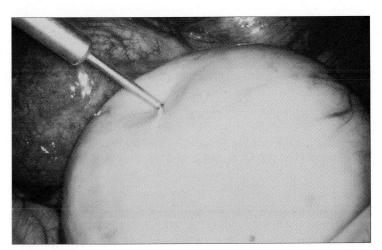

10.8 Needle aspiration of simple cyst.

Infertility, low parity, nulliparous
Middle of upper socio-economic class
Caucasian
Age over 50 years
Family history of ovarian, breast or endometrial cancer
No history of oral contraceptive use

10.5 Known risk factors for ovarian malignancy.

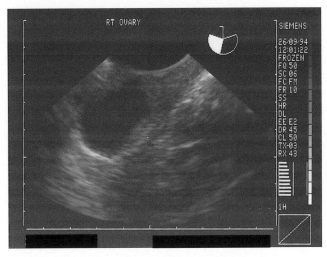

10.6 Ultrasound scan. Right ovarian simple cyst — unilocular.

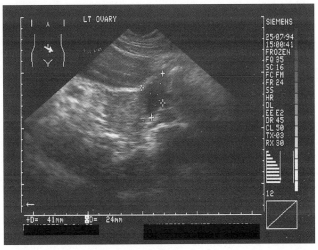

10.7 Dermoid cyst — mainly fluid.

Cysts may be aspirated under ultrasonic control. This procedure should be used with caution. Cytological examination of aspirated fluid is frequently unreliable. In a series reported in France in 1988, cytological examination corresponded to histological examination in just 22 out of 35 cases (**10.8–10.10**). There may also be a risk not only of missing a cancer but of disseminating malignant cells along the track of the needle. A newer technique of ultrasound guided cystosocpy with a 0.5 mm telescope is currently under evaluation.

Color doppler sonography may give a more accurate prediction. A pulsatile index of less than unity is indicative of a malignant lesion. In one series this criterion correctly identified 35 out of 36 benign ovarian tumors.

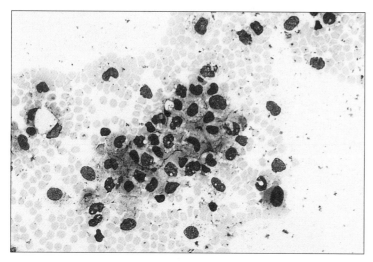

10.9 Lutenised follicular cyst. By courtesy of Dr C. A. Waddell.

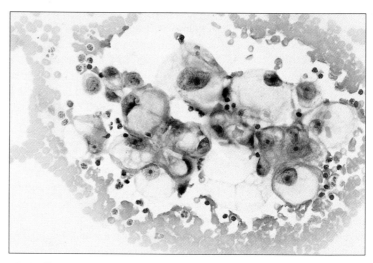

10.10 Clear cell adenocarcinoma (x 400). By courtesy of Dr C. A. Waddell.

Tumor Markers

The present serologic markers have variable specifity according to the nature of the ovarian neoplasm. They are relatively specific for ovarian germ cell tumors but these are rare. CA-125 is the most commonly used marker for epithelial ovarian tumors. Its value is limited because it is not sufficiently sensitive or specific except in postmenopausal women. In these patients, an elevated CA-125 level in association with an other positive diagnostic test has a positive predictive value approaching 100%. When CA-125 is used without other investigations it has a predictive value for women with a pelvic mass of 36% before the menopause and 87% after the menopause. In postmenopausal women the combination of ultrasound and CA-125 levels yields a sensitivity of 85% and a specivity of 97% in diagnosing malignant lesions.

In functional cysts the steroid concentration is usually raised while the CA-125 level is low. A correct diagnosis may usually be obtained by this combination of results when combined with the gross appearance of the cyst fluid.

LAPAROSCOPIC ASSESSMENT

It is still necessary to perform a laparoscopic evaluation even when an ovarian mass is thought to be benign as a result of the above preoperative investigations. This evaluation must be undertaken according to a definite protocol (**10.11**).

1. The cyst should first be inspected and fluid aspirated from the pouch of Douglas for cytological examination before it is contaminated by any other fluid.
2. The surface of the pelvic and abdominal peritoneum, bowel, omentum and liver must be carefully displayed and examined. Lesions such as endometriotic implants may be detected and treated laparoscopically (**10.12, 10.13**). The presence of other lesions suggesting or confirming malignancy should lead to immediate laparotomy.
3. The surface of both ovaries and tubes should now be examined. Adhesiolysis may be necessary to provide exposure. External papillae are easily identified. Elongation of the utero-ovarian ligament usually indicates a benign non-functional tumor (**10.14**). If there are features at the laparoscopic assessment or in the preoperative findings suggesting a malignant or borderline tumor, immediate laparotomy should be performed. If the lesion still appears benign, further laparoscopic examination should be carried out.

Laparoscopic assessment of ovarian neoplasms Procedures performed systematically
Aspiration of peritoneal fluid for cytology
Inspection of the abdominal cavity, omentum and liver
Inspection of the ovarian surface and ovarian ligaments
Puncture of the ovarian cyst
Cystoscopy
Frozen section

10.11 Laparoscopic assessment of ovarian neoplasms; procedures performed systematically.

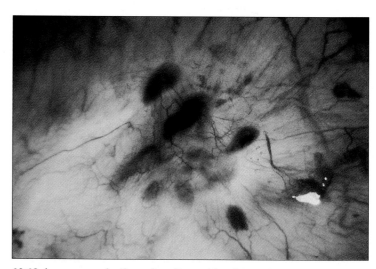

10.12 Laser vaporization of peritoneal implant.

4. The ovary should be grasped gently and mobilised to select the appropriate site for puncture. This should preferably be at the apex of the cyst and at a distance from the blood vessels of the central hilum. Provided ultrasound has excluded internal papillae, the cyst fluid can be aspirated through a fine needle (**10.15**). Spillage of fluid should be avoided. The appearance of the cyst fluid gives a good indication of the risk of malignancy.
5. If cystoscopy is planned it is preferable to introduce the trocar and cannula directly into the cyst instead of aspirating with a

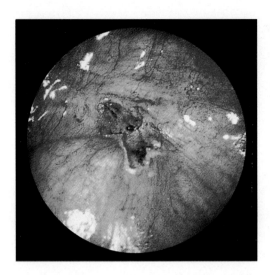

10.13 Peritoneal endometriosis.

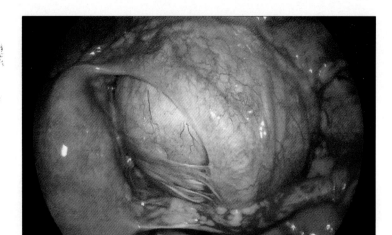

10.14 Benign cyst with stretched fallopian tube.

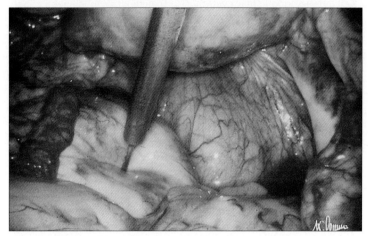

10.15 Aspiration of cyst fluid.

needle. The cyst may then be aspirated and lavage carried out before introducing a small endoscope. The entire internal surface of the cyst wall can be examined and any excrescence recognized. Alternatively the site of puncture can be enlarged with scissors and the interior of the cyst exposed with grasping forceps. The presence of a suspicious lesion is an indication to perform lavage of the pouch of Douglas and proceed to immediate laparotomy. Preliminary puncture should not be performed if it has been decided to perform oophorectomy or to remove the cyst intact, Occasionally it may not be possible to identify the nature of the cyst laparoscopically. In such cases:

6. Frozen section biopsy should be performed to establish a firm diagnosis.

Laparoscopic surgery should not be performed until the presence of malignancy has been excluded as far as possible. However, malignancy may be missed even when laparoscopic assessment has been negative (**10.16**). In four series in the literature totalling 3364 cases, nine of the 41 cases of malignancy did not appear malignant on gross inspection. However, in our own series of 735 cases of ovarian cysts, three patients who had laparotomy because they were thought to have malignant ovarian cysts had, in fact, benign lesions on histological examination. Other workers have reported similar false positive results from gross assessment.

Only cysts which appear to be macroscopically benign and are unilocular with smooth walls and cysts which can easily be defined as non-malignant such as endometriomas should be treated laparoscopially. The presence of severe dense adhesions may also make laparotomy preferable but this is not a problem specific to ovarian surgery. Thus all patients undergoing laparoscopy for ovarian cysts should also have given their consent to laparotomy.

TECHNIQUE OF OVARIAN CYSTECTOMY

After careful laparoscopic assessment has been performed and malignancy excluded as far as possible, the ovary should be gently mobilised with grasping forceps carrying out adhesiolysis if necessary. The size and location of the cyst within the ovary are determined in order to select the optimum site for incision of the tunica albuginea. The best site is on the antimesenteric border of the ovary at a distance from the blood vessels of the hilum and the fallopian tube.

Two different techniques may be used whether or not preliminary puncture or cystoscopy have been performed.

Prevalence of ovarian cancer in cysts which were not evident at the time of laparoscopy				
Author	Year	Number of cysts	Number of cancers	Malignancy not evident
Canis, Bruhat	1992	652	12	0
Nehzat	1992	1209	4	3
Mecke	1992	809	11	4
Audebert	1992	735	14	2
	Total	3364	41 (1.2%)	9 (21.9%)

10.16 Prevalence of ovarian cancer in cysts which were not evident at the time of laparoscopy.

OPEN CYST CYSTECTOMY

If the cyst has been punctured, the opening should be enlarged with scissors, unipolar needle or laser (**10.17**). The cyst wall is then grasped with forceps while the overlying ovarian wall is grasped with a second forceps (**10.18**). The length of the incision in the ovarian wall is determined by the size of the cyst. The wall of the cyst is then progressively stripped out of the ovary by traction and counter-traction with the forceps (**10.19**). The ease with which the cyst is removed depends on the strength of the wall. Functional cysts peel

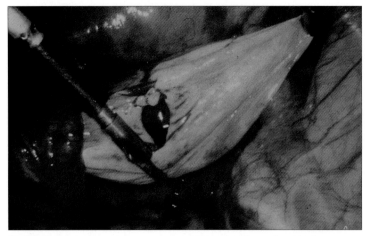

10.17 Ovarian cystectomy — part of the cyst is excised before destroying the remainder with laser.

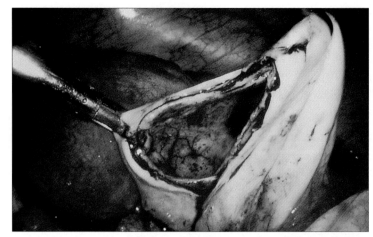

10.18 Ovarian cystectomy — cyst wall identified proior to removal.

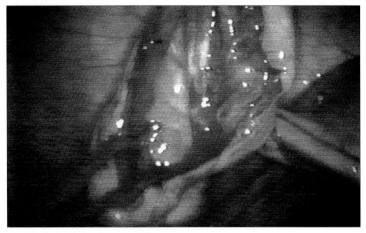

10.19 Stripping of cyst wall.

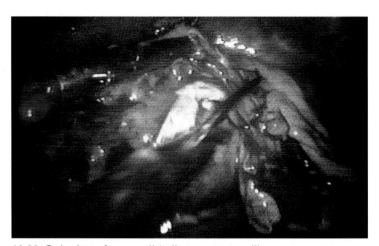

10.20 Stripping of cyst wall (adherent cyst wall).

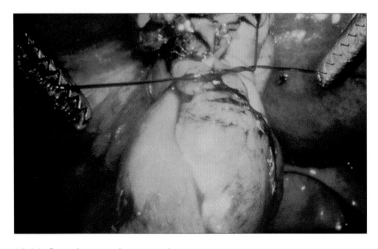

10.21 Suturing ovarian capsule.

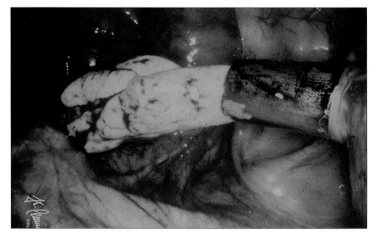

10.22 Removal of cyst wall.

out very easily because they are thin-walled and loosely attached to the ovarian stroma. Endometriomas may be very difficult to dissect free and the adjacent ovarian cortex may need to be excised to effect complete removal. Hemostasis should be achieved with fine bipolar forceps when necesary (**10.20**).

The dissection may also be performed with laser or facilitated with hydrodissection using an irrigating cannula. When the cyst has been completely excised, the ovary should be irrigated and complete hemostasis obtained with bipolar coagulation.

The incision in the ovary may usually be left open because the ovary inverts and allows primary healing to take place. Occasionally

apposition of the walls may be poor and the ovary should then be closed with a fine monofilament suture, the application of fibrin glue or by coagulating the ovarian cortex adjacent to the surface. This causes the ovarian cortex to retract and closes the opening (**10.21**).

The excised tissue should be removed from the abdominal cavity through a wider cannula (11 mm) using strong traction forceps or following morcellation with sissors or a tissue punch (**10.22**). The pelvis should be cleansed and all debris removed and copious lavage with warmed Ringer's lactate solution performed. The irrigation should be repeated if necessary until the fluid remains clear. Finally the operation field should again be checked for hemostasis and the abdominal incisions closed leaving a large amount of warm Ringer's lactate solution in the pelvic cavity to prevent adhesion formation.

All removed specimens must be submitted for histological examination.

CLOSED CYST CYSTECTOMY

This technique is appropriate if the cyst has not been punctured and allows the intact cyst to be removed from the ovary. It is the preferred technique if spillage of the cyst contents should be avoided as in teratomas or mucinous cysts.

The ovary should be exposed with great care to avoid rupture of the cyst. Grasping forceps should not be applied to the cyst but to the normal ovarian tissue. The incision in the tunica albuginea should be larger than in the previous technique. Dissection of the cyst from the ovarian cortex may be facilitated by hydrodissection.

Removal of the intact cyst from the abdominal cavity may present difficulties. The cyst may be removed by enlarging one of the abdominal incisions or through a posterior colpotomy incision but there is always a risk of the cyst rupturing with consequent spillage of its contents into the peritoneal cavity or the abdominal wall. It is preferable to place the unopened cyst in a disposable bag (**10.23**). The volume of the cyst can then be reduced by aspirating or morcellating it within the bag under direct vision. The bag can then be removed through an abdominal or vaginal incision. This avoids spillage and is probably safer than other methods of removal.

ALTERNATIVE TECHNIQUES

When difficulty is experienced in separating the cyst from the ovary or from the pelvic sidewall, the top of the cyst may be removed and the remaining part destroyed *in situ*. This technique is preferred by many laparoscopists instead of excision of an endometrioma.

Preliminary laparoscopy should be performed to confirm the nature of the cyst. If it is an endometrioma, the cyst should be aspirated and lavage of the cavity carried out. The patient should then be given medical suppressive drugs such as danazol, gestrinone or GnRH agonists for 3–6 months. The cyst volume should now be smaller.

A second laparoscopy is performed. The top of the cyst is removed and the contents aspirated before irrigating the cavity (**10.24**). The whole interior surface of the cyst should now be carefully inspected. The lining of the cyst may be ablated with laser or bipolar electro-coagulation. This may be difficult if the cyst is large but is essential that the ablation is complete to prevent recurrence. If the cyst is adherent to the pelvic sidewall, which is often the case with endometriosis, great care must be taken to avoid damage to underlying structures such as the ureter. The depth of destruction depends on the technique used. At completion of the procedure the operation field must be inspected carefully to ensure hemostasis and ablation are complete.

Another method of removing cysts is to bring the cyst outside the abdominal cavity by enlarging one of the secondary cannula incisions. The cyst may then be aspirated, excised and the ovary repaired by a standard laparotomy technique. This procedure is only possible if the adnexa can be fully mobilized. It is recommended when a meticulous repair of the ovary is necessary as in the case of a single ovary when it is necessary to save the maximum amount of ovarian tissue to preserve fertility.

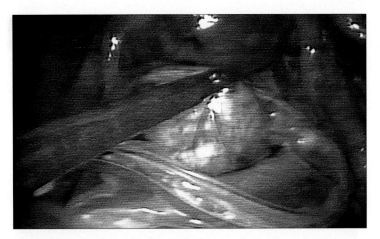

10.23 Cystectomy. Removal in a bag.

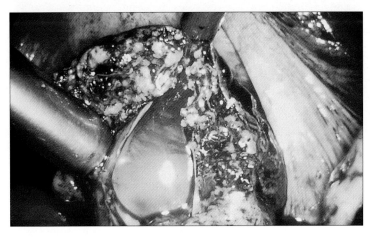

10.24 Dermoid cyst.

OOPHORECTOMY

Laparoscopic oophorectomy or salpingo-oophorectomy is preferred when the cyst appears to fill all of the ovarian tissue or routinely in postmenopausal women. the development of endoscopic suturing and stapling devices have made this procedure easier.

It is important first to mobilize the ovary or adnexa to ensure that the ovarian vessels can be easily exposed and skeletonized at a sufficient distance from the pelvic sidewall. Important structures such as the ureter must be identified. If mobilization is difficult the procedure may be aided by making a small incision in an avascular area of the anterior leaf of the broad ligament, inserting an irrigating cannula and dissecting the peritoneum away from the sidewall with hydrodissection using Ringer's lactate solution.

The vessels in the infundibulo-pelvic and utero-ovarian ligaments should then be skeletonized and ligated with sutures tied extracorporeally, staples or clips. The pedicles should then be transected and, for safety, a second endoloop applied. Alternatively the pedicle may be coagulated using a bipolar current or thermocoagulation. The forceps should be applied carefull at a safe distance from the pelvic sidewall and the pedicles divided when dessication is complete. This is our preferred technique. The fallopian tube may be removed by the same means.

Finally, hemostasis should be ensured, the specimen removed, preferably in a bag, and irrigation and lavage of the pelvic cavity performed.

RESULTS

FEASABILITY

All benign ovarian cysts, including ovarian endometriomas and teratomas, can be treated by laparoscopy depending on the experience of the surgeon and the availability of proper instruments and facilities. This approach offers all the advantages of laparoscopic surgery. Most of the conversions to laparotomy are due to suspicion of cancer.

The cause of most operative difficulty is the presence of dense adhesions usually secondary to previous surgery especially for endometriosis. Dermoid cysts over 8 cm in diameter are also responsible for some conversions to laparotomy because of the difficulty in extracting them, especially when solid portions are present. Apart from dermoids, the volume of the cyst does not present serious technical problems.

The prevalence of ovarian cysts presenting in pregnancy requiring surgery is about 1:2000. Laparoscopic surgery is possible up to 16 weeks gestation. Up to that time the size of the uterus does not hinder the introduction of trocars at the usual sites.

COMPLICATIONS

As in other laparoscopic surgical procedures, complications may occur but unfortunatley are rarely reported in the literature.

1) Immediate complications. During the operation there may be uncontrolled bleeding, injury to other structures or unsuccessful removal of the tumor. In our experience and in the experience of others amounting to about 1000 cases, no such complication occurred. Laparotomy was necessary in only one case of unsuspected ovarian malignancy. Rupture of the cyst with spillage of its contents may be deleterious in teratomas, mucinous cysts or endometriosis. Postoperative adhesion formation or the development of peritonitis may be prevented by prolonged, copious and meticulous lavage which should be continued until the irrigant fluid remains perfectly clear. In a large French study, severe complications necessitating laparotomy occurred in only 0.67% of cases mainly during surgery for endometriosis.

2) Delayed complications. Abdominal pain, ovarian abscesses, adhesions and loculated haematomas have been reported.

FOLLOW-UP

Patients who have had an ovarian cyst excised must be meticulously followed up by clinical examination and sonography. The incidence of postoperative adhesion formation has only been evaluated for endometriosis. The prevalence of adhesions depends on the technique used and is most common after excision (100%) followed by stripping of the lining (37%), laser ablation (30%) and drainage (28%). Fertility following laparoscopic surgery for ovarian cysts excluding endometriosis is 89%.

The incidence of recurrence of ovarian cysts depends upon their nature. Recurrence is more frequent with endometriosis, serous cysts, teratomas, para-ovarian cysts and cysts which have undergone malignant change. There is no proof that the use of supressive drugs lowers the recurrence rate of endometriomas.

RISK OF PERFORMING LAPAROSCOPIC SURGERY FOR UNIDENTIFIED MALIGNANT TUMORS

The largest published series of ovarian cysts managed laparoscopically reports very few unidentified malignant tumors were managed inappropriately. This optimistic view which is probably due in part to the expertise of the surgeons and in part due to a particular referral practice which limited the number of carcinomas, probably hides the reality. Several surveys have suggested that over 1% of borderline tumors and 0.3% of malignant tumors were treated inappropriately by laparoscopy even though in 20% of cases both preoperative and intraoperative assessment suggested the lesion was benign. There is a risk of dissemination of malignant cells if treatment has been inappropriate and this probably has an adverse effect on the course of the disease.

It is worth repeating that laparoscopic surgery should only be performed if malignancy has been excluded as far as possible. In case of doubt conversion to laparotomy is mandatory. In older women and those with large cysts, puncture and opening of the cyst should be avoided. The use of oophorectomy in a bag is advocated in all such cases and should give the same results as removal by laparotomy. There should be no delay in instituting conventional surgery when histological examination of the excised cyst has revealed an unexpected carcinoma.

CONCLUSION

Laparoscopic treatment of benign ovarian neoplasms can be achieved in the majority of cases. The advantages of laparoscopic surgery are well established. As always, proper instruments and training are essential. The techniques of oophorectomy and ovariotomy have been evaluated and give results comparable to conventional surgery.

Strict case selection is necessary to exclude malignant tumors which should be treated by conventional surgery. There is still a fear of unrecognized malignancy which makes meticulous preoperative and intraoperative evaluation essential. With present day facilities there is always a small risk of performing laparoscopic surgery on an unsuspected case of malignant ovarian disease. Closed cystectomy and removal of tissues in a laparoscopic bag should be used in high-risk patients.

FURTHER READING

Audebert AJM. Laparoscopic ovarian surgery and ovarian torsion. In: *Endoscopic Surgery for Gynaecologists* 1993. Eds: Sutton C and Diamond MP. WB Saunders, London, pp 134–141

Bruhat MA, Mage G, Bagory G, *et al.* Laparoscopic treatment of ovarian cysts. Indications, techniques and results. Apropos of 250 cases. Chirurgurie 1991; **117**: 300–307

Mage G, Caris M, Manhes H, et al. Laparoscopic management of adnexal cystic masses. *J Gynecol Surgery* 1990; **L6**: 71–79

LAPAROSCOPIC SURGERY FOR ENDOMETRIOSIS

11

John A Rock and Bradley S Hurst

The diagnosis and treatment of women with endometriosis is the subject of ongoing controversy in gynecology. The debate is due to the variability of symptoms associated with endometriosis, the variation in appearance of lesions, and the multiple choice of treatments available. For effective management of endometriosis, a knowledge of the pathophysiology of the disease, diagnosis, and all the treatment options is essential.

INDICATIONS FOR LAPAROSCOPY WITH SUSPECTED ENDOMETRIOSIS

Endometriosis is found in up to 50% of infertile women. In severe cases, anatomic distortion due to endometriomas or tubo-ovarian adhesions is present, which compromises oocyte pick up and transport, but the cause of infertility with minimal and mild endometriosis is not clearly understood. At present the leading hypothesis for subfertility associated with minimal endometriosis is based on studies of peritoneal fluid macrophage activity. A higher number of peritoneal macrophages and a higher concentration of activated macrophages are found in patients with endometriosis. Activated macrophages display greater phagocytic ability. As a result, there may be phagocytosis of sperm, eggs, or embryos, which might impair oocyte pick up, tubal transport, or implantation. Other mechanisms such as a compromise in the immune system, prostaglandin activity, and hormonal abnormalities have also been proposed to explain subfertility associated with minimal endometriosis.

Laparoscopy is performed to confirm the diagnosis. Prior to laparoscopy, a general examination of the male partner and a semen analysis should be performed. If no obvious causes for infertility are identified, laparoscopy is indicated.

Endometriosis can be identified in approximately 20–50% of women with chronic pelvic pain, dyspareunia, or dysmenorrhea. The pain may be a mechanical result of the endometriotic implant or mediated through prostaglandins. Laparoscopy should be considered if the chronic pain interferes with the patient's lifestyle and is not relieved with drugs such as prostaglandin synthetase inhibitors.

DIAGNOSTIC LAPAROSCOPY

TECHNIQUE

Laparoscopy is scheduled in the follicular phase of the cycle to avoid confusion between an endometrioma and a corpus luteum cyst. A patient with significant bowel symptoms should be evaluated before surgery with a barium enema or a colonoscopy. If operative laparoscopy is anticipated, a bowel preparation is initiated. An intravenous pyelogram may be helpful to evaluate ureteral involvement. If the pelvic examination is difficult because of pain or obesity, a pelvic ultrasound scan is helpful to evaluate ovarian cysts. The operating room is not the place to be surprised by finding extensive endometriosis.

APPEARANCE OF ENDOMETRIOSIS

Endometriosis can take on a variety of appearances (**11.1–11.8**). Most gynecologists are familiar with the brown 'powder burn' peritoneal lesions. In addition, reddish blue proliferative endometriotic nodules are commonly encountered. Red, raised peritoneal nodules

may also be present. Scarring or retraction of the peritoneum in a stellate pattern surrounding these lesions strongly suggests endometriosis. Endometriotic implants lacking hemosiderin have an atypical appearance and may be seen as white opaque peritoneal nodules or superficial peritoneal ecchymotic areas. Endometriosis is the most common cause of peritoneal windows or defects and isolated adhesions binding the ovary to the pelvic sidewall. Suspicious or atypical pelvic lesions should be biopsied for histologic confirmation of the diagnosis.

Ovarian implants may result in endometrial cysts or endometriomas which are usually dark brown, black, or blue. Rupture of the cyst will release a thick brown 'chocolate' fluid, although cysts may occasionally contain a yellow fluid if old blood is resorbed.

To complicate the difficulty in diagnosing endometriosis, investigators have identified microscopic endometriosis using scanning electron microscopy in normal appearing peritoneum. Although laparoscopy can magnify up to six times when the lens is in close contact, most authorities agree that all endometriosis may not always be visible in patients with the disease.

TREATMENT OF ENDOMETRIOSIS

The optimal treatment for endometriosis will depend on the symptoms, the extent of disease, and desire for fertility. Patients with

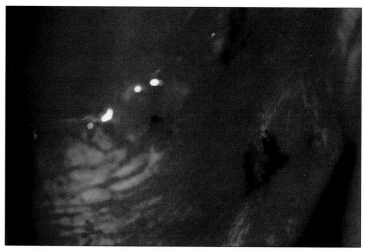

11.1 Appearance of endometriosis; brown 'powder burn'.

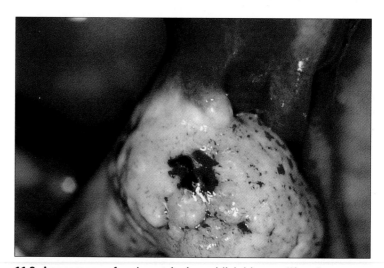

11.2 Appearance of endometriosis; reddish blue proliferative nodule.

infertility in whom there is no anatomic distortion are unlikely to benefit from medical or surgical therapy. On the other hand, infertile patients with anatomic distortion are likely to benefit from a surgical approach designed to restore normal anatomy. Unlike patients with infertility, most patients whose primary complaint is pain may expect to improve by surgical ablation of the endometrial implants. Medical therapy for endometriosis includes danazol, gonadotropin releasing hormone analogues (GnRHa), or progestogens, which usually produce a significant improvement of pain. Patients who do not want children and who have recurrent pain following laparoscopic or medical treatment will be cured by hysterectomy with or without bilateral salpingo-oophorectomy.

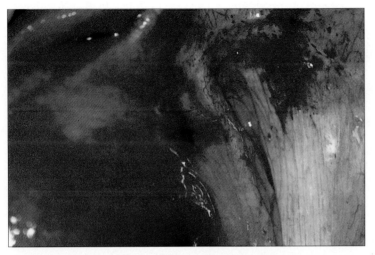

11.3 Appearance of endometriosis; red peritoneal implants.

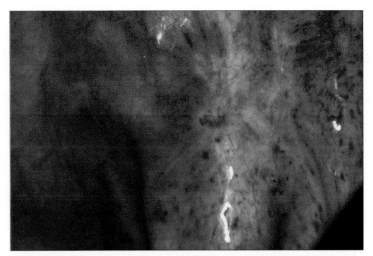

11.4 Appearance of endometriosis; stellate scarring of the peritoneum surrounding an endometriotic implant.

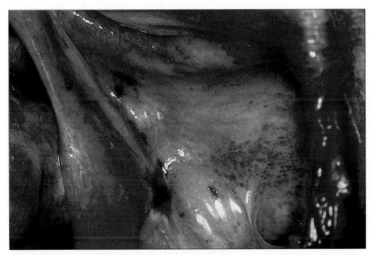

11.5 Appearance of endometriosis; superficial ecchymotic implants and peritoneal 'window'.

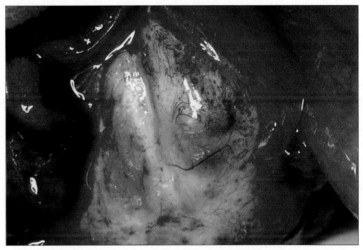

11.6 Appearance of endometriosis; blue endometrioma.

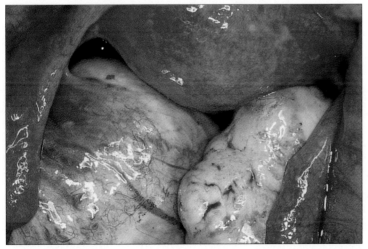

11.7 Appearance of endometriosis; large endometrioma left ovary.

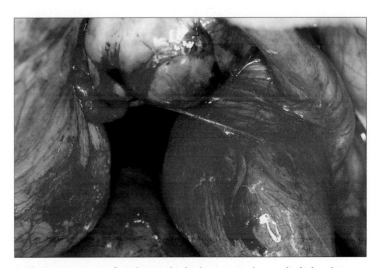

11.8 Appearance of endometriosis; brown endometriotic implant and ovarian surface neovascularization.

LAPAROSCOPIC TREATMENT OF MINIMAL OR MILD ENDOMETRIOSIS

Various methods and instruments are used to treat isolated endometriotic implants. The techniques include electrical coagulation, and laser or surgical excision. All these approaches have the same goal, which is the complete destruction of the endometriotic implant with minimal damage to surrounding tissues. No single technique or instrument has been shown to be superior to the other. Therefore, the instrument should be chosen on the basis of the experience of the surgeon. Other considerations include risks, benefits, and expense of the individual technique.

Coagulation is the simplest way to accomplish destruction of endometriosis. Monopolar cautery, bipolar cautery, or thermocoagulation may be used.

Monopolar coagulation is best performed with a needle tip or fine tip instrument. The power required to coagulate endometriotic implants depends on the size of the instrument used, but a fine tipped instrument generally should function at about 10–20 watts. Coagulation is accomplished by touching the implants with care to avoid contact with the bowel, bladder, or ureters, because a deep burn can occur. Monopolar electrosurgery offers the surgeon the ability to coagulate superficial and deep lesions, and can also be used as a cutting instrument.

Bipolar coagulation can be performed with a microtip instrument or paddles. The microtip forceps is ideal for coagulating superficial implants. The current passes directly from one tip to the other, resulting in coagulation between the two electrodes. A power setting of 10–20 watts is adequate to accomplish coagulation with forceps, but a higher power may be necessary with the paddles. Although the risk of distant conduction is less with bipolar than with monopolar electrocoagulation, care should be taken to avoid its use directly over ureters, on the bowel, or bladder. Bipolar coagulation is not effective for destruction of deep endometriotic implants.

Thermocoagulation is used by some surgeons to destroy endometriosis. The technique involves the direct application of a probe which heats tissue to 120°C, to cause local destruction. Thermocoagulation has a smaller risk of thermal injury to surrounding organs compared with monopolar electrocoagulation. However, as with bipolar coagulation, this technique is not effective for deep endometriotic implants.

Lasers are preferred by many laparoscopic surgeons to vapourise endometriosis. The carbon dioxide (CO_2) laser, neodynium, yttrium:aluminum-garnet (Nd:YAG) laser, the potassium-titanyl-phosphate (KTP), and argon laser have all been used.

The CO_2 laser is directed through an articulating arm system connected to an operating laparoscope or a wave guide used through the lower abdominal puncture sites (**11.9**). The CO_2 laser gives excellent vaporization of endometriotic implants, but little coagulation. The CO_2 laser requires a 'backstop' to limit the depth of vaporization and to avoid deep tissue injury. This is accomplished by injecting the retroperitoneal space with saline to elevate the peritoneum and endometriotic implant from the pelvic sidewall. The power density needed to ablate endometriotic lesions is dependent on the laser spot size. In general, a setting of 15–20 watts on a continuous superpulse mode is adequate. The CO_2 laser produces significant smoke and carbonization, and is used with a smoke evacuator and a high flow gas insufflator. CO_2 laser offers the advantage of allowing superficial coagulation, deep excision, and a cutting ability.

The Nd:YAG laser is directed through a fiber that can be placed directly through one of the secondary cannula sites. The Nd:YAG laser is best used with a sapphire tip. Coagulation is accomplished with the use of a flat or rounded tip, a combination of cutting and coagulation is accomplished with a chisel tip, and the needle tip is used to cut tissue. The probe is placed in direct contact with the tissue. Usually, l5–30 watts on the continuous mode is necessary for coagulation and 10-20 watts for cutting. Unlike the CO_2 laser, a backstop is not necessary. A major disadvantage of the Nd:YAG laser is the expense of the disposable fiber and the sapphire tip.

Surgical excision of endometriotic implants is safe and effective, but requires an experienced surgeon and well maintained equipment. Injection of saline into the retroperitoneal space aids identification of tissue planes. Scissors are used to make a small incision in the peritoneum. A circumferential incision is then made around the endometriotic implant. Hemostasis can be accom-

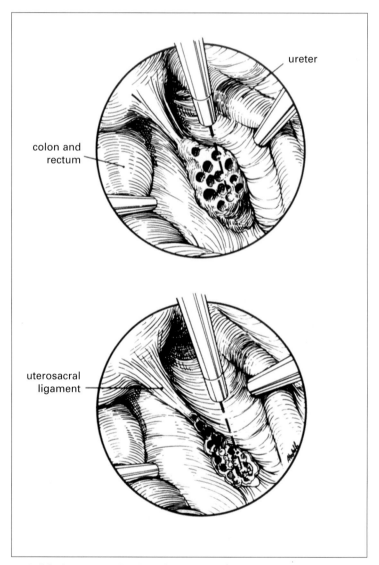

11.9 CO_2 laser vaporization of uterosacral endometriosis implant, using wave guide. The beam is applied until the implant has been completely destroyed. The course of the ureter must be identified before surgical ablation. (From Hesla JS, Rock JA. Endometriosis. In: Rock JA, Murphy AA, Jones HW, Jr., eds. Female Reproductive Surgery. Baltimore, Maryland: Williams and Wilkins, 1992:205–244, with permission)

plished with electrocoagulation, if necessary. Surgical excision is a useful method of confirming the diagnosis, especially when there is an atypical appearance of the implants. In addition, the surgeon can determine the depth of endometriotic implants to enable adequate removal of the lesion. Disadvantages of this technique include the greater potential for peritoneal damage than by simple coagulation. Additionally, there may be a higher risk of injury to underlying vessels.

Alternative therapy may be considered in patients with minimal and mild endometriosis. Expectant management for patients with infertility is likely to provide pregnancy rates of approximately 60%, which is comparable to surgical therapy. Superovulation combined with intrauterine insemination, *in vitro* fertilization, gamete intrafallopian transfer, and zygote intrafallopian transfer have all been used to augment fertility. Patients with pain are likely to experience significant improvement with medical therapy. Severe mid-line dysmenorrhea may improve with presacral neurectomy. Hysterectomy with or without bilateral salpingo-ophorectomy should be considered for symptomatic women who no longer desire to maintain fertility.

LAPAROSCOPIC TREATMENT OF MODERATE TO SEVERE ENDOMETERIOSIS

Operative laparoscopy is appropriate for patients with moderate to severe endometriosis and pain or infertility (**11.10**). The aim of the operation is restoration of normal anatomy, with minimal tissue injury. This may be accomplished by electro-dissection, laser, or sharp dissection.

Electro-dissection has the advantage of being able to cut and coagulate tissue at the same time. Using an insulated needle tip probe, cutting is accomplished with 10–30 watts of cutting current or a blend current if a combination of cutting and coagulation is desired. Adequate visualization of the adhesions, a knowledge of the anatomy, and protection of the bowel from current 'spray' and deep tissue injury are essential. Tissues are placed on tension to give optimal exposure and to identify the tissue planes. Adhesions are divided at their site of origin on both the proximal and distal surfaces and removed completely. Microsurgical principles should be observed and care should be taken to avoid damage to the normal peritoneal surfaces.

Generally the results are similar in the different surgical procedures available. An exception might be the case in which the fimbriae are adherent to the ovary. Sharp dissection is likely to result in unacceptable bleeding from the surfaces. Electro-dissection with monopolar current may result in incidental touching and damage of normal ovary or fimbriae. For this reason, the YAG laser is helpful since a hemostatic dissection of the fimbriae from the ovary can be performed with a chisel tip with minimal surrounding tissue damage.

ADHESION PREVENTION

Following adhesiolysis, attempts should be made to reduce the recurrence of adhesions. The current methods available to reduce adhesion formation include the use of Hyskon, Interceed, and GORE-TEX surgical membrane.

Hyskon is a high molecular weight dextran with the consistency of syrup. In some studies, Hyskon has been shown to reduce occurrence of severe adhesions. However, in most studies, no therapeutic effect is seen. Hyskon is applied by injecting 100 cc into the pelvis through an aspiration/irrigation portal. Hyskon should be avoided in patients with a known infection, gastrointestinal or urinary tract injury, or dehydration. Although Hyskon was quite popular in the 1980's, the lack of efficacy has led to reliance upon other methods of reducing adhesions.

Interceed (TC7) is a mesh-like adhesion barrier that reduces the recurrence of severe adhesions by 50% on the pelvic sidewall. Interceed is resorbable and dissolves within one to three weeks of use. To place Interceed, the fabric is cut to a size large enough to cover the denuded peritoneal surface. The Interceed is then rolled into a cylinder and held with forceps that have been inserted through the operating channel of a laparoscope. The entire laparoscope, forceps, and Interceed barrier are then introduced. The Interceed is placed on the pelvic sidewall and held in place on one end, and rolled towards the operator with a second instrument

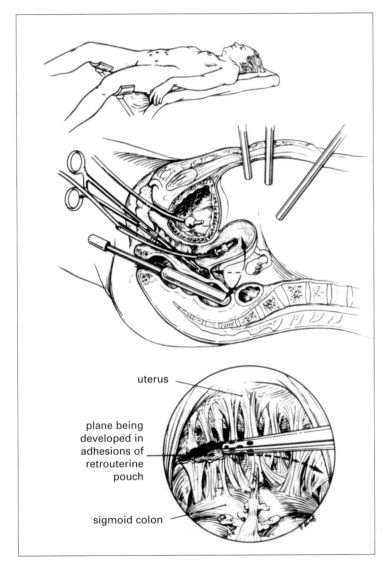

11.10 Laparoscopic treatment of endometriosis. The dorsal lithotomy position for surgery is shown in the upper diagram. Markings indicate puncture sites for ancillary instruments. Traction on bougie in rectum and sponge forceps in vagina mobilize the rectovaginal and perirectal spaces. Uterine cannula, bladder drainage and multiple transabdominal instruments aid exposure and facilitate safe dissection (middle diagram). CO_2 laser division of posterior cul-de-sac adhesions, using laser wave guide (lower diagram). (From Hesla JS, Rock JA. Endometriosis. In: Rock JA, Murphy AA, Jones HW, Jr., eds. Female Reproductive Surgery. Baltimore, Maryland: Williams and Wilkins, 1992:205–244, with permission)

uterus

plane being developed in adhesions of retrouterine pouch

sigmoid colon

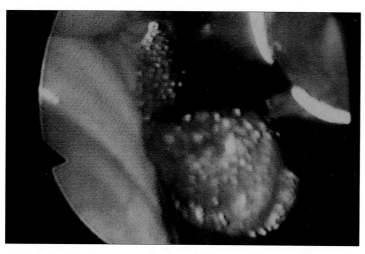

11.11 Placement of adhesion barrier. Prior to insertion, the barrier is rolled away from the surgeon. After placement on the pelvic sidewall, the membrane is rolled toward the surgeon to cover the denuded peritoneal surface.

(**11.11**). There is no need to anchor the Interceed barrier. Confirmation of hemostasis prior to placement is essential, since bleeding behind the Interceed may increase adhesions. Until data are available, Interceed should not be used on the uterus, fallopian tubes, or ovaries.

The GORE-TEX surgical membrane is a permanent barrier that prevents adhesion formation to the membrane. An overlap of the denuded peritoneal surfaces by at least 1 cm is required. The GORE-TEX surgical membrane is placed in the same manner as the Interceed, but requires fixation by a stapling device, permanent suture, or permanent clip. If desired, the GORE-TEX surgical membrane may be removed at a later date. As with Interceed, hemostasis should be established prior to placement of the GORE-TEX surgical membrane.

SURGICAL ADJUNCTS

Laparoscopic uterosacral nerve ablation (LUNA) has been used to treat women with dysmenorrhea. The procedure is performed by ablating the uterosacral ligaments with laser or electrocoagulation. Care should be taken to avoid damage to the ureters and the colon. Unfortunately, most women appear to have recurrent dysmenorrhea by 6 to 12 months following surgery. Because of the potential risk of bowel or ureteric injury with the procedure and the absence of a long-term benefit, the LUNA procedure should rarely, if ever, be performed.

Presacral neurectomy has been shown to provide excellent relief of midline dysmenorrhea in patients undergoing laparotomy. Adequate performance of the procedure requires dissection of the hypogastric plexus from the posterior peritoneum overlying the sacrum. The ureters and common iliac vessels are the lateral margins and the middle sacral vessels and periosteum of the sacrum are the posterior margins of dissection. Although laparoscopic presacral neurectomy is enthusiastically advised by some surgeons, long-term studies of patients undergoing the laparoscopic procedure are scant. The major risks involved in presacral neurectomy include damage to the iliac vessels, ureters, and middle sacral vessels. Further studies will be necessary to determine if the risk of laparoscopic presacral neurectomy warrants performance of the procedure.

CONCLUSION

Endometriosis should be considered in the differential diagnosis of a patient with infertility, chronic pelvic pain, dysmenorrhea, or dyspareunia. Visual documentation is necessary to confirm the diagnosis of endometriosis. Once the diagnosis is made, treatment should be initiated on the basis of the patient's symptoms, extent of disease, age, associated pelvic pathology, and desire for fertility. Operative laparoscopy may benefit infertile patients with anatomic distortion and patients with pelvic pain.

FURTHER READING

Cook AS, Rock JA. The role of laparoscopy in the treatment of endometriosis. *Fertil Steril* 1991; **55**:663–80

Hesla JS, Rock JA. Endometriosis. In: Rock JA, Murphy AA, Jones HW, Jr., eds. Female Reproductive Surgery. Baltimore, Maryland: Williams and Wilkins. 1992: 205–44

Hurst BS, Rock JA. Endometriosis: Pathophysiology, diagnosis and treatment. *Obstet Gynecol Survey* 1989: **44**:297–304

Martin DC. Laparoscopic treatment of endometriosis. In: Azziz R, Murphy AA, eds. Practical Manual of Operative Laparoscopy and Hysteroscopy. New York: Springer-Verlag, 1992: 101–9

Vancaillie T, Schenken RS. Endoscopic surgery. In: Schenken RS, ed. Endometriosis: Contemporary Concepts in Clinical Management. Philadelphia, JB Lippincott Company:1989: 249–66

LAPAROSCOPIC MANAGEMENT OF LARGE OVARIAN ENDOMETRIOMAS

12

**Michelle Nisolle, Françoise Casanas-Roux,
Françoise Clerckx and Jacques Donnez**

OVARIAN ENDOMETRIOSIS

Endometriosis should be suspected when the ovary is fixed to the posterior aspect of the broad ligament by adhesions. These adhesions should be dissected so that the entire ovarian surface can be seen. The posterior surface near the hilus is the typical location of an endometrioma, but the disease may occur anywhere. A deep endometrioma within an ovary may be perfectly free of adhesions, and the surface may look normal.

The three types of ovarian endometriosis are classified as superficial hemorrhagic lesions; hemorrhagic cysts (endometriomas); and deep infiltrating ovarian endometriosis, which are less common.

SUPERFICIAL LESIONS

Superficial ovarian endometriosis consists of small vesicular lesions on the ovarian cortex or small implants, usually found on the lateral surface of the ovary. Adhesions between the ovary and the broad ligament are common.

From a histopathological aspect, the endometrial cysts may be lined by free endometrial tissue (**12.1**) that is similar histologically and functionally to eutopic endometrium. Active ectopic endometrial tissue may cover the inner surface of a small cavity in the ovary. In some instances, atypical epithelium with ciliated (**12.2**) cells may be found.

ENDOMETRIOMAS

The term 'chocolate cysts' was introduced by Sampson to describe the endometrial cysts of the ovary.

In large endometriomas, the cyst is often lined by a flattened endometrial epithelium (**12.3**). The cyclical changes in these enclosed lesions are less significant than those in the free-growing lesions, and late secretory changes and menstrual bleeding are absent. When cysts are mobilized they may rupture, with subsequent spillage of their contents into the abdomen. The internal surface of a chocolate cyst is really the external surface of the ovary; the ovarian cortex is identifiable by the presence of primordial follicles. Ovarioscopy, as described by Brosens, demonstrates dark fibrotic areas with hemosiderin pigmentation alternating with highly vascularized areas with focal bleeding. The vessels in these areas are often congested and tend to be larger at the hilus of the ovary. According to this hypothesis, the hemorrhagic content of many 'chocolate cysts' may originate from chronic focal bleeding from congested blood vessels rather than from endometrial shedding.

Three months after drainage of an endometrial cyst followed by gonadotrophin-releasing hormone (GnRH) agonist therapy (to induce amenorrhea), chocolate-colored fluid may still be present. This proves that endometrial shedding is not responsible for the chocolate-colored fluid. In our opinion, it could arise from exudate in the cyst wall, the congested blood vessels in the cyst or inflammation around persistent endometrial foci which have resisted medical therapy.

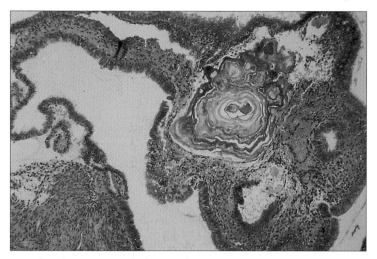

12.1 Ovarian endometriotic cyst: free endometrial polypoid structure (Gomori's trichrome x 110).

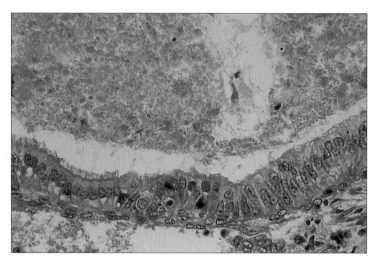

12.2 Ovarian endometriotic cyst: area of oviduct-like epithelium (Gomori's trichrome x 110).

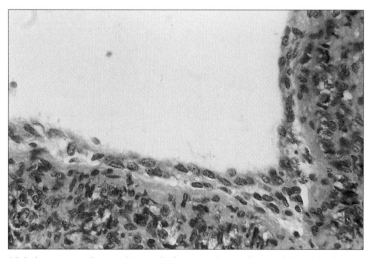

12.3 Large ovarian endometriotic cyst: the endometrial epithelium is flattened.

DEEP INFILTRATING ENDOMETRIOSIS

Deep infiltrating endometriosis is characterized by the presence of very active endometrial glands which invade the ovarian cortex. In this type of ovarian endometriosis, areas of normal-looking endometrium with ciliated cells can be demonstrated in 62% of cases. Endometriotic lesions were considered active when typical glandular epithelium was seen. This is found in 84% of cases. The mitotic index was calculated in typical glandular epithelium and its value was 3.9%. Deep endometriotic implants do not show the normal cyclical endometrial changes.

RATIONALE FOR SURGERY

EVALUATION OF HORMONAL THERAPY

In the last decade, three new drugs, danazol, gestrinone and GnRH agonist, have offered further options in the hormonal treatment of endometriosis. In one of our studies, we compared the effects of these drugs on deep endometriosis over a six-month period. Ovarian endometriosis regressed in only 30% of cases after danazol therapy as opposed to the effect of danazol on peritoneal and superficial ovarian endometriosis. The results obtained with lynestrenol were slightly better but the results obtained with gestrinone were similar to those obtained with danazol. The GnRH agonists are more effective and often the ovarian endometriotic lesions regressed even in severe endometriosis.

When the scores before and after hormonal therapy were compared in moderate and severe endometriosis, the most important difference was found in women treated with GnRH agonists. These data agree with a previous study in which a lower mitotic index was found in ectopic glandular epithelium after buserelin therapy than that observed after either lynestroenol or gestrinone therapy. Thus, medical oophrectomy with GnRH agonists allows temporary suppression of ovarian function. Within two weeks of the first injection, the production of gonadal steroids falls to castrate-like levels – less than 30 pg/ml.

As suggested in our previous studies, the advantage of an effective hormonal treatment is a reduction in pelvic vascularity and inflammation, which is often present around endometriotic foci. The improved pelvic environment makes surgery easier and reduces the risk of postoperative adhesion formation.

Despite its superior efficacy compared with other drugs, GnRH agonists are unable to suppress endometriotic cells completely because the ectopic foci are not influenced by the normal control mechanisms that regulate the uterine endometrial glands and stroma. Therefore, surgical removal of invasive ovarian endometriosis is necessary.

We reported a histological study of residual endometriotic ovarian lesions after hormone treatment (either danazol, lynoestrenol, gestrinone, buserelin nasal spray, or buserelin subcutaneous implant). Glandular epithelium was usually found. These findings did not agree with other published reports which give a recurrence rate of only 30–40% after hormone treatment. A high incidence of active endometriosis without signs of degeneration was found in all groups except after GnRH agonist implant. Mitotic figures were discovered although others described the absence of mitosis in such implants. Histologic study showed that a lower mitotic index of ovarian endometrial epithelium was observed in the GnRH agonist group.

Mitotic processes account for the persistence of ovarian endometriosis despite the administration of hormonal therapy. The ectopic foci are more or less autonomous, and are not governed by the normal control mechanisms that govern the uterine endometrial glands and stroma.

The precise reason why a number of implants or cells do not respond to hormone therapy is unknown, but several hypotheses have been proposed:
- The drug does not gain access to the ovarian endometriotic foci because fibrosis surrounding the foci prevents local access.
- Endometriotic cells may have their own genetic programming. An endocrine influence appears to be secondary and dependent on the degree of differentiation of the individual cell.
- The low number of endometriotic steroid receptors and their different regulatory mechanisms in ectopic and eutopic endometrium may result in deficient endocrine dependency. The nuclear oestrogen-binding sites seen in foci of endometriosis do not appear to change during the menstrual cycle, whereas these sites in the uterine endometrium downregulate during the secretory phase.

TECHNIQUES OF ENDOSCOPIC SURGERY

Preoperative evaluation should include transvaginal sonography and measurements of CA. 125 serum level.

LASER SURGERY

The endoscopic use of the laser is not new in gynecology, and several types of operative procedures have been carried out with the carbon dioxide (CO_2) laser laparoscope for the treatment of disease in the reproductive tract. The most frequent indication is endometriosis, which can be vaporized by means of CO_2 laser laparoscopy with high pregnancy rates. Laser surgery allows destruction of endometriosis with great precision.

Between 1982 and 1991, 6,250 laser laparoscopies were carried out in our department, almost 3,000 of which were for endometriosis.

Peritoneal Endometriotic Implants
Usually, a power setting of 40-50 watts is used. The debulking of endometriotic implants is best performed using a continuous firing mode. If a lesion overlies a vital structure such as the ureter, urinary bladder, colon, or larger blood vessels, a retroperitoneal injection of fluid (aquadissection and aquaprotection) can be used to act as a backstop for the CO_2 laser. When an endometriotic implant is treated with laser, old blood first bubbles out, followed by a curdy white material produced by vaporization of the stromal layer. Retroperitoneal fat is then encountered, and when this is seen, complete vaporization of the lesion is confirmed.

Ovarian Endometriotic Implants Less Than 3 cm in Diameter
Ovarian endometriosis can be treated at the time of diagnostic laparoscopy if the cyst does not penetrate more than 3 cm into the ovary and if its diameter is no larger than 3cm (**12.4**).

Endometriotic implants of less than 1 cm in diameter can be vaporized until fluid-filled follicles are seen or no further pigmented tissue is left. Large endometriomas of 1–3 cm diameter are treated differently. An area of 3–4 mm of the top of the cyst is first

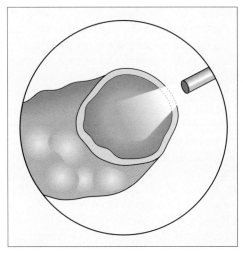 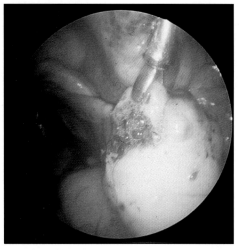 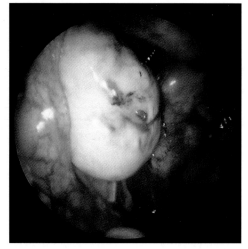

12.4 Small ovarian endometriotic cyst (less than 3 cm): the vaporization is performed during the first-look laparoscopy.

12.5 Ovarian endometrioma (greater than 3 cm).

excised, the chocolate-colored material aspirated, and the cyst then washed out with irrigation fluid. The interior wall of the cyst is now examined carefully to confirm the absence of any suspected intra-cystic lesion (ovarian cystoscopy). The laser is set to 40 watts and with continuous mode, the interior wall of the cyst is vaporized to destroy the mucosal lining. The vaporization is continued until no further pigment is seen. The pelvis is irrigated, and the ovaries are left open without suturing.

Ovarian Endometriotic Implants More Than 3 cm in Diameter

In our series of 2,192 patients with endometriosis, ovarian endometriomas more than 3 cm in diameter were found in 481 patients (**12.5–12.9**).

During diagnostic laparoscopy, these endometrial cysts were washed out with irrigation fluid and biopsied. A GnRH analogue was then administered for 12 weeks to decrease the cyst size. A sec-ond-look laparoscopy was then carried out, and if the diameter of the residual endometrial cyst was less than 3 cm, the interior wall of the cyst was vaporized as previously described.

If the diameter of the residual cysts was more than 3 cm after GnRH agonist therapy, another technique was used. In this series, the range of the ovarian cyst sizes was 3–8 cm. A portion of the ovarian cyst was first removed by making a circular incision with CO_2 laser over the protruding portion of the ovarian cyst. Partial cystectomy was then carried out. Ovarian cystoscopy was per-formed for evaluation of the interior cyst wall, and a biopsy was taken. The residual endometrial cyst wall was then vaporized. The ovary was left open in the first 20 patients. In a further group of 62 patients, the ovary was closed with fibrin glue injected transab-dominally into the cyst bed. The edges of the ovarian cyst were approximated with atraumatic forceps for 2–3 minutes. At the end of the procedure, copious irrigation of the pelvic cavity was car-ried out to prevent deposits of carbon and glue. Finally, 100–200 ml of 32% dextran 70 was instilled into the peritoneal cavity.

The component parts of the fibrin glue must be thoroughly mixed and kept at a temperature of 37°C. The tissue surfaces must be dry. The sealant can be applied as a thin film through a needle insert-ed through the abdominal wall.

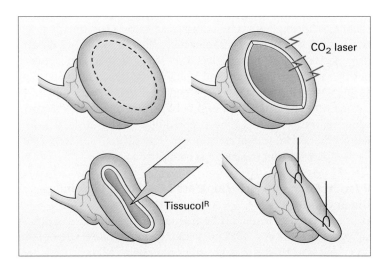 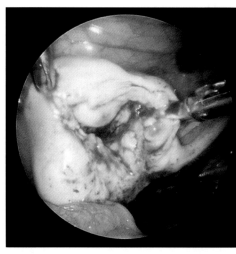

12.6 Scheme of endoscopic therapy of large endo-metrioma. (left) Large ovarian endometrioma – a circular cut over the protruding portion of the ovarian cyst and partial cystectomy are carried out (right).

RESULTS

The operating time varied from 45 minutes to 80 minutes. Vaporization of the mucosal lining was easier if the GnRH agonists were administered preoperatively. The interior wall of the endometrial cyst seen during ovarian cystoscopy was found to be less hemorrhagic and more atrophic than before therapy. These data were confirmed by ovarian biopsy. An endometriotic lesion was considered 'active' when typical glandular epithelium appeared either proliferative or unresponsive to hormone therapy with typical stroma. These active lesions were found more often (84% of cases) before GnRH agonist therapy than after GnRH agonist therapy (44% of cases) ($P < 0.001$).

In a first series of 20 patients with residual ovarian cysts larger than 3 cm in diameter, CO_2 laser surgery was used successfully to vaporize the endometriotic ovarian lesions, and the ovary was left open. A third-look laparoscopy was performed three months later in nine patients. We found dense and fibrous adhesions between the vaporized area of the ovary and the broad ligament, the bowel, and the fallopian tube were found in eight out of nine patients, which necessitated laparoscopic salpingo-ovariolysis.

In a second series of 62 patients with residual ovarian cysts greater than 3 cm in diameter, vaporization of the mucosal lining was performed, and fibrin glue was used to close the ovary. Fifteen of these women underwent a laparoscopy three months later. In all cases, peri-ovarian adhesions were absent, and the healing of the ovarian closure was good. There was no inflammation.

To date, we have used this technique successfully in 482 patients with endometriomas greater than 3 cm in diameter.

OVARIAN CYSTECTOMY

Ovarian cystectomy can be accomplished laparoscopically in most cases (**12.10–12.12**).

The procedure begins with adhesiolysis. When the cyst is mobilized, the cortex is grasped with a forceps introduced through a second cannula. The cortex is incised with laser or scissors, and the cyst wall is exposed. The incision is enlarged with scissors. Aquadissection can be used to separate the cyst wall from the ovarian stroma. If the cyst is opened and spill occurs, peritoneal irrigation must be performed to remove the chocolate-colored fluid. Ovarioscopy, and careful evaluation of the internal cyst wall, allow the surgeon to exclude malignancy. The ovary usually does not require suturing.

CONCLUSION

CO_2 laser laparoscopy offers advantages over electrosurgery. With the CO_2 laser, the laparoscopist is able to control the process of vaporization precisely.

In a previous study, significantly different pregnancy rates were found in the different grades of endometriosis. Severe endometriosis had the poorest prognosis in terms of pregnancy rates. For this reason, preoperative GnRH agonist therapy was given to patients with very large ovarian endometriomas (greater than 3 cm). The release of a GnRH agonist by a biodegradable implant is effective in reducing endometriotic size to a greater extent than danazol or progesterone and GnRH agonist decreases pelvic inflammation. Treatment by sustained release is an effective alternative to using

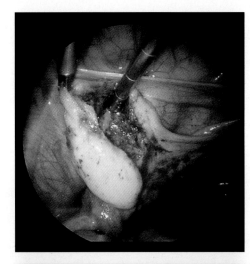

12.7a Large ovarian endometrioma: the residual endometrial cyst is vaporized.

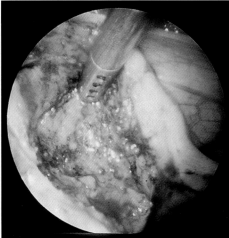

12.7b Close-up of the vaporized area.

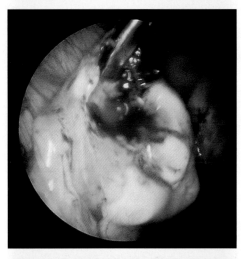

12.8 Fibrin glue is injected transabdominally into the intra-ovarian vaporized area.

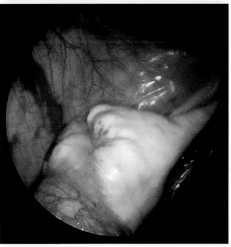

12.9 Final appearance of the ovary.

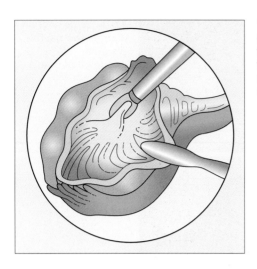

12.10 Ovarian cystectomy. The cyst wall is separated from the ovarian cortex using atraumatic forceps.

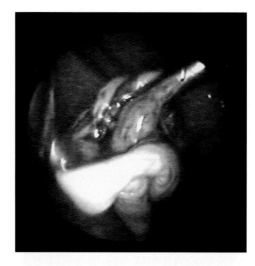

12.11 Laparoscopic view of ovarian cystectomy.

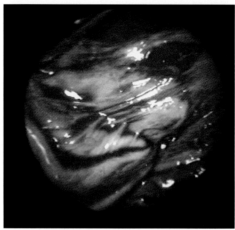

12.12 Close-up of the cleavage plane.

steroid hormones before laser laparoscopy. A subcutaneous GnRH agonist implant causes a substantial reduction in size of large ovarian cyst and a decrease in pelvic inflammation so that a second-look laser laparoscopy can be performed for laser vaporization of residual endometriomas. During the ovarian cystoscopy, the interior ovarian wall was found atrophic, vascularity was decreased, and the vaporization was thus made easier.

In endometriotic cysts over 3 cm in diameter, we found the risk of postoperative adhesions was high if the ovary was left open. Dense fibrous peri-ovarian adhesions were usually seen during subsequent laparoscopy. These findings are in conflict with results reported by others.

In conclusion, our results demonstrate that the use of fibrin glue permits the laparoscopic closure of the ovarian cyst cavity and reduce the risk of the postoperative adhesions in cases of vaporization of severe ovarian endometriosis.

FURTHER READING

Brosens I, Gordon A. Endometriosis: ovarian endometriosis. In: *Tubal Infertility* 1989. Eds: Brosens I, Gordon A. Gower Medical Publishing, London, pp313–17

Buttram V, Reiter R, Ward S. Treatment of endometriosis with danazol: report of a 6-year prospsective study. *Fertil Steril* 1985; **43**:353

Donnez J. CO_2 laser laparoscopy in infertile women with adhesions or endometriosis. *Fertil Steril* 1987; **48**:390–94

Donnez J, Nisolle M, Casanas-Roux F. Endometriosis-associated infertility: Evaluation of preoperative use of danazol, gestrinone and buserelin. *J Fertil* 1990; **42**:128

Donnez J, Nisolle M. Laparoscopic management of large ovarian endometrial cysts: use of firbrin sealant. *J Gyn Surg* 1991; **7**:163–67

Nezhat C, Crowgey SR, Garrison CP. Surgical treatment of endometriosis via laser laparoscopy. *Fertil Steril* 1986; **45**:778–83

ECTOPIC PREGNANCY   13

Hubert Manhes and Salil Khandwala

INTRODUCTION

The management of ectopic pregnancy has undergone a 'radical' change towards a more conservative approach. With improved diagnostic aids, ectopic pregnancies should be diagnosed very early and, hence, mortality should no longer be a problem. Instead, it is conservation of fertility and minimizing patient morbidity that are of primary importance in minimally invasive surgery. Laparoscopy has a triple role to play and provides a stategy for the diagnosis, treatment and management of extrauterine pregnancy.

DIAGNOSIS

The clinical presentation of ectopic pregnancy is variable. The patient may present with typical symptoms, non-specific symptoms or no symptoms. This variation in clinical presentation depends upon the time when the diagnosis is made. With the present attitude of 'think ectopic' in any woman of childbearing age who complains of abdominal pain and with high-resolution ultrasonography and beta human chorionic gonadotropin (ßHCG) estimations, the diagnosis of ectopic pregnancy can be made with a high degree of certainty. However, laparoscopy remains the final arbiter as it allows visual confirmation.

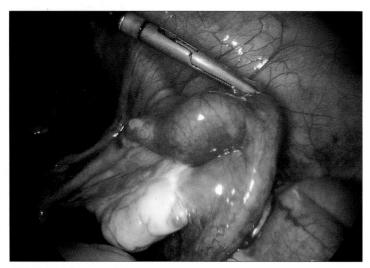

13.1 Ampullary ectopic pregnancy.

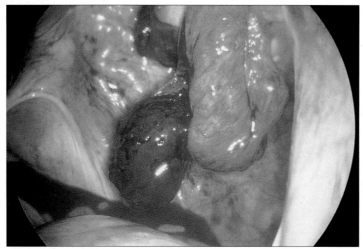

13.2 Fimbrial ectopic pregnancy.

DIAGNOSTIC LAPAROSCOPY

Diagnostic laparoscopy enables not only visualization of the ectopic pregnancy but also recognition of the site of the ectopic pregnancy **(13.1–13.3)**, its size **(13.4a,b)**, the state of the tube containing the ectopic sac, that is, whether it is ruptured **(13.5a)** or intact , the condition of the contralateral tube, and the presence and volume of the haemoperitoneum **(13.5b)**. Once the diagnosis is confirmed, the next step is to proceed with operative laparoscopy to treat the ectopic pregnancy.

Our policy has always been to perform linear salpingotomy in all cases including those in whom at first glance, conservation seems futile. This is because when the ectopic pregnancy has been removed we have often been able to change from a radical to a conservative approach. The operator now has sufficient time and is better placed to carry out a detailed assessment of the prognostic factors. Moreover, even if the final decision were to be in favor of salpingectomy, the removal of the ectopic pregnancy makes the operation easier than if the tubal pregnancy is *in situ*.

LAPAROSCOPIC SALPINGOTOMY

The immediate problem is to remove the ectopic gestation. In addition to the usual instruments used at operative laparoscopy, the authors also use a special instrument adapted exclusively for treating ectopic pregnancies. This is the Triton, which is a 7 mm diameter instrument consisting of a 5 mm aspiration canal, a 2 mm lavage channel and a retractable monopolar needle. Thus, it enables the three key functions required for extraction of the ectopic: incision, aspiration, and lavage **(13.6–13.9)**.

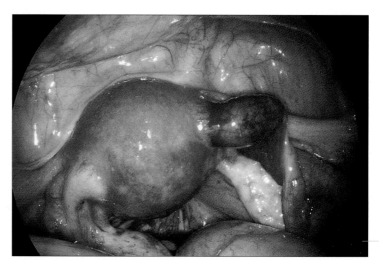

13.3 Isthmic ectopic pregnancy.

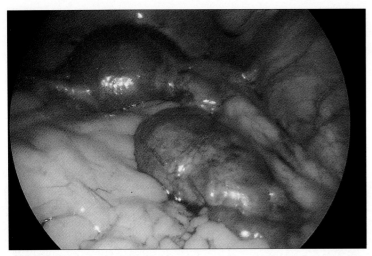

13.4a Small ampullary pregnancy.

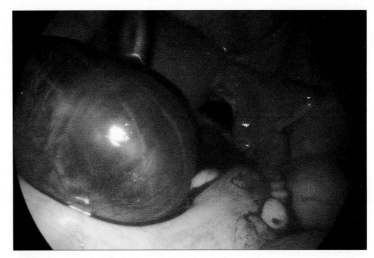

13.4b Large ampullary pregnancy.

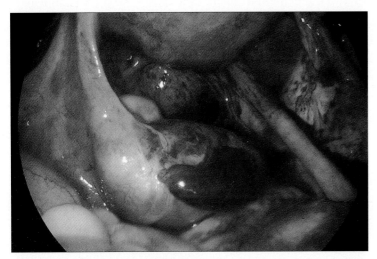

13.5a Rupturing ectopic pregnancy.

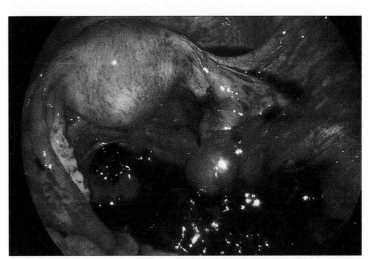

13.5b Hemoperitoneum.

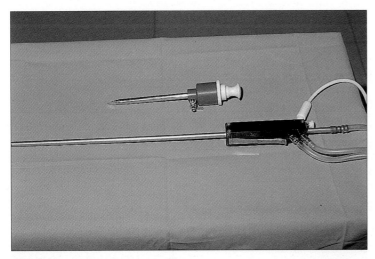

13.6 Triton with an 8 cm cannula.

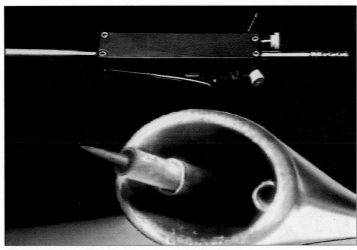

13.7 Triton with end-on view.

TECHNIQUE

Two suprapubic secondary portals are inserted on either side of the midline within the safety triangle delineated inferiorally by the bladder fundus and laterally by the obliterated umbilical arteries.

The Triton is introduced into the abdominal cavity through the contralateral 8 mm cannula so that it approaches the site of the ectopic perpendicularly. The grasping forceps (**13.10, 13.11**) is inserted through the ipsilateral trocar, and holds the tube proximal to the ectopic thereby steadying it. The procedure of laparoscopic salpingotomy is then carried out systematically.

The first step is to examine the ectopic pregnancy after peritoneal lavage has removed blood clots. In the second step, hemostasis is achieved by injecting a vasoconstrictive agent such as vasopressin into the mesosalpinx (**13.12**). This step reduces bleeding during the procedure. Ornithine 8 vasopressin (POR-8; Sandoz) is a synthetic polypeptide with the vasoconstrictive properties of vasopressin. Five international units should be diluted in 50 ml normal saline. About 10 ml of solution should be injected into the mesosalpinx. The injection is performed with a 15 cm 18 gauge needle inserted directly through the abdominal wall. The puncture site of the needle should be selected so that the injection is performed between the two leaves of the broad ligament adjacent to the ectopic pregnancy. It is imperative that the anesthetist be informed and his permission obtained prior to the injection. Because of the increased vascularity near the ectopic pregnancy, care should be taken to avoid an intravascular injection. Ectopic pregnancies should now be diagnosed very early when they are small and therefore injection of vasoconstrictor agents is only necessary in 5–10% of cases.

The third step involves the performance of the salpingotomy (**13.13**). The salpingotomy incision is made with the monopolar retractable needle on the proximal part of the antimesenteric border of the tube. If it were to be made on the mesenteric border, this would jeopardize the blood supply to the tube and would result in greater bleeding. Of still greater importance is incising the proximal part of the swelling as the pedicle of the ectopic formed by the invading trophoblastic tissue is situated at this site (**13.14–13.16**). The authors have realized that most failures occur when this principle is not respected and the incision is made distally. A distal incision risks leaving behind a part of the active trophoblastic tissue.

Thus, a proximal antimesenteric incision provides the best access for the complete extraction of the ectopic pregnancy. However, the incision should be precise — large enough to allow passage of the Triton, but small enough to enable a tight fit around

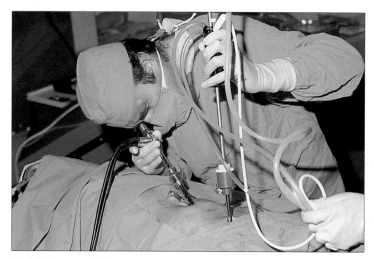

13.8 Triton used through a second puncture.

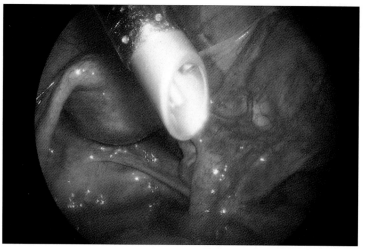

13.9 Triton viewed through the laparoscope.

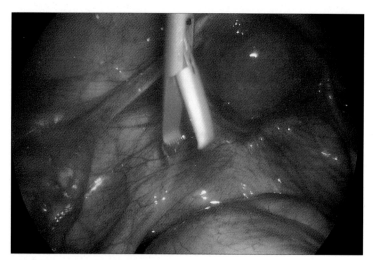

13.10 Grasping forceps approaching the tube.

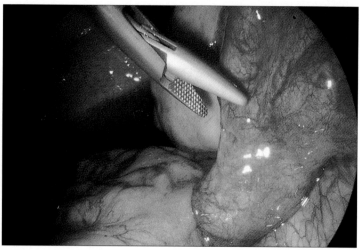

13.11 Forceps grasping the tube proximal to the ectopic.

the instrument so as to permit aspiration and lavage of the trophoblastic tissue without leakage. Once the Triton is introduced through the salpingotomy incision, the ectopic pregnancy is aspirated and extracted (**13.17**). Repeated aspiration and lavage results in complete extraction of all the trophoblastic tissue. In some cases of large ectopic pregnancy, extraction of the entire trophoblastic tissue may not be possible because it is embedded in the tubal wall. In these cases, grasping forceps may be required to remove residual tissue (**13.18a,b**).

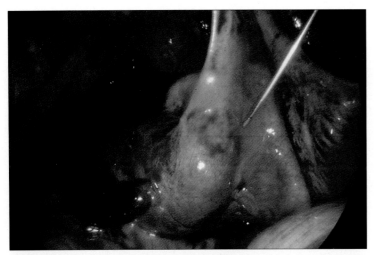

13.12 Prophylactic hemostasis with vasopressin.

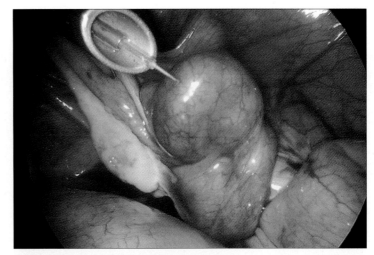

13.13 Salpingotomy with microneedle.

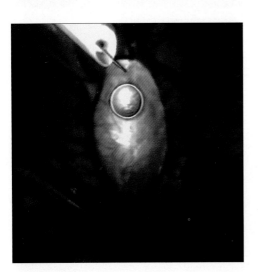

13.14 The ectopic gestation is implanted at the proximal end of the tubal swelling (the incision should be at this point).

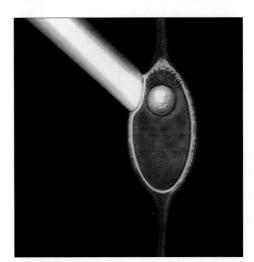

13.15 Triton is inserted into the incision followed by lavage and aspiration.

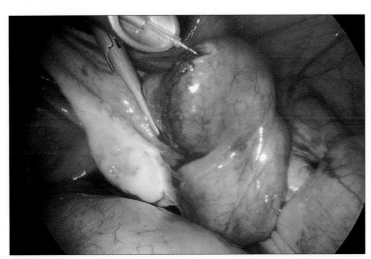

13.16 Proximal incision.

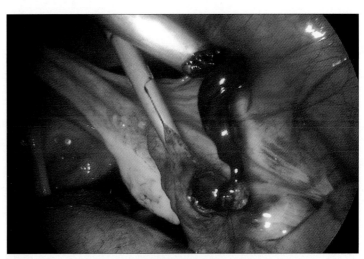

13.17 Extraction of the ectopic pregnancy.

Once the ectopic has been extracted, meticulous hemostasis is carried out. In most cases, repeated washing **(13.19)** of the pregnancy bed with warm saline at 40°C aided by the hemostatic effect of the positive intra-abdominal pressure succeeds in stopping the bleeding. If bleeding persists, selective coagulation of the bleeding vessel can be carried out using fine bipolar forceps at low power.

The authors do not believe in suturing the salpingotomy incision. Their policy is to leave the incision open **(13.20)**. Once the ectopic pregnancy has been extracted and the overlying tubal wall collapses, the two edges of the incision fall together and are thus held by a serum seal, thereby making suturing superfluous. Moreover, studies have shown that suturing the salpingotomy results in greater postoperative adhesion formation.

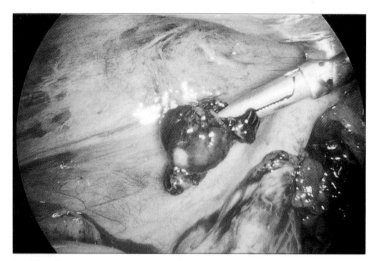

13.18a Grasping forceps removing tissue.

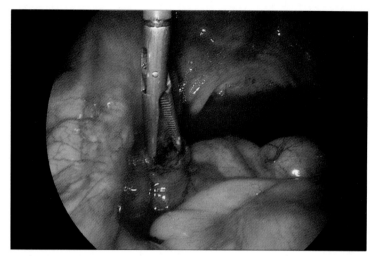

13.18b Exploring the tube for retained products.

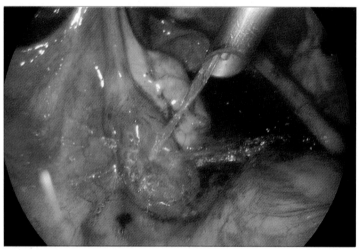

13.19 Lavage.

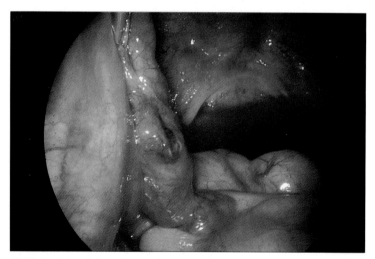

13.20 Incision left unsutured.

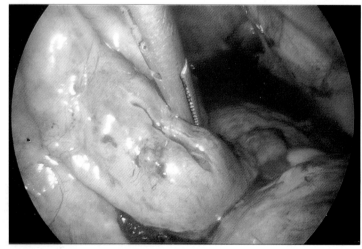

13.21a Early second-look laparoscopy.

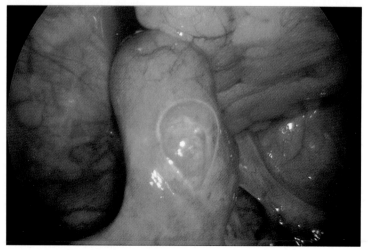

13.21b Healed tube at later second-look laparoscopy.

The authors have had the opportunity to perform a second-look laparoscopy in some of those patients who had undergone laparoscopic salpingotomy (**13.21a,b**). A slight bulge was seen at the site of the salpingotomy incision. Biopsies of these bulges indicated the presence of endosalpingeal mucosa and serosa with the muscular layer absent. This indicates that healing is associated with herniation of the mucosa through the defect in the muscularis. In fact, this herniation is advantageous since it prevents constriction of the tube at this site, which, by itself, could predispose to another ectopic pregnancy.

Once the extraction of the ectopic pregnancy has been accomplished, a thorough assessment of the adnexa and the pelvis is carried out.

MANAGEMENT STRATEGY

Several studies have demonstrated that laparoscopic salpingotomy has a definitive place in the conservative surgical treatment of ectopic pregnancy. It protects subsequent fertility and gives results comparable with those of laparotomy and microsurgical techniques. Intrauterine pregnancy rates following laparoscopic salpingotomy range from 50 to 70%. However, the question arises whether all cases of ectopic pregnancy should be treated conservatively and whether conservative treatment in some patients would not expose them to an unacceptably high risk of recurrent ectopic. The authors have carried out a study to determine the factors that influence future fertility and the risk of recurrence. The prognostic factors included the age of the patient, her parity and obesity, and whether the tube was intact or ruptured and the site of the ectopic. The presence of peritubal adhesions and a past history of salpingitis, ectopic pregnancy, salpingectomy or tubal infertility were also considered.

The results showed that age, parity and the type of ectopic pregnancy had little influence on subsequent fertility. Peritubal adhesions or damage to the contralateral tube significantly reduced future fertility and increased the risk of recurrence. From these results, a scoring system was proposed so that the most appropriate treatment to preserve fertility and reduce recurrence rates could be selected. These treatment options range from conservative surgery to laparoscopic salpingectomy with contralateral sterilization.

In order to select the best management, each of the above factors was carefully assessed and given a score. Treatment was planned depending on the score (**13.22**).

A score of 0 to 3 indicates a conservative approach. Peritoneal lavage is performed, and the pelvis examined for adhesions (**13.23, 13.24**) and endometriosis (**13.25**) which if found, should be treated.

The treatment of a patient with a score of 5 must take into account the availability of an *in vitro* fertilization (IVF) program. If IVFET is not available, salpingectomy with conservation of the contralateral tube should be performed.

Risk factors and therapeutic score of ectopic pregnancy	
Score data	Score
One previous ectopic pregnancy	2
For each additional ectopic pregnancy[a]	1
Previous laparoscopic adhesiolysis[b]	1
Previous tubal microsurgery[b]	2
Solitary tube	2
Previous salpingitis	1
Homolateral adhesions	1
Contralateral adhesions[c]	1

a If the ectopic occurred in both tubes just count 'solitary tube'
b Only one is taken in count
c If the tube is blocked or absent count 'solitary tube'

Score 0 to 3: laparoscopic conservative treatment,
Score 4: laparoscopic salpingectomy,
Score 5 or more: laparoscopic salpingectomy and contralateral conservation

13.22 The risk factors and therapeutic score of ectopic pregnancy.

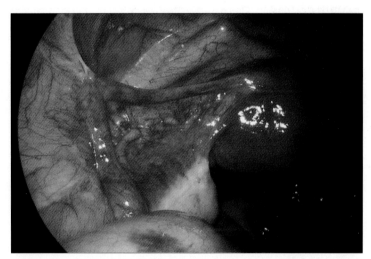

13.23 Adhesions between the tube and the pelvic sidewall.

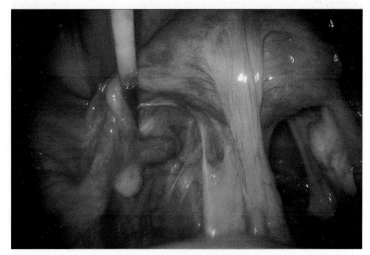

13.24 Adhesions between the tube and the floor of the pouch of Douglas, and between the bowel and uterus.

Serial ßHCG estimations should be performed postoperatively, to confirm complete removal of the trophoblastic tissue and to recognize operative failure because of incomplete removal. Complete removal of the ectopic pregnancy is indicated by a ßHCG level in zone A. If ßHCG level is in zone B, serial estimations should be carried out if the initial level is high. If ßHCG level is in zone C, serial estimations should be performed irrespective of the initial level. If ßHCG is in zone D, it is likely that the trophoblastic tissue has not been completely removed (13.26).

For a score of 4, laparoscopic salpingectomy would be the treatment of choice.

LAPAROSCOPIC SALPINGECTOMY

TECHNIQUE

Laparoscopic salpingectomy should be carried out in a retrograde manner from the isthmus to the fimbriae (13.27). Grasping forceps is introduced through the ipsilateral cannula and the tubal isthmus is grasped so that the proximal end of the tube can be coagulated with bipolar forceps introduced through the contralateral cannula. The coagulated tube is then divided with scissors. Successive coagulation and cutting of the mesosalpinx adjacent and parallel to the tube enable salpingectomy to be performed. The two leaves of the mesosalpinx are sealed with bipolar forceps used at a low power output (13.28). The tube is either removed through an 8 mm trocar or in a bag.

Retrograde salpingectomy (i.e. from the isthmus to the infundibulum) is preferable to the antegrade technique because the latter requires the trocars to be placed at a higher and more lateral position with resulting visible scars.

CONTRA-INDICATIONS TO CONSERVATIVE LAPAROSCOPIC TREATMENT

- Laparotomy should be carried out in cases of severe hemorrhage with shock (13.29, 13.30).
- Large hematoceles are difficult to evacuate laparoscopically using the Triton or any other aspiration–irrigation system. In such cases, laparotomy may also have to be performed.

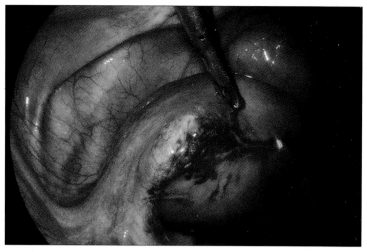

13.25 Endometriosis: salpingitis isthmica nodosa.

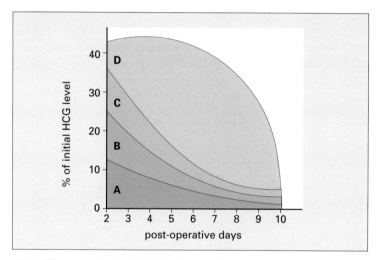

13.26 The rate of fall of ßHCG after treatment.

- If ectopic pregnancy is surrounded or hidden by dense adhesions, or in cases of gross obesity, when access is difficult, laparotomy is preferable.
- Finally, laparotomy is indicated in all cases of cornual pregnancy.

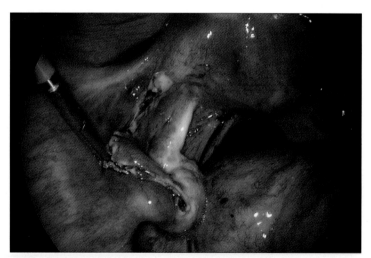

13.27 Salpingectomy using bipolar electrocoagulation.

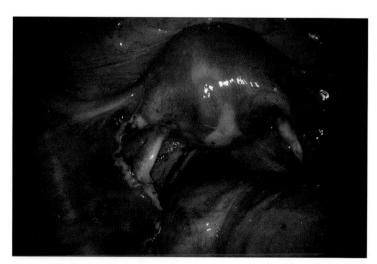

13.28 Salpingectomy completed.

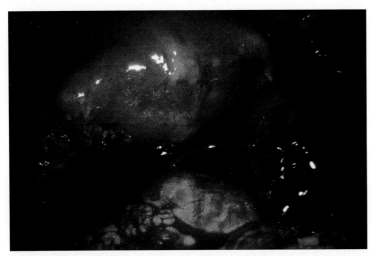

13.29 Hemorrhage from a right ampullary ectopic pregnancy.

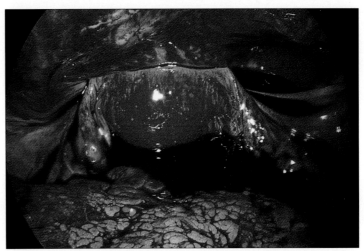

13.30 Large hemoperitoneum with over 500 ml blood loss.

Fertility rate following conservative treatment of ectopic pregnancy by laparoscopy		IUP		EP	
Authors	n	n	%	n	%
Conventional laparotomy					
Timonen	185	98	53	22	12
Sherman	47	39	83	3	6
Querleu	129	67	52	36	30
Tuomivaara	86	57	66	12	14
Makinen	42	29	69	12	29
Langer	118	83	70	12	11
Total	607	373	61.5	98	16
Microsurgery					
Janecek	10	6	60	2	20
De Cherney	9	5	55	0	0
Oelsner	51	26	51	13	25
Total	70	37	53	15	21

13.31 Fertility rate after conservative treatment of ectopic pregnancy by laparotomy.

Fertility rate after conservative laparoscopic treatment of ectopic pregnancy			IUP		EP	
Authors	Year	No.	n	%	n	%
De Cherney	1987	69	36	52	7	16
Donnez	1990	38	70	51	14	10
Pouly	1990	223	149	67	27	12
Total		607	430	255	59	48	11

13.32 Fertility rate after conservative laparoscopic treatment of ectopic pregnancy.

RESULTS

Pregnancy rates after conservative laparoscopic treatment are comparable with those after conventional laparotomy or microsurgery (**13.31,13.32**).

CONCLUSION

Until recently, the classic treatment of tubal pregnancy was salpingectomy at laparotomy to remove a ruptured and bleeding tube. The object of such practice was the preservation of the patient's life. Such practice has been changed to procedures that favor the conservation of the tube. This conservative approach has been made possible thanks to improved methods that enable early diagnosis of ectopic pregnancy prior to rupture, and also to improved surgical equipment that allows the procedure to be performed laparoscopically.

Laparoscopy is the only technique that enables diagnosis, management and assessement of prognosis at the same time.

Conservative laparoscopic surgery must now be considered to be the optimum treatment for ectopic pregnancy because it is effective and preserves fertility.

FURTHER READING

Bruhat MA, Mage G, Pouly JL, Manhes H, Canis M, Wattiez A: *Operative laparoscopy* 1991. Medsi/Mc Graw-Hill Publishers, New York

Pouly JL, Manhes H, Mage G, Canis M, Bruhat MA: Conservative laparoscopic treatment of 321 ectopic pregnancies. *Fertil Steril* 1986; **46**:1093

Bruhat MA, Manhes H, Mage G, Pouly JL: Treatment of ectopic pregnancy by means of laparoscopy. *Fertil Steril* 1980; **33**:411

Nagamani M, London S, St Amand P. Factors influencing fertility after ectopic pregnancy. *Am J Obstet Gynecol* 1984; **149**:533

Pouly JL, Chapron C, Manhes H, Canis M,Wattiez A, Bruhat MA: Multifactorial analysis of fertility following conservative laparoscopic treatment of ectopic pregnancy through a 223 case series. *Fertil Steril* 1992; **56**:453–460

Sherman D, Langer R, Sadovski G, Bukovski, Caspi E: Improved fertility following ectopic pregnancy. *Fertil Steril* 1982; **37**:497-502

Tuomivaara L, Kaupila A: Radical or conservative surgery for ectopic pregnancy? A follow-up study of fertility of 323 patients. *Fertil Steril* 1988; **50**:580–583

Makinen JI, Salmi TU, Nikkanen VPJ, Koskinen EYJ. Encouraging rates of fertility after ectopic pregnancy. *Int J Fertil* 1989; **34**(1):46–51

Langer R, Raziel A, Ron-el R, Bukovski I, Caspie E. Reproductive outcome after conservative surgery for unruptured tubal pregnancy. A 15 year experience. *Fertil Steril* 1990; **53**:227–231

Janecek J. Résultats de la chirurgie reconstructive dans les grossesses extra-utérines non rompues. *Rev Med Suisse Romande* 1979; **99**:603

De Cherney AH, Polan ML, Kort H, Kase N. Microsurgical technique in the management of tubal ectopic pregnancy. *Fertil Steril* 1980; **34**:324–327

Oelsner G, Morad J, Mashiach S, Serr DM. Reproductive performance following conservative microsurgery. *Br J Obstet Gynaecol* 1987; **84**:1078–1083

Donnez J, Nisolle M. Laparoscopic treatment of ampullary tubal pregnancy. *J Gynecol Surg* 1989; **5**: 157-162

ADVANCED LAPAROSCOPIC SURGERY 14

Maurice A Bruhat and Arnaud Wattiez

INTRODUCTION

What is advanced laparosopic surgery? Most gynecologic operations can be performed using the laparoscope. These procedures include myomectomy, total and radical hysterectomy with lymph node dissection, and pelvic reconstructive surgery. The questions are not whether the operation can be performed laparoscopically but how the technique and instruments may be improved, whether the technique is as safe as the classic approach by laparotomy and to show that this new type of management improves patient care. The time for publishing case reports and techniques is over – the time for careful prospective studies is just beginning.

For many years it has been established that salpingostomy and salpingectomy by laparoscopy is as safe, efficient and cost-effective as by laparotomy. Laparoscopic surgery is now the 'gold standard' for the treatment of ectopic pregnancy. However, the relative indications for radical or conservative surgery for tubal pregnancy have not yet been established fully. The decision to conserve or remove the tube is made on the patient's past history and the gross appearance of the tube and not as a result of well documented prospective studies.

Although there have been many hundreds of laparoscopic hysterectomies performed throughout the world since 1989, there have been few prospective studies of the value of the technique in the peer–review literature. Laparoscopic hysterectomy is still to be confirmed to be the method of choice. Its place in surgical practice compared with vaginal hysterectomy or endometrial ablation has yet to be fully assessed by prospective randomized studies to ascertain the optimum management of dysfunctional uterine bleeding and other benign uterine diseases. Extensive laparoscopic procedures, which are technically possible, must be compared with the conventional operations, which take much less time in the operating room and give known results in terms of recovery and complications. Many of the newer laparoscopic procedures, which are difficult and time–consuming, and are performed with cumbersome instruments, cannot be compared with conventional surgery at the present time. Operating times and clinical results are likely to improve with increased experience and the development of better instruments.

Scientific data are needed to convince the traditionalists that laparoscopic surgery is the surgery of the future and not merely a technical gimmick. Such proof will not come from demonstrations by videos at scientific meetings, but as a result of prospective clinical trials with long-term follow-up.

CONTROVERSIES IN LAPAROSCOPIC SURGERY

Many laparoscopic techniques have evolved as a result of the development or modification of new instruments by surgeons with vision and skill. Too often, they have become accepted without well controlled studies to prove their efficacy. Controversies have arisen regarding their value and safety, and their influence on the standard of patient care.

ECTOPIC PREGNANCY: SALPINGOTOMY OR SALPINGECTOMY?

Several reports, from both the author's group in Clermont-Ferrand (France) and others, have established that fertility following conservative laparoscopic surgery for ectopic pregnancy compares favorably with conventional or microsurgical techniques. However, the author found that, in some groups of patients, conservative surgery was associated with an unacceptably high risk of subsequent infertility or recurrent tubal pregnancy. Fertility following laparoscopic treatment of ectopic pregnancy depends on the patient's previous medical history, the presence of adhesions involving the ipsilateral tube and the status of the contralateral tube. It is not influenced by age, parity, or the size or location of the pregnancy. On reviewing the results of a large number of cases, the author has devised a scoring system to assist in decision–making (14.1). Conservative surgery should be performed if the score is 0–3. When the score is 4, laparoscopic salpingectomy is the correct treatment.If the score is 5 or more, salpingectomy should be combined with contralateral tubal obstruction and the patient referred for *in vitro* fertilization (IVF). As most of the factors comprising the scoring system may be derived from the patient's history, the management can be discussed in detail preoperatively. The final decision on treatment will also depend on the availability and ease of referral to an IVF unit.

It should be emphasized that the size of the hematosalpinx, the volume of hemoperitoneum and the occurrence of tubal rupture have no influence on postoperative fertility. It is possible to treat conservatively large (over 6 cm) hematosalpinges in patients with a favorable previous medical history.

ADNEXAL CYSTS: IS LAPAROSCOPIC SURGERY EVER JUSTIFIED?

Laparosopic management of large adnexal cysts is still not accepted by many gynecologists. Review of the literature suggests that this simple and common operation is considered by many to be an advanced and hazardous procedure of questionable merit. The author's group is convinced that, when properly indicated and performed, laparoscopic management of adnexal cysts is a valuable and safe alternative to the conventional approach by laparotomy. However, strict guidelines must be observed, and the ability to convert immediately and effectively to open surgery for ovarian cancer is a prerequisite for the laparoscopic approach.

The risk of spilling cancer cells during laparoscopic puncture remains controversial even after 10 years of experience. Several recent reports from the UK and France suggest that the prognosis of Stage 1A epithelial ovarian cancer may be made worse by inadequate laparoscopic surgery. The risk of tumor cell dissemination appears to be more significant when laparoscopic surgery is per-

Therapeutic scoring system for ectopic pregnancy	
Prior history of one ectopic pregnancy	2
For each additional ectopic pregnancy	1
Prior history of laparoscopic adhesiolysis	1
Prior history of tubal microsurgery	2
Solitary tube	2
Prior history of salpingitis	1
Ipsilateral adhesions	1
Contralateral adhesions	1

14.1 Therapeutic scoring system for ectopic pregnancy.

formed several days or weeks after the original laparoscopic diagnosis is made. It is possible that this could be avoided by careful preoperative selection and efficient laparoscopic surgery.

Patients with adnexal masses that appear suspicious or frankly malignant should have laparotomy. However, malignant change may be found in non-echogenic tumors and in patients with normal CA125 levels. Similarly, malignancy may be found in dermoid and parovarian cysts and in endometriosis. There is therefore no perfect method of case selection. It is still necessary to demonstrate the safety of laparoscopic surgery for ovarian tumors.

The risk of intraoperative rupture or puncture of a stage 1 epithelial ovarian cancer, which is then removed immediately by laparotomy, is uncertain. Using multivariate analysis, two recent reports suggested that there was no significant increase in the risk of dissemination when there had been intraoperative rupture, or when there was macroscopic or microscopic invasion of the ovarian cortex. As yet, there are too few data available from patients in whom the diagnosis of ovarian carcinoma has been made laparoscopically to come to firm conclusions. Provided that the laparoscopic diagnosis is reliable and there is facility to proceed to immediate and effective laparotomy, laparoscopic management of an ovarian cyst is a valuable alternative to conventional laparotomy.

The author's practice of laparoscopic management of ovarian cysts was established over 10 years ago, and includes immediate laparotomy if evidence of malignancy is found. From the author's data, the laparoscopic diagnosis of malignancy appears reliable and safe. Laparoscopic diagnosis of benign tumor was always confirmed histologically, and the negative predictive value was 100%. The sensitivity of malignancy diagnosis was also 100%. They had 53.8% false positives, which reflects their cautious approach. The value of laparoscopic diagnosis might have been anticipated, because the technique of macroscopic evaluation by laparoscopy is similar to that used by the pathologists to select which part of the ovarian tumor to study histologically.

It is advised that, when posible, the ovarian cyst be dissected from the ovary without puncture to prevent intraperitoneal dissemination. The ovarian cortex should be incised with a unipolar microneedle, scissors or Nd:YAG laser. Once the plane of cleavage has been opened, blunt dissection of the cyst is performed using atraumatic forceps, 5 mm probes or hydrodissection. The cyst is then placed in a laparoscopic bag, punctured and emptied. (This technique of 'oophorectomy in a bag' is also useful for dermoid cysts to avoid chemical peritonitis.) However, because malignant tumors are invasive or adherent to the remaining ovarian tissue, cystectomy without previous ovarian puncture will usually be impossible. The dissemination produced by tumor rupture is probably more significant than if needle aspiration is performed. The choice of surgical technique should be determined by careful and complete laparoscopic examination including inspection of the cyst lining. Excision of ovarian cysts without puncture is frequently only possible by oophorectomy, which is the optimum management in postmenopausal women but would not be acceptable as a routine in young patients.

The laparoscopic treatment of early stages of ovarian carcinoma including lumbo-aortic lymph node sampling will soon be reported. However, large studies wil be required to establish the safety of this approach.

ADNEXAL CYSTS IN POSTMENOPAUSAL PATIENTS: HOW SHOULD THEY BE MANAGED?

The author has been using the laparoscope to manage selected ovarian cysts in postmenopausal women since the early days of the author's work in this field. The data suggest that patients who are over 50 years old or who are postmenopausal should have bilateral oophorectomy. Three of the patients who were over 50 years old developed recurrence of ovarian carcinoma following complete cystectomy carried out over 5 years previously. They had all been followed up clinically and by ultrasound. The author assumed that these malignant recurrences were different from the tumors excised at the first laparoscopy. Postmenopausal patients and those older than 50 years are now treated by bilateral oophorectomy because:

- The incidence of malignant recurrence was high among the few postmenopausal patients who were followed up for more than 5 years after conservative management of a serous cyst.
- Previous reports in the literature of malignancy in recurrent ovarian neoplasms following unilateral oophorectomy. In a series of 345 patients there were 24 recurrences, four of which were malignant. The patients were aged 46, 47, 56 and 68 years old at the time of oophorectomy.
- Ovarian carcinomas, especially serous carcinomas, are often bilateral.
- Ovarian dysplasia is often bilateral and occurs in a macroscopically normal ovary.
- Normal postmenopausal ovaries are small and can be removed with minimal operating time and postoperative morbidity.

The author does not remove the uterus in these patients because the prevalence of uterine carcinoma in screening programs in asymptomatic postmenopausal women is low. Hysterectomy would add to the operating time and postoperative morbidity. However, the uterus should be removed in patients at risk of endometrial and/or cervical cancer. The author has now created a new epidemiologic group – postmenopausal women with an intact uterus but loss of ovaries – for benign ovarian disease. Long-term follow-up is needed to ensure that this management is correct.

TECHNIQUES OF ADVANCED LAPAROSCOPIC SURGERY

GENERAL GUIDELINES

Extensive laparoscopic surgery is now possible as a result of the development of new instruments, but it takes longer to perform and is more difficult than simple laparoscopic procedures such as the treatment of ectopic pregnancy. Certain criteria must be fulfilled when performing advanced laparoscopic surgery.

- Surgery cannot be performed without a video camera, which makes operating more comfortable for the surgeon and allows better understanding and cooperation from all the operating - room staff, including the assistants, nurses and anesthetists. Two video cameras, monitors and light sources should be available so that the operation can be completed even if one breaks down.
- Several complete sets of instruments should be available. These should include three large bipolar forceps, several straight and curved laparoscopic scissors, a powerful lavage system and efficient needle holders.

- A laparoscopic retractor, an automatic insufflator capable of delivering CO_2 at 9 liters/minute, a shoulder brace for prolonged, steep Trendelenburg position, and an efficeint uterine cannula are all required.
- Trocar and cannula sites should be chosen carefully, taking into account the size of the uterus and the operation to be performed. The distance between the secondary cannulas should be great enough for instruments not to impede each other. They should be sited high enough in the abdomen to allow easy access to the pouch of Douglas. Most procedures can be performed through two 5 mm cannulas, inserted suprapubically laterally to the deep inferior epigastric vessels, and one 5, 10 or 12 mm cannula inserted medially.
- Knowledge of conventional surgery, laparoscopic surgery, electrosurgery, endoscopic suturing techniques and the use of all the instruments is mandatory.
- The patient should have had preoperative bowel preparation.

LAPAROSCOPIC HYSTERECTOMY

Laparoscopic hysterectomy was first performed by Harry Reich in January 1988 and reported by him in 1990. The authors have been performing this operation since 1989. Their current technique is as follows.

The patient should be under general anesthesia with endotracheal intubation and positive pressure respiration. A Foley catheter should be inserted into the bladder, a long curette or cannula is inserted into the uterus and two cervical tenaculums applied to the cervix. The uterine cannula is the only way by which the uterus can be manipulated and retracted when performing laparoscopic hysterectomy. It is used to push the uterus upwards and to twist it to allow better exposure of its pedicle. The cannula must be longer than those used in conventional laparoscopic surgery because, as the procedure progresses, the uterus becomes more and more mobile and a shorter cannula would not allow satisfactory exposure towards the end of the operation.

The pelvis should be inspected as at laparotomy. The sigmoid and/or abnormal bowel adhesions are divided to obtain perfect exposure of the pelvis. The bowel should be pushed above the pelvic brim and it is then possible to reduce the Trendelenberg tilt to 10° or less. This reduced Trendelenberg tilt may be important when treating older patients.

Several methods may be used to achieve hemostasis of the infundibulo-pelivc ligament. Whichever technique is used, it is important first to confirm the line of the ureter either by inspection or by dissection. The most common method used by our group is bipolar coagulation with or without previous skeletonization of the vessels. The instruments are inserted through the secondary cannulas as follows: (1) atraumatic forceps through the contralateral cannula. (2) Laparoscopic scissors through the ipsilateral cannula. (3) Bipolar forceps through the midline. Two or three applications of the coagulating forceps are necessary to produce complete haemostasis. Endoclips are not suitable for the control of haemostasis in these pedicles even after skeletonization. Endoloops or extracorporeal knots are a satisfactory alternative to bipolar electrocoagulation. The EndoGIA is effective but too expensive to use routinely. The remainder of the broad ligament and the round ligament may then be coagulated and divided.

When the adnexa are preserved, the tube and utero-ovarian ligament may be coagulated and divided without previous skeletonization. This is time consuming because of the large uterine veins which may be encountered. The EndoGIA therefore appears to be the best instrument to secure this pedicle. The multifire stapling device is introduced through a third 12mm cannula placed in the midline. The round ligaments should be divided and the bladder mobilized before application of the EndoGIA to prevent ureteric injury. Once again, the line of the ureters should be carefully ascertained especially in patients with endometriosis or pelvic adhesions.

Before commencing dissection of the bladder the uterus must be pushed backwards towards the sacral promontory. The peritoneum of the utero-vesical fold should be opened starting at the round ligaments as at laparotomy. The vesical peritoneum should then be lifted up using one or two grasping forceps placed laterally to the uterine pedicles. The vesico-uterine space is then developed using scissors and bipolar coagulation. Hydrodissection is not necessary in patients who have not had previous surgery. However it may be helpful to instill 100 ml of saline into the bladder to help define its margins.

The uterine vessels are then dissected lateral to the uterine isthmus. The uterus should be pushed towards the opposite pelvic sidewall and rotated and the adnexal pedicle grasped and traction applied with forceps introduced through the contralateral cannula. This allows the uterine vessels to be clearly identified. When feasible, the artery should be skeletonized and occluded with endoclips. Dissection of the uterine artery is easier when carried out 1–2 cm below the uterine isthmus but this puts the ureter at risk of thermal damage if electrocoagulation is required to control incidental bleeding. Hemostasis may be ensured with bipolar coagulation when skeletonization of the vessels is difficult. Hemostasis may also be achieved using endoscopic sutures. When suturing the uterine artery it should be ligated lateral to the isthmus using a straight needle and extracorporeal knots.

The hysterectomy is then completed using an intrafascial technique. A transverse incision 1-2mm deep should be made on the anterior and posterior surfaces of the uterine isthmus and the cervico-vaginal vessels coagulated and divided inside the fascial cuff. This should be performed systematically dealing with the left, anterior, right and posterior aspects of the cervix sequentially. This may be carried out using a monopolar current. In most cases the uterosacral vessels may be occluded with bipolar coagulation. The vagina should be disinfected again and a wet sponge placed in the anterior vaginal fornix. The vagina can now be opened using a unipolar knife and cutting current. The uterus is delivered through the vaginal vault which is sutured through the vaginal route. The operation is completed by copious peritoneal lavage, a careful check of haemostasis and inspection of both ureters for peristalsis. In our department all patients are given prophylactic antibiotics (Ampicillin with B Lacatamase Inhibitor, 3g/day).

Laparoscopic hysterectomy is especially valuable in patients with a normal or slightly enlerged uterus who would otherwise have abdominal hysterectomy because of adnexal disease or who require an associated procedure. A large fibroid uterus may also be removed laparoscopically depending on the location of the fibroid and the mobility of the uterus. Preoperative treatment with GnRH analogues may be used to reduce the size of the uterus and the uterine vessels. The limits and the indications for laparoscopic hysterectomy have yet to be defined.

Laparoscopic hysterectomy should only be performed by well trained laparoscopic teams. The development of new instruments will make it more acceptable but its value as compared to vaginal hysterectomy must be assessed by prospective studies. Several of the potential advantages of laparoscopic over abdominal hysterectomy such as reduced physical stress, shorter hospital stay and reduced cost apply equally to vaginal hysteretomy. The value of laparoscopy to assist vaginal hysterectomy is obvious. Associated procedures such as adhesiolysis, lymphadenectomy, bladder neck suspension or the treatment of ovarian cysts can be performed thus increasing the rate of vaginal hysterectomy and reducing the number of laparotomies.

The advent of laparoscopic or laparoscopically assisted vaginal hysterectomy has resulted in a resurgence of the performance of total hysterectomy. However, it must be remembered that the majority of hysterectomies can be avoided. The optimal surgical treatment of dysfunctional uterine bleeding is endometrial ablation. Hysteroscopic surgery also needs to be fully assessed as it is far less expensive than any laparoscopic or conventional surgical technique.

LYMPH NODE DISSECTION

Laparoscopic pelvic lymph node dissection was first described by Harry Reich but the largest series have been reported by Querleu et al and Schlussler and Vancaillie. The technique is especially valuable in men with bladder or prostatic cancer in whom staging is normally used. However, most gynecologic surgeons do not routinely evaluate the lymph nodes in cervical or endometrial cancer. The value of routine staging in these cases must be determined by prospective studies. Histologic assessment of pelvic lymph node involvement is more reliable than computed tomography or magnetic resonance imaging.

Laparoscopic lymphadenectomy may be of value in the following:
- To avoid surgical treatment for small Stage 1B carcinomas of the cervix which can be treated by brachytherapy when the pelvic lymph nodes are not involved.
- To decide the best preoperative radiotherapy protocol in patients with large cervical carcinomas of more than 3cm diameter.
- To decide the best protocol for patients who will be treated with radiotherapy only. In such patients evaluation of the para-aortic nodes could be valuable.
- As part of laparoscopic hysterectomy for Stage I endometrial carcinoma.

Bilateral lymphadenectomy is performed using scissors, atraumatic grasping forceps and bipolar electrocoagulation. The ipsilateral adnexa is grasped on its medial aspect with atraumatic forceps. A peritoneal incision parallel and medial to the external iliac vessels is made between the round and infundibulo-pelvic ligaments. The umbilical artery should then be first identified and fully dissected up to the internal iliac artery. Using the umbilical artery as the main landmark, the paravesical fossa will be easily identified and the ureter can be pushed medially away from the field of dissection. When the umbilical artery is fully dissected, the upper limit of the lymph node dissection is clearly identified ensuring that a complete clearance can be achieved. In some patients, the dissection of the upper internal iliac lymph nodes may be difficult when the axis of the external iliac vessels is almost parallel to the direction of the laparoscope. This problem may be solved by introducing the laparoscope through a suprapubic cannula.

The umbilical artery is identified more easily by laparoscopy than by laparotomy. At laparoscopy this vessel is often visible when the posterior aspect of the abdominal wall is inspected. It can be recognised on the pelvic sidewall when it grasped and moved in its course on the anterior abdominal wall. The umbilical artery should be grasped with atraumatic forceps and the paravesical space developed with scissor dissection. The external iliac lymph nodes

may now be removed from the bifurcation of the common iliac artery to the inferior epigastric artery. The nodal tissue is then detached from the posterior aspect of the external iliac vein, the obturator nerve and the pubic bone. Thereafter cephalad dissection of the lymph nodes is performed up to the junction of the external iliac vein and the obturator nerve. When extracting the lymph nodes from the abdomen care should be taken to avoid dissemination of malignant cells into the abdominal wall. Although uncommon, surgically induced abdominal wall metastases have been reported in studies of lymphadenectomy performed by retroperitoneoscopy. Two techniques may be employed to extract the lymph nodes. (1) The small lymph nodes can be removed using 10 mm disposable cannulas and 5 mm forceps. (2) Large lymph nodes should be removed using a laparoscopic bag. Finally, the pelvis should be irrigated copiously and the abdominal incision closed without drainage.

A similar technique may be used to perform dissection of the common iliac lymph nodes. From the authors preliminary experience and reports in the literature, they feel that para-aortic lymph node dissection will soon be accepted as a reasonable laparoscopic procedure.

Because of the magnification provided by the laparoscope and because the position of the internal iliac vessels is much better when observed through the umbilicus, laparoscopic lymphadenectomy appears to be a promising procedure. However, the disadvantages should be emphasized.
- At the present time there is no effective method of suturing vessels. Although it is uncommon, vascular laceration may occur during laparoscopic surgery. Conversion to laparotomy must be immediately available and the instruments ready in the operating room before surgery commences. Vascular injury should be less common during laparoscopic lymphadenectomy than at laparotomy because visualization is better.
- As at laparotomy, the dissection of clinically malignant lymph nodes is more difficult. In such cases one should remove enough tissue for histological confirmation. Hydrodissection may facilitate recognition of the correct plane of cleavage along the iliac vessels because the nodes are difficult to grasp with laparoscopic forceps. Despite these problems, every effort should be made to achieve complete removal of the nodes because simple biopsy or incomplete removal may increase the risk of dissemination.
- When performing this procedure as part of a pre-treatment staging, one should be aware that during radical hysterectomy, dissection of the uterine artery is more difficult after laparoscopic lymphadenectomy. Because postoperative fibrosis induced in the retroperitoneal space by laparoscopic surgery is similar to that induced by conventional procedures.

RADICAL HYSTERECTOMY

The authors first radical hysterectomy was performed in November 1989 and reported in 1991. Similar procedures have been reported by Nehzat in 1991. It is now apparent that almost any surgical procedure may be performed laparoscopically. However, the value of the procedure remains to be fully established.

Conventional surgery for stage 1 cervical and endometrial carcinoma results in 5 year survival rates of about 90%. Given such good results, one must therefore be cautious about advocating a new approach. Laparoscopic surgery for carcinoma should not be considered a viable alternative to conventional surgery until the results of long-term prospective studies become available.

When performing radical laparoscopic hysterectomy the uterine artery is dissected and ligated at its origin using endoclips or bipolar coagulation. The arteries are then retracted medially with forceps and the ureter dissected. The ureteric dissection is more easily performed when the rectovaginal space has been developed and the utero-sacral ligaments divided. Once the ureter, bladder and rectum have been fully mobilized, the vagina is opened and hemostasis of the paracervical ligaments obtained vaginally.

DEEP INFILTRATING ENDOMETRIOSIS

It is more common to find deep infiltrating endometriosis in patients complaining of chronic pelvic pain than infertility. The optimum treatment is complete excision of the lesion. Laparoscopy for deep endometriomas should be considered like an oncologic procedure in that all endometriotic tissue and fibrotic lesions must be excised. When deep infiltrating endomtriosis is suspected, bowel preparation should be routine the day before surgery.

These lesions are mainly retroperitoneal. The diagnosis is confirmed by vaginal and/or rectal examination during laparoscopy. It may also be necessary to use rectal or vaginal probes during the dissection to identify tissue planes. As with all surgical procedures, these probes should be moved slowly under continuous visual control to avoid bowel laceration.

The rectum should first be clearly identified. Similarly both ureters should be visualized whenever the uterosacral ligaments or the pelvic side wall are involved. The endometriotic tisue should then be dissected from the rectum and the uterosacral ligaments using scissors and bipolar coagulation. It is often necessary to completely excise lesions infiltrating the vagina. The operation may be completed either laparoscopically or vaginally depending on whether or not a satisfactory pneumoperitoneum can be maintained. Vaginal examinations and palpation should be carried out frequently to ensure that excision of all endometriotic tissue is complete. These operation can be prolonged and tedious. Nevertheless it is always necessary to ensure hemostasis since even minimal bleeding may completely obscure the operative field in the pelvis.

At the end of the procedure the pelvic cavity is irrigated using saline or Ringer lactate solution to decrease the risk of vaginal contamination and to detect bleeding. The ureters should be visualised and peristalsis observed. The uterus should be returned to its normal position and the pelvis again checked for bleeding which may have been hidden when it was elevated and anteverted. Prophyllactic antibiotics should be given and supressive medical therapy such as danazol, oral contraception in LH/RH analogues administered for 3–6 months to reduce the risk of recurrence.

BLADDER NECK SUSPENSION

Laparoscopic surgery offers a possible alternative to open surgery for bladder neck suspension. Attempts have been made to use fibrin glue similar to Stamey's technique, but a modified Burch operation appears to be more promising. The vaginal wall is fixed laterally to Cooper's ligament using non-absorbable sutures and extracorporeal knots. A retroperitoneal approach can be used similar to some of the approaches for lymph node dissection. The best technique still has to be decided but the following points are important: (1) This procedure should be performed using the clasical laparoscopic approach when combined with an intra-abdominal operation such as hysterectomy. (2) It can also be performed using a retroperitoneal approach which gives a better view than the similar procedure by laparotomy. (3) When the intraperitoneal technique is used, the peritoneum should be closed at the end of the operation. (4) The final position of the vagina may be more accurately ascertained by laparoscopy than by laparotomy because visualisation of the retropubic space is better by laparoscopy. (5) Finally, when using Roeder's knot one is able to vary the degree of elevation of the vagina while the knot is being tightened. At completion, the knot is locked by inserting an intracorporeal knot. Long-term follow-up is needed.

PELVIC RECONSTRUCTIVE SURGERY 15

Jeremy T Wright and Robert Hawthorn

INTRODUCTION

Advances in laparoscopic suturing and stapling techniques together with the ability to endoscopically visualize the cave of Retzius has led to the development of laparoscopic procedures to elevate the bladder neck and alleviate genuine stress incontinence (GSI).

The 'gold standard' operation for the management of GSI remains the Burch colposuspension, described in 1968, which has been adopted with modifications throughout the Western world. As such, studies of the effectiveness of laparoscopic surgery would have to be compated with those of the open Burch procedure. There are as yet no randomized controlled studies published although initial results of studies published by Liu and Nezhat are encouraging.

The investgation of a patient's suitability for surgery for GSIs essentially the same as that for the open procedure. Ideally patients should undergo urodynamic assessment although this is not always possible. In the USA this may also be prohibitively expensive. Various alternatives to urodynamic assessment have been proposed particularly for younger patients in whom stress incontinence is only provoked during exercise, these include weighed pad tests with provocation exercises and fluid charts. A particularly cheap and simple test is described in the US literature in which patients are treated with pyridian, which stains the urine, and are then sent away with a pad to perform the exercises that provoke stress incontinence, staining of the pad confirming the diagnosis. A useful test to confirm descent of the bladder base is the 'Q tip' test in which a sterile cotton wool tipped swab on a small stick literally or a 'buddy' is placed in the distal urethra while the patient is in the dorsal postion with her legs abducted. She is then asked to cough and significant descent of the bladder base will be seen as extensive movement of the arm of the Q tip. This is an easy test performed in the office both before and after surgery to assess support of the bladder neck.

PATIENT PREPARATION

Laparoscopic surgery is associated with a considerably shorter in-patient stay than open surgery and thus patient preparation and counselling about postoperative care is particularly important and should always be backed up by written literature to which they can refer. The surgeon needs assure himself the patient will have adequate backup at home with easy access to advice and help from the unit carrying out the surgery, rather than via a general practitioner, or primary care physician as this advice is more likely to be informed and helpful. Most patients will only be in hospital for 36–48 hours and in the USA it is frequently performed in a 24-hour-stay unit. Patients should also be made aware that the rapid recovery towards normal activities would be exepcted and encouraged. There is little point in undertaking laparoscopic Burch colposuspension for a patient who is not well motivated and keen to make the most of a rapid recovery. Patients may require to be discharged with either a suprapubic or urethral catheter in place so adequate counselling is necessary to ensure that they will not be too distressed if this happens and that they would be able to care for it adequately. There thus needs to be a strict polivy of catheter management to be agreed by all those concerned such as the nursing and medical staff both in the community and the hospital.

Transient detrusor instablility occurs following laparoscopic bladder neck suspension with approximately similar frequency to that following the open procedure, but responds well to bladder retraining and if necessary treatment with oxybutinin particularly if the history suggests a mixed picture of stress and urge incontinence.

EQUIPMENT

As with every other form of advanced laparoscopic surgery it is essential to have the proper equipment available and clear vision is necessary particularly when undertaking suturing techniques. In addition to the usual laparoscopic instruments suture carriers, knot pushers and Roeder knots will be necessary depending on the surgeon's preference. Pleglets should only ever be introduced attached to a length of thread that is left outside the abdominal cavity so that retrieval is easy. Although the authors are able to routinely perform these procedures in under an hour, early attempts may be time consuming and frustrating so a realistic time schedule should be allowed. As the surgeon becomes more adept at the procedure, coversion to open surgery becomes much less likely, but both the patient and the theatre should be prepared for an open operation should this be necessary. Both authors cover their procedures with prophylactic antibiotics, but this is a matter for individual decision.

APPROACH TO THE CAVE OF RETZIUS

The cave of Retzius can be approached either by using an intraperitoneal or extraperitoneal approach, the extraperitoneal approach most closely mimicking that of the classical Burch colposuspension procedure. The advantages of the extraperitoneal approach are as follows:-

- There is less risk of perforation of the dome of the bladder, the most common site of bladder injury during this procedure.
- Less risk of injury to large vessels especially the inferior epigastric vessels.
- Less risk of bowel herniation.
- Less risk of damage to other intraperitoneal viscera.

The extraperitoneal approach is particularly useful when there has been previous pelvic or abdominal surgery with the liklihood of intraperitoneal adhesions and colposuspension has been successfully performed by the authors using the extraperitoneal route in patients who have undergone laparotomies for Crohn's disease and bowel obstruction in the past.

The intraperitoneal approach is advantageous in two circumstances:

- When other laparoscopic abdominal surgery is being carried out such as laparoscopic hysterectomy or oophorectomy.
- So that surgery to minimise the risk of enterocele can be carried out simultaneously.

Procedures that have been described to reduce enterocele consist of uterosacral ligament plication, McCaldoplasty or Moschcowitz's procedure as well as other cul-de-sac obliterative operations all of which may be accomplished laparoscopically. Surgeons undertaking laparoscopic surgery for GIS should become adept at both the extra- and intraperitoneal approach. As with the open procedure many patients will require hysterectomy at the same time for menstrual problems. As these patients will usually have good vaginal access they are ideally suited for laparoscopically assisted vaginal hysterectomy, which can then be combined with bladder neck suspension procedure. Once the cave of Retzius has been opened and adequately deflected the procedures for elevating the bladder neck are essentially the same and it is thus appropriate to describe the method for entering the cave of Retzius using either the extraperitoneal or transperitoneal approach before describing the various procedures that are available to elevate the bladder neck.

EXTRAPERITONEAL APPROACH

The difficulty with the extraperitoneal approach to colposuspension is finding the space in a logical, consistent and safe manner. The patient's legs should be placed in Lloyd Davis stirrups and a generous Trendelenburg lift after the bladder has been emptied. A Foley catheter should be left in the bladder with the balloon distended to allow easy identification of the bladder neck. Dilute methylene blue (60 ml) can be instilled and the catheter spiggotted, as is the preference of JT Wright. However, R Hawthorn attaches the catheter to a 500 ml bag of saline with methylene blue. This can be raised or lowered to empty or distend the bladder. Both these techniques allow rapid diagnosis of bladder perforation should this occur. Various techniques have been described to facilitate entry of the cave of Retzius, but in our experience the simplest and most direct methods have proved the easiest.

The pubic symphysis should be palpated and a Veress needle inserted one finger breadth above at an angle towards the middle of the back of the symphysis pubis. The tactile sensation is similar to placing the Veress needle intraperitoneally and often a pop is also heard as the needle passes through the rectus sheath in the tendinone part of the rectus muscles. The Veress needle is now in the cave of Retzius which is a low pressure space similar to the peritoneal cavity. The space is insufflated at 1–2 liters/minute with a preset pressure of 12–5 mmHg. The slow rate of 1–2 liters/minute is usually all that is necessary. If the catheter is draining freely and the bladder is perforated the bag of saline will distend. An intraumbilical incision is made in the usual fashion, the trochar advanced subcutaneously for 1–2 cm and placed through the rectus muscle into the cave of Retzius. Most gynecologists have found themselves on occasion in the cave of Retzius at some time inadvertently doing routine laparoscopic surgery. The appearance of the spiders web of filmy adhesions are instantly recogniseable. An optical trochar (Visiport, Auto Suture) instead of a reuseable trochar allows the operator some visual control over the placement of the primary trochar. After an abdominal incision is made, the laparoscope is placed in the optical trocar and the near focus checked. The blunt trochar is then tunnelled subcutaneously above the rectus sheath from the umbilical insertion to half way between the umbilicus and the pubic symphysis in the midline. The trigger handel of the Visiport activates a small blade and with the trochar now directed through the rectus sheath is cut in small portions by the blade. Continued pressure is applied to the trochar and with repeated cuts the trochar advances through the sheath and muscle and into the cave of Retzius. This process is easily followed as the sheath appears very white and the muscle between it looks red. As soon as the muscle has been traversed the trochar is in the cave of Retzius. The trochar and laparoscope are now removed leaving only the 10 mm cannula *in situ*. The laparoscope is now reinserted.

DISSECTION OF THE CAVE OF RETZIUS

Ths initial dissection is performed by the CO_2. The tip of the laparoscope can also be used to perform some dissection which is advanced onto the symphysis pubis and gently moved from side to side. The laparoscope may be palpated through the abdominal wall to confirm its position on the symphysis pubis. A good landmark is the Veress needle if this is left in place and will clearly identify the cave.

A balloon dissector (General Surgical Innovations Inc., Portola Valley, California, USA) has also been developed. This consists of a cannula, a guide rod and a balloon system. The dissector inserted through a 1 cm infraumbilical incision. This is advanced between the rectus muscle and the anterior surface of the posterior rectus sheath to the symphysis pubis. The dissectors external sheath is removed and the balloon is inflated with approximately 950 ml saline solution. During inflation the balloon unrolls sidways and exerts a perpendicular force to separate tissue layers. Blunt dissection of the connective tissue occurs as the balloon expands taking about a minute. When maximum volume is reached the balloon is deflated and removed through the incision. The resected space is insufflated with CO_2 at a pressure of 8 to 10 mmHg. The predefined shape of the balloon and the non-elastometric material together with an incompressable character of the saline ensure a large relatively bloodless working space of predictable size and shape. The spare is adequate for identifying the appropriate landmarks and to allow manipulation of the surgical instruments.

INTRAPERITONEAL APPROACH

Laparoscopy is performed in the normal way and then two lateral cannulas are placed so as to avoid the epigastric vessels and above the anterior/superior iliac spine. Placing of the lateral cannulas too low will make dissection of the anterior wall and peritoneum difficult and subsequent suture placement will be complicated by the dissection flap of the peritoneum impinging on the edge of the trochar and the cannula possibly snagging the sutures as they are placed. For extracorporeal suturing soft plastic valves are essential. Trumpet valves will snag the sutures and reducing sleeves will allow too much escape of gas. The cave of Retzius may be approached either using laser energy or laparoscopic scissors. An assistant is asked to identify the area 3 cm above the symphysis pubis in the midline (2 finger breadths) by downward palpation. The peritoneum at this level is grasped and pulled down through one of the lateral cannulae. A transverse incision is made at this point extended to between the two umbilical ligaments above the anatomical landmarks of the round ligament from the internal ring to avoid bladder entry. Blunt dissection and hydrodissection together with a sharp dissection are used to expose the retropubic space. It is important to stay close to the back of the pubic bone dropping the anterior wall and urethra downwards. Dissection is limited over the urethra in the midline to approximately 2 cm lateral to the urethra to protect its delicate musculature. This connective tissue is cleared until there is a good view of the cave of Retzius.

DISSECTION OF THE CAVE OF RETZIUS

Having entered the cave of Retzius by either route further dissection is necessary before suturing can begin. The iliopectineal (Cooper's) ligament on both sides can be easily identified as strong white structures on either side of the pelvis. Loose fatty tissue needs to be cleared off the ligament and bipolar diathermy may be necessary to control any venous ooze particularly from vessels lying below the ligament. As with the open procedure the bladder has to be dissected medially off the vagina. This can be greatly helped by a finger placed either side of the balloon or the urethral catheter in the bladder either by the operator of an assistant. As with the open procedure dissection is achieved by the use of gauze swabs and counter traction on the vagina until the glistening white of the vaginal fascia is seen. Instead of gauze swabs the tip of the sucker can be used or blunt nosed grasping forceps. However, metal instruments are more likely to cause damage to the edge of the bladder and bleeding or possible perforation than gauze, although better dissection and traction can be obtained. Both sides can be prepared for suture or each side can be prepared and sutured individually depending on the surgeons preference. Preparing both sides before suturing can lead to some bleeding that will not be arrested until the sutures are tied which may impede vision and thus the operation. On the whole however bleeding is considerably less at laparoscopic surgery as it is as open surgery and haemorrhage is rare. For the extraperitoneal approach three further ports will have to be placed under direct vision. A 5 mm trochar can be inserted in the midline replacing the Veress needle. This marks the position of the midline and allows scissors or grasping forceps to be inserted and dissection of the loose tissue in the cave of Retzius to be completed. Lateral trochars are inserted about 6 mm in the midline at the same level as the lower midline trochar. These should be 12 mm trochars (Premium Surgiport, Auto Suture) with the attached reducing device. Other operators may prefer to perform the dissection with scissors and in these circumstances 5 mm ports may suffice assuming straight needles are used for suturing. If the patient had undergone laparoscopic hysterectomy the ports used for this procedure can be facilitated to allow suturing in the cave of Retzius.

SUTURING THE VAGINA TO THE ILIOPECTINEAL LIGAMENTS

Various suturing techniques have been employed to suture the vagina to the iliopectineal ligament. There is a choice of suture material. The number of sutures on each and the needle holder is operator dependant as is the tension in the suture and the closeness of apposition of the vagina to the iliopectineal ligament that the operator wishes to achieve. However, it is the authors' view that they should most closely mimic what they set out to achieve at the open operation.

R Hawthorn uses a straight needle on Ethibond and a simple needle holder inserting two sutures on each side. The needle is grasped and passed through the ipsilateral port and is dropped and regrasped before being passed through the vagina. The needle is then grasped again at an angle and pulled through the medial aspect of the ilio-pectineal ligament. The suture is then withdrawn through the ipsilateral port and knotted extraperitoneal using a modified Roeder knot. This is then pushed down with the vagina elevated and the suture then cut. A second suture is then passed through the elevated 'dog-ear' of the vagina before being tied and cut. The suture is then repeated on the other side commencing with the exposure of the iliopectineal ligament. JT Wright prefers using the O-ethibond or Goretex and a curved needle. The abdominal cannula is removed and the suture backloaded in the cannula. The thread is then grasped via the needle holder about 2 cm from the needle and passed through the abdominal cavity followed by the trochar. The needle is then grasped by grasping forceps placed through the cannula on the other side and repositioned on the needle holder. The needle is then passed through the vaginal wall either as a single or a figure of eight stitch in which case it is important to ensure the position of the thread is pulled through to allow this to be withdrawn through the cannula again to facilitate extra-

corporeal knotting. The needle is then passed through the iliopectineal ligament and secured on the peritoneal edge so it does not get lost. The thread can then be cut about 2 cm from the needle and withdrawn through the cannula. Knotting is achieved using series of half hitch knots which are then accurately placed using a Clark–Reich knot pusher. The stitch is then cut and the needle retrieved by delivering it from the abdominal cavity by pulling it out having removed the trochar. As many stitches as are required can be placed either side and the operation is then complete. The modification of this technique has been described by Carter, in which a Nottingham needle is passed through a small stab wound suprapubically. This is then passed through the Cooper's ligament allowing a substantial bite to be taken atraumatically. The thread is then passed through a hole in the tip of the needle. The needle is then withdrawn through Cooper's ligament and the thread retrieved and passed through the cannula to facilitate extra corporeal knotting. With either technique extra corporeal knotting is preferred to intra corporeal knotting as it is much easier to assess the tension. The suture that is used is very much due to the preference of the various surgeons. A mono filament suture is best used as a significant number of sutures will penetrate the entire vaginal mucosa. This presents no problem as long as a mono filament suture is used as the vaginal mucosa will usually re-epithelialize within 10 days.

Various other techniques have been described for elevating the bladder neck at laparoscopic surgery and will be reviewed briefly.

PROLENE MESH

Effective elevation can be achieved by passing a 1 cm x 3 cm strip or Prolene mesh into the cave of Retzius. This can be laid across the vagina at the level of the urethra and stapled into place using 2 mm Endo hernia staples. The vagina is then elevated to the desired level and the mesh placed across the Cooper's ligament where it is stapled into place. The procedure is quick and easy, but the use of Prolene mesh and clips more expensive. However, there is no need to learn stapling techniques if a stapling technique is to be used. Another approach has been to pass the needle laparoscopically through the vagina where it is grasped by the vaginal surgeon and returned into the cave of Retzius thereby ensuring a good bite of vaginal tissue. There have however been complications particularly with granulation tissue and infection and a very high rate of detrusor instablity.

RESULTS

There are as yet no published formal double-blind control studies on the outcome of laparoscopic Burch colposuspension and a test of cure has ideally to be at five years although if the operation has not failed at 18 months the prognosis is good. Initial results published by Nezhat and Liu show that there is an over 90% improvement and similar results have been reported by various other authors all of whom have considerable enthusiasm for this technique. It should be remembered, however, that the second-line treatment for stress incontinence is technically difficult as there is considerable scarring of the cave of Retzius whether the procedure is performed by open surgery or laparoscopic surgery.

LAPAROSCOPIC HYSTERECTOMY 16

Jeffrey H Phipps

INTRODUCTION

No other operation in minimal access surgery (MAS) in gynecology has generated the same degree of controversy and debate as the laparoscopic approach to hysterectomy. 'Is laparoscopic hysterectomy a waste of time?' was the academic gauntlet cast down in an article which occupied several pages of 'The Lancet' recently. Yet the advantages of avoiding laparotomy seem irrefutable. The problem which causes so much argument surrounding laparoscopic hysterectomy is that a substantial proportion of hysterectomies can be accomplished using simple vaginal surgery. Vaginal hysterectomy is safer compared with the abdominal approach, and has considerable advantages for the patient. The absence of an abdominal wound and the reduced pain, hospital stay and convalescence, together with a lower reported incidence of accidental injury to the urinary tract, especially the ureter, has made vaginal hysterectomy the first choice for many gynecologists when removal of the uterus is indicated.

Why is it then, that the ratio of abdominal hysterectomies performed in the UK outnumber those accomplished by the vaginal route by a factor of four? Over 80% of hysterectomies both in the UK and the USA are performed abdominally, although it may not be so in Europe. Vaginal surgeons will answer: 'what is required is better training in vaginal surgery, not the substitution of a safe and inexpensive technique by a high-tech' gimmick for lack of adequate training'. Indeed, it is their contention that laparoscopic hysterectomy has served but one useful purpose – to raise awareness of the paucity of good vaginal surgery.

Such a simplistic view is not supported by critical analysis of studies 'comparing' vaginal to laparoscopic hysterectomy.

Those in favor of the laparoscopic approach to hysterectomy would not subscribe to an extreme view which suggests that this group of techniques should be performed almost exclusively, and certainly few would argue the laparoscopic choice should be first in all cases. Laparoscopic hysterectomy should form only one technique of several from which a surgeon will select the most appropriate for each individual case. 'Why not simply make ourselves more versatile vaginal surgeons?' Professor Sheth of Bombay, for example, is able to remove the uterus and ovaries per vaginum with ease. Individual variation means some surgeons are more skilled in particular aspects of surgery when compared to others. It is this

fact that makes the argument 'is laparoscopic hysterectomy a waste of time?', meaningless. The correct response to this question is 'it depends upon whom it is carried out, and by whom'.

Reference has been made to comparisons between laparoscopic and vaginal hysterectomy. Provided patients are selected appropriately, there should be no need to compare the two operations. They are different procedures with different indications. There is no doubt that those who merely staple the upper pedicles in what should have been a straightforward vaginal operation in an effort to append the word 'laparoscopic' to 'vaginal hysterectomy' have imposed a serious disservice on the whole concept. One surgeon's series may show vaginal hysterectomy is quicker, safer and cheaper than his laparoscopic operations, but this merely means that the surgeon is either not comparing like with like, or he/she is good at vaginal surgery and not so good with the laparoscope.

The central feature of the use of the laparoscope in removing the uterus is it should enable open abdominal hysterectomy to be avoided. At the present time, there is no evidence to substantiate the contention that laparoscopic hysterectomy carries any advantage at all over unassisted vaginal surgery.

In women undergoing laparoscopic total hysterectomy where no descent is coupled with narrow vaginal access, the utero-sacral/transverse cervical ligaments can be divided laparoscopically, although in the author's experience this is nearly always unnecessary.

The possibility of facilitating vaginal hysterectomy by laparoscopic resection of the adnexa and parametrial structures has generated considerable interest over the last few years. Since the early demonstration of the feasibility of laparoscopically assisted vaginal hysterectomy (LAVH), the laparoscopic approach has gained an increasingly wide acceptance throughout Europe and North America.

The majority of gynecologists will select abdominal hysterectomy when:
- the uterus is over 12 weeks' gestational size
- there is a combination of poor vaginal access (due to narrow pubic arch) and zero uterine descent
- there is a co-indication for oophorectomy
- there are known or suspected adhesions in the pelvis (**16.1, 16.2**)
- there exists a combination of these factors

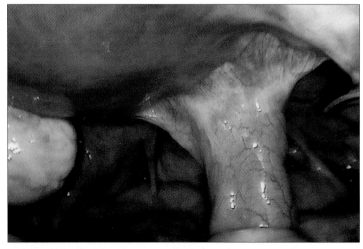

16.1 Dense adhesion of small bowel to the right posterior surface of the uterus due to a uterine perforation two years previously. Vaginal hysterectomy may have caused bowel injury.

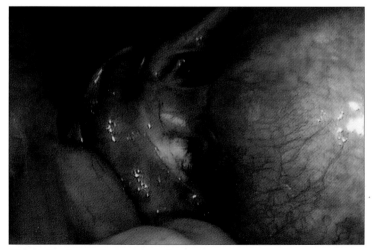

16.2 Adhesions of uterus to adnexa.

NOMENCLATURE

Some confusion exists concerning terminology, and the following is included here to clarify nomenclature.

'Laparoscopic hysterectomy' and 'laparoscopically assisted vaginal hysterectomy' (LAVH) tend to be used interchangeably, but this should not be the case, since they refer to different operations. A pre-operative check of the pelvis (to exclude and, if necessary, divide adhesions) followed by a vaginal hysterectomy when the pelvis is 'clean' is the simplest way in which the laparoscope is able to aid vaginal surgery. There are cases when a laparoscopic examination of the pelvis may help to avoid serious injury to bowel where adhesions are dense (**16.1**). The next 'level' is that of LAVH. In this operation, the upper pedicles are dissected free, but the laparoscopic approach ceases above the level of the uterine arteries. The rest of the dissection is completed vaginally. However, when the uterus is large (>16 weeks gestational size) and when descent is poor, it may sometimes be difficult to safely secure the uterine arteries from below without risking loss of hemostasis, and under these circumstances it is preferable to divide and secure the uterine arteries from above. This requires more dissection through the laparoscope, especially in respect of the urinary tract, and special precautions must be taken to protect the ureters (see below). Such an operation is referred to as a laparoscopic hysterectomy. The lower part of the utero-sacral/transverse cervical ligaments are dissected vaginally.

Laparoscopic total hysterectomy is a term which has been used to describe an operation where the laparoscopic dissection is continued to free the uterus/adnexa, including dividing the utero-sacral ligaments and the vagina. Such an operation is useful where vaginal access is difficult or impossible.

A major concern about these new operations is the length of time needed to complete surgery, and one hears of laparoscopic hysterectomy and bilateral salpingoophorectomy requiring two, three or more hours to complete. However, with practice, the operation can usually be completed in around one hour or less in uncomplicated cases, provided the precepts of Doyen are adhered to. The minimum number of instruments consistent with safe and efficient surgery should be employed. There is never any need, for example to coagulate with one modality (e.g. YAG laser), and cut with another (e.g. CO_2 laser or harmonic scalpel). Straightforward application of endoscopic staples, sutures or bipolar diathermy coagulation and combined cutting/coagulating diathermy-armed instruments are all that is required. Bipolar diathermy and sutures are cheaper, but may prolong operation time and in the case of 'diathermy-only' operations the possibility of lateral thermal conduction and excessive tissue necrosis must be considered. Also of relevance to operation time is the safety of the ureters. Regrettably one of the common complications of laparoscopic hysterectomy is ureteric injury. Laparoscopic identification of the ureters by dissection and isolation is time consuming. In those cases where ureteric anatomy is distorted, placing transilluminating ureteric stents for identification is safe, effective and can be quickly performed. We routinely stent the ureters in all cases of hysterectomy.

Hysterectomy techniques where the cervix is conserved in constitute less of a risk to the ureter, since the dissection does not proceed lower than the cervico-isthmic junction. The anatomical course of the ureter is variable, however, and great care must be taken not to damage it when securing hemostasis, particularly with diathermy.

The alternative method of ensuring ureteric security is to dissect out the structure, either laparoscopically (as in the original classic technique described by Reich), or in the case of laparoscopically assisted Doderlein's type procedure described by Garry by doing so transvaginally, as it passes below the uterine artery.

What follows is a personal view of the subject of laparoscopic hysterectomy. The first technique described ('staples and stents') has been developed in our unit over four years, in over 500 cases. Our complication rate (i.e. significant, when blood transfusion and/or return to theatre is required) is less than 1% (4/445 cases). Three techniques are described here, and comprise the basic approaches currently in use. I have not included the original description of the technique by Harry Reich, but there is little doubt that in large part we owe the concept of avoiding laparotomy for the purpose of hysterectomy to Reich.

TRAINING AND PATIENT SELECTION

It is of paramount importance that every step possible should be taken to minimize complications. Adequate training of gynecologists (as in other surgical specialties) in the skills necessary for safe practice in endoscopy is absolutely essential. Training in endoscopic surgery is the subject of other chapters.

The other pre-requisite to successful endoscopic surgery is patient selection. Patients must be offered operations which are both appropriate to the disease entity and to the ability of the surgeon at that particular stage of his training. Attempting a laparoscopic hysterectomy in the presence of severe endometriosis, or where the uterus is over 12 weeks' gestation size until the learning curve has been completed is poor practice with high risk. Laparoscopic hysterectomy is probably not appropriate for the treatment of malignant disease with the exception of stage I endometrial carcinoma, although this subject is the subject of current discussion. The indications for a laparoscopic approach to hysterectomy include:

- A valid indication for removing the uterus and/or ovaries
- When simple vaginal hysterectomy is likely to prove difficult, dangerous or impossible
- A uterine size which is (until experience has been gained) 12 weeks gestation or less (the author's upper limit is approximately 18 weeks gestation size)

Contraindications are relative to the practice and experience of the surgeon, but broadly speaking include:

- Malignancy (other than stage I endometrial carcinoma)
- Uterine size greater than (or about) 18 weeks gestation
- The presence of severe adhesive disease involving bowel or urinary tract (unless the surgeon is expert and is absolutely satisfied at the end of the operation that the bowel is intact)

In the case of the latter, it may be noted that in cases where large bowel is involved in adhesions below the level of the proximal sigmoid colon, it may be gently transilluminated with any illuminated 'scope, guided by the exploring finger transrectally, if integrity is in question. This manoeuvre is only for the experienced, however, since the bowel may easily be perforated if explored in this way. Examining the bowel after dissection of adhesions by looking for bubbles of escaping bowel gas 'underwater' in the abdomen or pelvis is a test of bowel integrity which is unreliable. First, sections of small bowel in particular may be empty of gas, hence a defect in the bowel integrity will be missed. Second, severe abrasions to the serosa and muscularis of the bowel, which require oversewing, will likewise be missed if the mucosa itself has not been penetrated. If there exists the slightest doubt, a laparotomy should be performed immediately and the bowel examined 'inch by inch'.

TECHNIQUES OF LAPAROSCOPIC HYSTERECTOMY AND LAVH

'STAPLES AND STENTS' TECHNIQUE

The standard technique we use is as follows.

A 10 mm trochar and cannula (metal) is inserted beneath the umbilicus to allow passage of the 10 mm laparoscope.

The abdomen is filled with CO_2 using a high flow insufflator unit. Two 12 mm trochar and cannulae are passed into the abdominal cavity under direct vision, lateral to the rectus sheaths (**16.3**). The inferior epigastric vessels are avoided by by direct laparoscopic inspection of the interior abdominal wall. The large vessels of the abdominal wall are almost always visible, and lie just lateral to the peritoneal folds of the obliterated umbilical vessels. **16.4** shows the left inferior epigastric vessels. It is vital that transillumination of the abdominal wall is not relied upon to avoid damage to the inferior epigastic vessels. It is absolutely vital that the lateral trochar/cannulae are introduced under direct vision, even if they are self-guarding, since the sharp point remains exposed inside the abdomen for a significant time interval before the shield locks down to cover the tip (**16.5**). An assistant cannulates the cervix using either a Hegar dilator and Vulsellum or one of the commercially available purpose built instruments.

If the uterus is enlarged with fibroids (**16.6**), a fourth entry point in the midline, about 4 cm below the laparoscope may be made (5 mm) for the introduction of a laparoscopic myomectomy screw (**16.7**). An instrument with a universally-jointed operating screw greatly facillitates manipulation of the uterus (**16.8**, Rocket of London, Watford, UK).

The uterus is then deviated by the assistant to one side. The ovarian ligament on the contralateral side is grasped using laparoscopic forceps via the lower cannula, and the ovary and tube placed 'on stretch' to expose the infundibulopelvic ligament. A staple gun (e.g. Endo GIA 30, Auto Suture Company, Conn. USA) is fitted with the 1.0 mm closure height staple cartridge (white coded), and the infundibulopelvic ligament clamped up to, and preferably over, the round ligament. If the gun jaws fail to close with only moderate pressure on the closure handle, the volume of tissue trapped is excessive, and the gun must be removed from the abdomen, and fitted with a blue coded cartridge (1.5 mm closure height). The use of the tissue thickness gauge, or similar devices is not recommended.

At this stage it is important to thoroughly examine the tissues clamped (**16.9**). The distal tip of the staple gun must be in the 'clear'

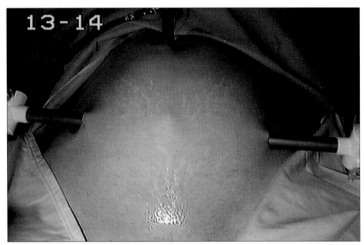

16.3 Laparoscopic port cannulae in situ. Note metal cannula for the laparoscope, and absence of plastic skin grips from the lower (metal) cannulae. Bowel burns due to capacitative coupling or accidental shorting of diathermy to the laparoscope cannot occur.

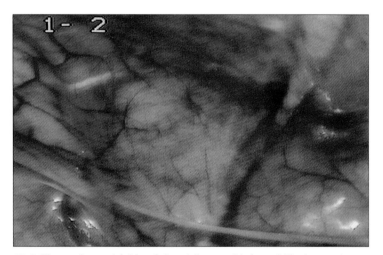

16.4 The peritoneal folds of the obliterated left umbilical vessels, and (lateral), the inferior epigastric vessels.

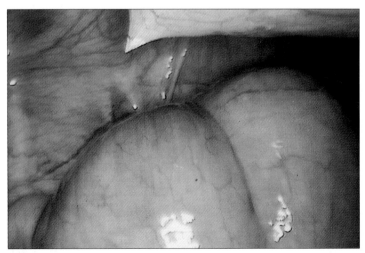

16.5 Exposed end of the self-shielding trochar/cannula inside the abdomen and close to bowel. Insertion under direct vision is essential.

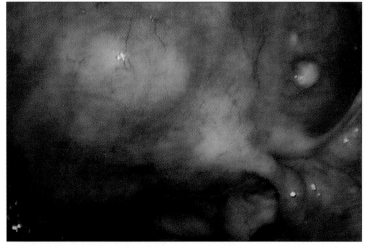

16.6 Fibroid uterus demonstrating difficult laparoscopic access to right adnexal dissection site.

area of the broad ligament to avoid partial transection of blood vessels and bleeding. Care must be taken to avoid the bladder edge and 'tenting' of the pelvic side wall peritoneum to exclude damage to the bladder or ureter. There is rarely need to dissect the round and infundibulopelvic ligaments separately. If, however, the round ligament is excluded from this first stapling, it may be included in the diathermy/scissors dissection for the bladder. Ensuring that the tip of the staple gun does not extend below the 'bare area' of the broad ligament, and that the jaws of the instrument are closed immediately lateral to the ovary (i.e. as far from the pelvic side-wall as possible) ensures the ureter is clear of the operative site. We routinely insert transilluminating ureteric stents ('Uriglow', Rocket of London Ltd, UK;) cystoscopically, at the beginning of the operation which means that the ureter is easily identified as a row of glowing points (**16.10, 16.11**). A 25–30 degree operating cystoscope with an operating channel at least 2 mm in diameter, without manipulation bridge, should be used. The stents should be handled with care to avoid kinking and damage to the fibre optic strands which may cause 'spillage' of light from cracks and thus a loss in light intensity inside the ureter. The stents should be lubricated with sterile water-soluble jelly to facilitate easy insertion and minimise trauma to the ureters. They are graduated with blue lines

at 10 mm intervals so that depth of insertion may be judged. There is also a red marker which should lie at or close to the urethral meatus. 'Fine tuning' of the stent position may be accomplished under laparoscopic control. Occasionally, hematuria may be noted for a few hours postoperatively. The light points running parallel to the utero sacral ligaments must be fully mobile when the staple gun is fully closed over the uterine artery. It is this mobility of the lights which guarantees ureteric freedom from injury.

The broad ligament is opened using monopolar diathermy-armed scissors, and the bladder freed from the anterior surface of the uterus. The dissection is contunued as far as the uterine artery, taking care not to damage the vessels (**16.12**).

When the surgeon is satisfied the gun is placed correctly, it may then be fired. The bladder is next freed and displaced inferiorly and laterally, and the gun placed over the uterine arteries (**16.13**).

The jaws of the staple gun should remain in the clamped position on the uterine arteries for one minute prior to firing to allow the entrapped tissues to be compressed. This ensures good staple fixation and therefore hemostasis. Adequate tissue compression may be judged when the tissues either side of the jaws of the staple gun appear white. Premature firing of the gun may lead to loss of hemostasis. The process is repeated on the opposite side.

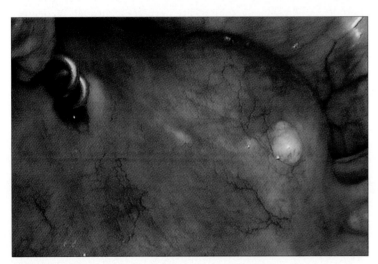

16.7 The laparoscopic myomectomy screw used to gain access to the parametrium in the presence of large fibroids.

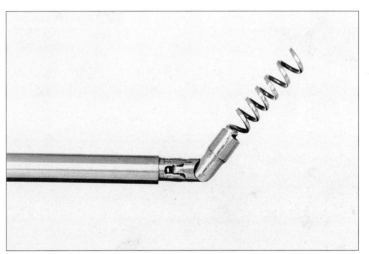

16.8 Detail of operating end of lockable universally jointed laparoscopic myomectomy screw (Rocket of London, Watford, UK).

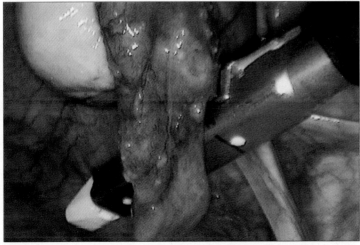

16.9 EndoGIA staple gun applied to right infundibulopelvic ligament.

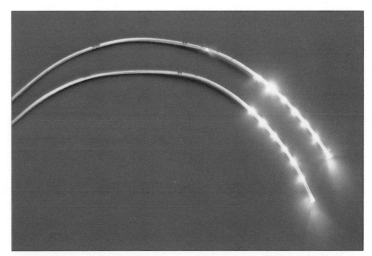

16.10 'Uriglow' cold transilluminating ureteric stents (Rocket of London Ltd, Watford, UK).

The bladder is then freed from the anterior wall of the uterus using non-self locking forceps and scissors, uniting the inferior ends of the incisions achieved with the staple gun. Bladder dissection then continues until the vaginal wall is seen, which may be confirmed by the assistant with a finger in the anterior fornix – the vagina, stripped free from bladder, is easily identified by the surgeon. It is important not to incise the vaginal wall at this stage because of loss of pneumoperitoneum.

The laparoscopic dissection is now complete. Although it is possible to divide the uterosacral ligaments and the vagina from the cervix via the laparoscope, this is more easily achieved vaginally. Moreover, completing the operation vaginally obviates the need to use further endoscopic staples or suturing techniques, reducing operative time and cost.

The laparoscopic ports should be left *in situ* to allow inspection of the uterine bed at the end of the procedure to ensure hemostasis, and wash the pelvis.

The vaginal dissection may then be commenced, noting the surgeons assistants should avoid excessive traction on the uterus. Without the support of the round and infundibulopelvic ligaments, the smaller branches of the uterine artery are easily sheared off from the lateral aspect of the body of the uterus, leading to bleeding which may be very difficult indeed to control. The ureteric

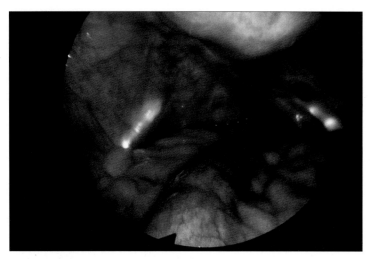

16.11 'Uriglow' ureteric stents *in situ.*

stents should remain in place until the vaginal dissection is finished. The reason for this is that if hemostasis is not secure by the time the uterus is completely removed, and extra sutures are needed to control bleeding from the uterine artery pedicles, the ureter can be damaged.

The cervix is grasped using two pairs of Vulsellum forceps, and the dissection proceeds as for vaginal hysterectomy, although certain aspects require emphasis. The pouch of Douglas is opened using a knife to incise the posterior fornix vaginal skin and peritoneum. Circumcision of the cervix is then completed, and the uterovesical pouch opened to unite with the laparoscopic bladder dissection. Once entry is gained to the peritoneal cavity both anteriorly and posteriorly, the bladder (and therefore the ureters) should be swept digitally laterally and superiorly to ensure the lower urinary tract is clear of the operative field. With ureteric stents in situ the ureters may be easily palpated.

The exploring finger is then placed through the peritoneum anteriorly, into the uterovesical pouch, and curled around the remaining tissue (mostly comprising the transverse cervical ligaments). A long, curved-on-the-edge non-toothed clamp (ideally a 12 inch Zeppelin clamp) is then placed over the tissue in a single manoeuvre. Occasionally this volume of tissue will prove excessive for a single clamp, and may have to be dealt with in two 'bites'. The uterus is then delivered vaginally, taking care to rotate it through 90 degrees to avoid snagging the lateral pelvic side wall staples (see below). If the uterus is enlarged, it may be bisected and morcellated.

The pedicles should then be inspected vaginally for bleeding. Sometimes it is possible to see the whole dissection, including the staples in the infundibulopelvic ligament, but more often the latter requires laparoscopic inspection, which should be performed in all cases.

One circumstance deserves special mention. If the uterus is significantly enlarged by fibroids to an extent that extracting the uterus through the pelvis is likely to prove 'tight', the possibility 'snagging' the hemostatic staples on the infundibulopelvic and uterine artery pedicles must be considered. The sides of the isolated uterus are of course also studded with staples, which may catch and even avulse those securing the pedicles, leading to severe arterial bleeding. This can be avoided by rotating the isolated uteus

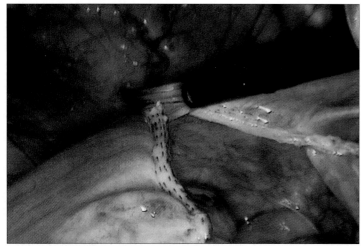

16.12 Continuation of the laparoscopic dissection line beyond the round ligament with diathermy scissors.

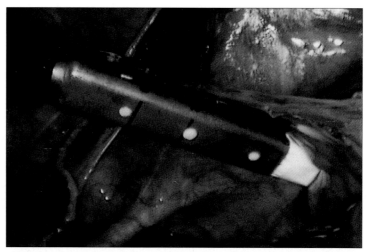

16.13 EndoGIA staple gun applied to left uterine artery. Note the ureter with 'Uriglow' stents. Movement of the lights indicates the ureter is free of the staple line.

through 90 degrees prior to extraction. The two lines of staples on the uterus and pelvic sidewall are thereby separated, and snagging avoided.

There is no need to close the peritoneum separately, although it should be included in the vaginal skin stitch posteriorly to prevent bleeding from the vascular space between the layers of the vaginal skin/peritoneum. We use a transvaginal tube drain, through the vault for 24 hours. A pack in the vagina makes laparoscopic inspection of the uterine bed easier, since it 'tents' the vault, exposes the dissection line and seals the vagina against loss of gas for the final inspection. Bladder catheterization for 24 hours is helpful.

Finally, the abdomen is re-insufflated with CO_2, and the pelvis checked for bleeding. Insufflation pressure should be kept to a minimum consistent with good visualization because high pressures may conceal venous leakage. Any leaking vessel may be sealed with monopolar or bipolar diathermy, although the proximity of the ureters must always be kept in mind. Unipolar diathermy should not be applied to tissue bearing staples. If current is applied directly to the staple line, the tissue surrounding each staple will necrose resulting in possible bleeding. A final check should be made without CO_2 using the 'C' abdominal wall retractor. Finally, the port sites are closed with a 'J' peritoneal closure needle (**16.14, 16.15**).

Results
n = 446, 1990–1994
Operation time: 28–74 min (median 36 min)
In patient stay: 1– days (median 36 h)
Return to normal activity: 1–9 weeks (median 3 weeks)

Major complications
1/445 (0.002%) small bowel hernia (before routine use of 'J' peritoneal closure needle)
2/445 (0.004%) primary haemorrhage requiring blood transfusion and return to operating theatre; bleeding was controlled laparoscopically.
Ureteric injuries: 0/445
Bladder injuries: 0/445

SUPRACERVICAL LAPAROSCOPIC HYSTERECTOMY

This is a modified Semm's 'CASH' (Classic Abdominal Semm Hysterectomy) operation. The main difference is staples are used instead of endoscopic sutures for securing the parametrial tissues. At the beginning of the operation, the cervicouterine canal is cannulated, and a coaxial 'boring bar' instrument is used to core out the cervix to just above the level of the isthmus. This removes the transformation zone, and is an answer to the problem of possible future development of malignancy in the cervical stump. Once this is achieved, the infundibulopelvic and broad ligaments are dealt with laparoscopically, to just above the uterine artery. The uterus is then divided either with a laser, harmonic scalpel or diathermy, and the fragments removed by morcellation through one of the abdominal ports.

The vagina is not opened which has the advantage of sterility. Other advantages are the ureters are safer, since they are not at risk from the staple gun, and the cervix is conserved.

The operative time for this procedure is around an hour and a half, but this depends upon the size of the uterus and how much morcellation is performed. Despite the ingenious developments in motorizing morcellation devices, the procedure is time-consuming. Nevertheless, this technique has been used with success.

CLASSIC ABDOMINAL SEMM HYSTERECTOMY (CASH)

The original operation described by Semm is much the same as that described above, except that extracorporeally knotted sutures are used to secure the pedicles instead of staples, which is cheaper. Semm recommends that diathermy should never be used inside the abdomen under any circumstances to avoid the risk of burns. Bleeding is controlled only with a thermal coagulating device ('cold coagulator', which in fact operates at around 100° C) and sutures.

LAPAROSCOPICALLY ASSISTED DODERLEIN'S HYSTERECTOMY

This operation is a variation of the original operation described by Doderlein approximately 85 years ago, and involves uterine inversion to allow access to the uterine arteries and vaginal identification of the ureters.

The laparoscopic approach deals with adhesions and allows division of the infundibulopelvic and broad ligaments as far as the uterine artery. When the upper pedicles are secured by bipolar

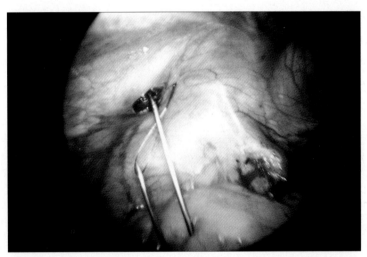

16.14 Closure of lateral port wounds with 'J' peritoneal closure needle (Rocket of London Ltd, Watford, UK).

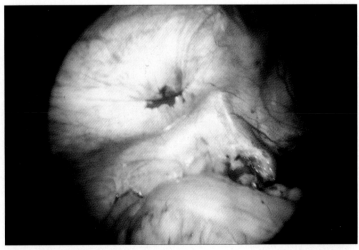

16.15 Closed peritoneal port incision.

diathermy (or extracorporeally knotted sutures), the remainder of the operation is then performed vaginally. An incision is made on the anterior vaginal wall from 9 o'clock to 3 o'clock. The bladder is dissected free from the anterior surfaceof the uterus, and mobilised laterally with the ureters. A Wertheim's retractor is next inserted between the bladder and uterus and the anterior surface of the uterus is grasped with a Vulsellum, as cephalad as possible, and traction applied. Simultaneously, a Vulsellum on the posterior lip of the cervix is pushed upward, to create a 'rocking' movement of the uterus to deliver the fundus of the uterus into the vagina through the utero-vesical pouch. The uterine arteries are then exposed, and lie inferior to the ureters.

Good results have been reported for this technique. Saye *et al* and Garry claim a mean operating time of about an hour, with most patients leaving hospital within 24 hours.

A fairly large uterus can be removed using this technique, which has the great advantage of low cost because no disposable instruments are used.

CONCLUSION

Hysterectomy techniques should never be 'in competition', but should be complimentary. The flexible and able surgeon is familiar with all available techniques so that the best operation can be selected for individual patients.

Laparoscopic hysterectomy is a good operation, both for the patient and the surgeon, which may save women from laparotomy but it must always be remembered: 'first, do no harm'. Training, experience and patient selection are the keys to safe practice.

FURTHER READING

Phipps JH. Laparoscopic Hysterectomy and Oophorectomy: A Colour Atlas and Practical Manual, 1993. Edinburgh, Churchill-Livingstone

Garry R, Reich H. Laparoscopic Hysterectomy, 1994. Blackwell, London

LAPAROSCOPIC LYMPHADENECTOMY 17

Joel M Childers and Amir Nasseri

Lymph nodes from the abdominal aorta to the pelvic floor can be the primary site of metastases in gynecologic malignancies. Part of the International Federation of Gynecology and Obstetrics' (FIGO) surgical staging of vulvar, endometrial, and ovarian malignancies includes sampling of these regional lymph nodes. While cervical cancer is not a surgically staged malignancy, surgical management of patients with this disease often includes removal of lymphatic tissue. It is therefore not surprising that the burgeoning field of operative laparoscopy has included feasibility studies involving lymphadenectomy in patients with gynecologic malignancies.

Initial feasibility studies of laparoscopic lymphadenectomy originated in Europe and the USA. It was an extraperitoneal approach that ushered modern operative endoscopy into the world of gynecologic oncology. This technique was first investigated by Daniel Dargent in France. Dargent uses this technique on patients with early cervical carcinoma. The pelvic lymph nodes are sampled endoscopically prior to radical vaginal hysterectomy (Schauta procedure). The first reported laparoscopic transperitoneal lymphadenectomies also came from France. Like Dargent, Querleu and his colleagues use this technique for staging patients with early cervical cancer. The first reports on para-aortic lymphadenectomy came from the USA, where patients with early and advanced cervical carcinoma underwent this procedure. Soon reports from the USA and Europe surfaced in which patients with cervical, endometrial, and ovarian carcinoma were being managed with laparoscopic lymphadenectomy including bilateral sampling of the infrarenal para-aortic lymph nodes.

Thus far, all reported para-aortic lymphadenectomies have been performed transperitoneally, but a completely retroperitoneal endoscopic approach to these nodes may help avoid the limitations of obesity and the potential complications in patients subsequently being treated with radiation. Feasibility studies have yet to be published on this technique.

SURGICAL PHILOSOPHIES

The extent of gynecologic lymphadenectomies is defined by the area of lymph nodes sampled and the radicality of this sampling. Worldwide, gynecologic oncologists have not agreed upon the extent of the lymphadenectomy necessary for each malignancy. Opinions differ on many aspects. A few examples include whether: (1) para-aortic lymphadenectomy should be performed on patients with early endometrial and cervical cancer; (2) left-side para-aortic lymph nodes should be sampled in endometrial cancer; (3) bilateral lymphadenectomies should be performed on unilateral adnexal malignancies; (4) lymph nodes between the inferior mesenteric artery and the renal vessels should be sampled on adnexal malignancies; (5) selective lymphadenectomy (lymph node sampling) or therapeutic (complete) lymphadenectomy should be performed in instances of endometrial and ovarian carcinoma.

This chapter will not enter the debate on the extent of lymphadenectomy necessary in gynecologic malignancies. We choose to emphasize only that philosophies regarding this issue should be unaffected by the surgical modality. Laparoscopy and laparotomy should be merely words to describe the size of the abdominal incision. Whether one chooses several 5- or 10 mm 'ports' or one 15- to 25 cm 'port' should not affect the extent of the lymphadenectomy that a particular surgeon believes is necessary. We believe strongly that surgeons should not compromise the surgery because laparoscopic techniques are being employed.

With this in mind, the advantage of laparoscopy is the avoidance of an abdominal incision. This translates to a shorter hospitalization and a more rapid recovery for the patient. Therefore, when endoscopic techniques are employed in the management of gynecologic malignancies, it should be done with the intent of performing the procedure entirely laparoscopically, or of converting an abdominal procedure to a vaginal procedure. If a radical hysterectomy is indicated in a patient with cervical cancer who has undergone laparoscopic lymphadenectomy, ideally the hysterectomy should be performed entirely laparoscopically, entirely vaginally, or by using a combination of these two approaches. Likewise, patients with adenocarcinoma of the endometrium should be managed with a combined laparoscopic and vaginal approach. For these patients, operative laparoscopy is used to assess the intraperitoneal cavity for metastatic disease, obtain washings, and perform a regional lymphadenectomy, and the hysterectomy and oophorectomy are performed vaginally, laparoscopically, or using a combined approach. With adnexal malignancies, the operative laparoscopist must be more versatile. Management of these malignancies may require omentectomies, diaphragm biopsies, removal of large masses, and sampling of infrarenal para-aortic lymph nodes. The ultimate goal in all cases is to accomplish an uncompromised surgical procedure while avoiding an abdominal procedure.

Laparoscopic lymphadenectomies can be accomplished in a number of ways. Surgeons differ on many aspects of the procedure, including the number, location, and size of ports; which energy modality to use (monopolar or bipolar electricity, argon-beam coagulator, or laser); and where the operating surgeon stands and in which port the telescope is placed. This chapter outlines the technique for pelvic and para-aortic lymphadenectomy developed at the University of Arizona.

We use a transperitoneal approach and mimic laparotomy techniques by utilizing monopolar electricity, traction and countertraction, blunt and sharp dissection, and proper use of surgical planes. No lasers are used and no aqua-dissection is performed. Mini-laparotomy pads are placed into the abdomen for pressure, 'cleaning up', and identifying 'bleeders'. We recommend that changing of instruments during the procedure be minimized. Ideally, a pelvic and/or para-aortic lymphadenectomy will be completed using graspers and scissors only, the irrigation–aspiration device never being placed in the abdomen. Adoption of this 'laparotomy' style has helped us lower our operative times dramatically and we believe will assist oncologic surgeons in their metamorphosis from laparotomists to laparoscopists.

PATIENT SELECTION

Several patient considerations are important to both the neophyte and the experienced laparoscopist. Each surgeon must weigh these considerations relative to his/her experience and skill level. While there are many relative contraindications, such as multiple prior abdominal surgeries, previous abdominal radiation, history of peritonitis or intraperitoneal chemotherapy, there are few absolute contraindications. The absolute contraindications to laparoscopic lymphadenectomy are identical to those that preclude any abdominal surgery in general, and are usually medical problems.

While not a contraindication, obesity is certainly a limiting factor, especially when sampling of para-aortic lymph nodes is required. Para-aortic lymphadenectomies are difficult to perform in heavy, short patients, dependent, of course, upon the patient's height relative to her trunk size and fat distribution.

PREOPERATIVE CONSIDERATIONS

Having the large and small bowel evacuated facilitates the laparoscopic approach to the para-aortic nodes. This is easily accomplished by having the patient on a liquid diet for two days prior to the procedure and administering one bottle (240 cc) of magnesium citrate one and two days prior to the procedure. This is routinely performed on our patients prior to laparoscopic surgery. Psychological preparation of the patient begins preoperatively. The patient should anticipate a short hospitalization or outpatient procedure. This process is facilitated if the patient expects to be able to eat, ambulate, and be discharged from the hospital within a short time.

ANESTHESIA CONSIDERATIONS

General anesthesia is used, an endotracheal tube is placed, and end-tidal CO_2 is monitored. A pulse oximeter is placed, the bladder is drained continually, and the stomach contents are evacuated prior to placement of the primary trocar or Veress needle. The patient's arms are tucked to the sides with consideration for padding of the ulnar nerve. The supine position is preferred except for patients on whom a hysterectomy is to be performed. Use of antithrombotic stockings should be considered, and the anesthesiologist should decide whether arterial and/or central venous access is necessary.

OPERATING ROOM CONSIDERATIONS

The instruments required for this procedure are simple and few, yet crucial. Utilizing the techniques described in this chapter, it is absolutely necessary to have: (1) sharp, curved, blunt-tipped scissors with monopolar electrocautery capability; (2) two 5 mm graspers; (3) a large grasping forceps (spoon-shaped or tri-pronged) that fits through a 10- to 12 mm laparoscopic sleeve; and (4) an irrigation suction device. A 10 mm laparoscopic telescope with a 0°lens is preferable for most cases. Special instruments such as needle drivers, knot pushers, clip applicators, and stapling devices are not absolutely necessary for the lymphadenectomy but may be required to avoid or manage complications. Bipolar electrocautery can be useful and should be available. Mini-laparotomy pads that can be placed through a 12 mm port are often more useful than irrigation and aspiration, and surgeons should be familiar with what pads/gauze are available at their hospitals.

Port Placement

Four laparoscopic ports are needed to perform this procedure (**17. 1**). The primary port is placed in the umbilicus and should be 10 mm in size for use with the 10 mm telescope and camera. The three ancillary ports are placed under direct laparoscopic visualization. Two 5 mm trocars and sleeves are placed lateral to the inferior epigastric vessels and the rectus muscles bilaterally in the mid lower abdomen. Ports should be placed perpendicular to the anterior abdominal wall; angling medially during placement can cause injury to the epigastric vessels. The third ancillary port is placed in the midline above the symphysis and should be 12 mm in size to allow removal of the nodal tissue, which at times can contain sizeable specimens. This port can be placed midway between the symphysis and the umbilicus if an infrarenal lymphadenectomy or radical hysterectomy is to be performed.

Operating Room Set-up

The basic premise of the technique described is to allow an 'oriented' surgeon to operate with both hands. Standing to one side of the patient, using scissors placed in the lateral port and graspers placed through the suprapubic port, the surgeon performs the lymphadenectomy on the side of the patient opposite to where he is standing. With a grasper in the 12 mm suprapubic port, lymphatic tissue can be grasped and extracted easily after both left- and right-side lymphadenectomies have been completed, and only one large ancillary port (suprapubic) is required. With 5 mm scissors placed through the lateral ports, the lateral ports are kept small and the scissors need not be removed during the entire unilateral lymphadenectomy. We believe that keeping both the size and the number of ports to a minimum reduces both the morbidity of the procedure and the recovery time for the patient. One drawback of this approach is that the surgeon is obligated to use scissors in his/her non-dominant hand while operating on one side of the patient. This task is simplified by using scissors with a pistol grip. However, some experience is required before a satisfactory 'comfort zone' is reached.

The assistant will need to acquire new haptic skills as well before he or she can become a good assistant. Using our technique, the assistant surgeon manages the laparoscope/camera (umbilical port) and a grasper (lateral port) (**17.1**). The two primary functions of the assistant are to (1) provide visualization of the surgical field (camera operator) and (2) provide surgical assistance such as retraction of tissue, countertraction of tissue, etc.

Learning to be a good assistant can be an arduous task. First, there is a tendency for many surgeons to want to do the operation when their primary goal is to be an assistant. Further, it is even more difficult to learn to be a good 'cameraman'. The laparoscope must be held as if on a tripod so that the image on the monitor does not move. The surgical 'action' should be in the center of the monitor. The surgeon, not the camera operator, should be oriented, and the distance of the camera from the surgical 'action' should be at the surgeon's discretion. Maintaining proper orientation is made possible by having the surgeon look in the direction in which

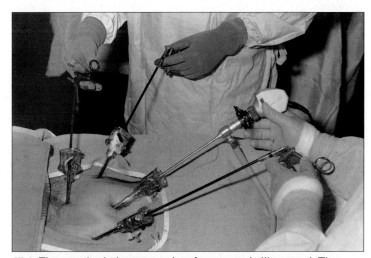

17.1 The standard placement sites for trocars is illustrated. The midline ports are placed in the umbilicus and suprapubically and the lateral ports are placed in the mid lower abdomen lateral to the epigastric vessels and rectus muscle. The patient's head is to the right and the surgeon, on the right side of the patient, is performing a left-side pelvic lymphadenectomy.

he/she is operating. Therefore, monitors are placed at the foot of the patient when operating in the pelvis, and at the patient's head when operating in the upper abdomen (**17.2, 17.3**). If monitors are placed on carts that roll, this orientation requirement is accomplished easily. The assistant (camera operator) must adapt to the surgeon's orientation. This becomes most difficult when the mid-abdomen is being operated upon.

LAPAROSCOPIC PELVIC LYMPHADENECTOMY

If the obturator, external iliac, hypogastric, or distal common iliac nodes are to be dissected, this can be performed in the following fashion. The peritoneum is incised over the psoas muscle between the round ligament and the infundibulopelvic ligament. The round ligament and infundibulopelvic ligament can be left intact, but if a hysterectomy or oophorectomy is to be performed, better exposure can be gained if these structures are transected prior to the lymphadenectomy being performed. The peritoneum is opened and the paravesical/obturator space is opened. It is imperative to isolate the obliterated umbilical artery and retract it medially. It can easily be identified in the pelvis by pushing on it at the anterior abdominal wall and watching for its movement in the pelvis. It is always near the external iliac vein. The paravesical space between the obliterated umbilical artery and the external iliac vein is easily opened. This is a key maneuver.

The obturator nerve is identified and the anterior nodal tissue is dissected off of the nerve by blunt and sharp dissection. The nodal tissue along the medial aspect of the external iliac vein is then bluntly dissected off along the length of the vein. In performing this dissection, one should be aware of aberrant or accessory veins that empty into the external iliac vein (**17.4**).

The nodal bundle is transected at the pelvic wall using monopolar electricity as needed. Clipping and cutting nodal chains is virtually never necessary. Once this is completed, the only remaining attachment of the obturator nodal package is at the junction of the hypogastric and external iliac arteries. This is usually the most difficult part of removing the obturator nodes, as the ureter crosses the iliac vessels near this junction, adequate visualization can be difficult to obtain, and the nodal bundle starts to course laterally. The nodal bundle is transected bluntly or with monopolar electricity and is removed intact through the lower 10-12 mm port using the large forceps.

The external iliac nodes are dissected by creating a plane in the adventitia of the external iliac artery and dissecting it up to the circumflex iliac artery (**17.5**). This is easily and simply performed using sharp, curved, blunt-tipped scissors and monopolar electrocautery. Effort should be made to avoid damaging the genitofemoral nerve laterally. The dissection can be extended proximally to the point where the ovarian vessels and/or the ureter cross the iliac vessels (**17.6**). Through this same peritoneal incision, the assistant can retract the ureter in a cephalad direction and the nodal dissection can be continued up the distal common iliac artery (**17.7**).

When performing the pelvic lymphadenectomy on the left side, the rectosigmoid generally needs to be taken down from the left pelvic sidewall. This can be accomplished by incising the peritoneum in this area along the white line of Toldt, which will give access to the retroperitoneal space. If mobilization of the rectosigmoid is not required, a peritoneal incision over the psoas muscle is made between the round ligament and the ovarian vessels. The surgeon stands on the right side of the patient and uses graspers through the midline port and scissors through the left lateral port (**17.1**).

If a therapeutic (complete) lymphadenectomy is required, a more thorough procedure can be accomplished by separating the external iliac vessels from the psoas muscle (**17.10**). Following completion of the lymphadenectomy, the operative site can be irrigated and should be inspected to ensure that hemostasis is adequate (**17.8, 17.9**). The peritoneum is left open and no drains are used.

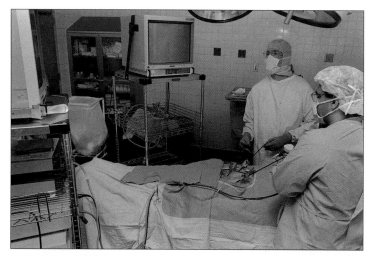

17.2 When pelvic surgery is performed, the monitors are placed at the foot of the patient. This helps orient the surgeon by allowing him/her to look in the direction in which he/she is operating. The surgeon on the right side of the patient performs left-side pelvic surgery. The assistant, on the left side of the patient, operates the camera through the umbilicus and uses the left lateral port.

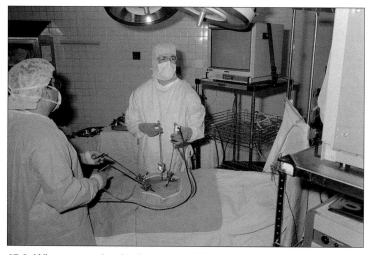

17.3 When operating in the upper abdomen, the surgeons orient themselves by placing the monitors at the patient's head (the right side of this figure). In this figure, the surgeon is standing on the left side of the patient, performing a right-side para-aortic lymphadenectomy, using graspers placed through the suprapubic port and scissors placed through the right lateral port. The assistant, standing on the patient's right side, manipulates an instrument through the right lateral port and the telescope placed through the umbilicus.

Preparation for the Para-aortic Lymphadenectomy

Key to successful removal of the para-aortic nodes is proper placement of the small bowel into the upper abdomen. This is facilitated by temporarily placing the telescope through the suprapubic port. This allows a more 'panoramic' view of the mid and upper abdomen. Initially the surgeon may require a monitor at the head of the patient during this step, but eventually this step will be achievable regardless of location of the monitors. When a para-aortic lymphadenectomy is to be performed, a monitor should be placed at the head of the patient (17.3). In some patients, the omentum will have to be placed on top of the liver before the small bowel is manipulated. The mesentery of the small bowel should be flipped in a cephalad direction and splayed out across the abdomen. This will place the small bowel into the upper abdomen, exposing the para-aortic area. Trendelenburg position, good bowel preparation

and placement, and, occasionally, lateral tilt of the operating table assist in keeping the bowel in the upper abdomen. It is during this process that the small bowel and both sides of its mesentery can be inspected for metastatic disease. 'Packing' of the bowel is extremely important and time should be taken to accomplish this correctly lest time be lost later. Occasionally, the use of additional ports to keep the bowel in the upper abdomen may be required to accomplish a para-aortic lymphadenectomy, especially in heavier patients. The aorta, right common iliac artery, and the ureter as it crosses the right iliac vessels are landmarks that should be identified prior to beginning the dissection if possible. Depending on its location, the transverse duodenum can often be visualized as it crosses the vena cava and aorta. Lifting the mesentery of the small bowel as it crosses the aorta will aid in visualizing the third portion of the duodenum.

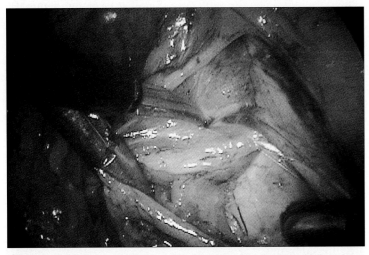

17.4 The assistant retracts the right external iliac vein as the surgeon grasps the right obturator nodal bundle and retracts it medially. Scissors are used to separate the nodal bundle from the medial aspect of the external iliac vein. Note an accessory obturator vein traversing through this nodal bundle to empty into the external iliac vein.

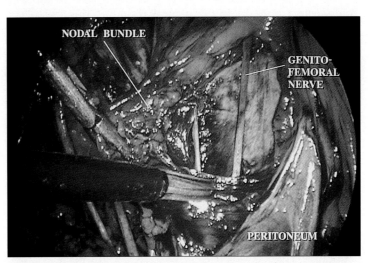

17.5 The right external iliac lymph node package is grasped and retracted medially, allowing the surgeon to safely remove the nodes between the genitofemoral nerve and the external iliac vessels.

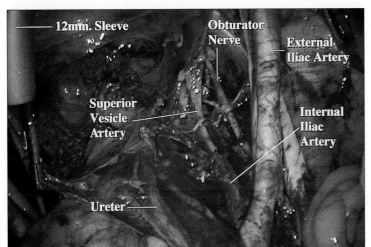

17.6 Following completion of the lower pelvic lymphadenectomy, major retroperitoneal structures should be easily identifiable, as seen in this photograph of the right pelvic retroperitoneal space.

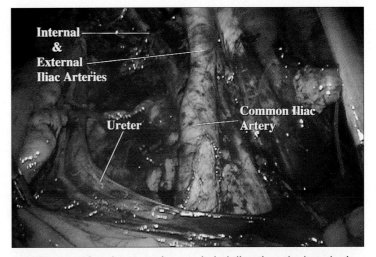

17.7 By retracting the ureter in a cephalad direction, the lymphatic tissue around the distal common iliac artery and its bifurcation can be adequately removed, as demonstrated on this right-side pelvic lymphadenectomy. These nodes can also be dissected through an incision in the peritoneum medial to the ureter over the proximal common iliac artery with the ureter retracted in a caudad direction.

RIGHT-SIDED PARA-AORTIC LYMPHADENECTOMY

The surgeon, on the left side of the patient, performs the procedure with graspers in the lower midline port and scissors in the left lateral port. The assistant holds the camera in the umbilical port and uses graspers in the right lateral port. An incision is made in the peritoneum over the aorta and right common iliac artery. The peritoneum is lifted with graspers, and blunt dissection is performed laterally toward the right psoas muscle. The right ureter is identified and lifted away from the underlying psoas muscle. The right psoas and tendon of the psoas should be easily seen.

The assistant then places his/her grasper (in the right lateral port) underneath the right ureter and ovarian vessels to retract them anteriorly and laterally out of the operative field. This also creates a small 'tent' which helps prevent small bowel from falling into the operative field.

The surgeon then dissects the nodal and fatty tissue off the aorta by dissecting in the adventital plane of the aorta. This arterial dissection is continued in a cephalad and caudad direction, up the aorta and down the common iliac artery, using the scissors and electrocautery as needed. Dissecting in the arterial adventital planes prior to 'grasping and removing nodes' is a key step in completing a thorough lymphadenectomy. There is a tendency to grasp the nodal tissue that is visible over the vena cava and begin dissection here. A safer and more complete dissection is accomplished by starting the dissection over the aorta and right common iliac artery. This allows development of the natural plane between the nodal tissue and the vena cava and dissection from medial to lateral direction, which aids in visualization of any perforating veins from this nodal bundle to the vena cava. Lateral dissection is then performed toward the psoas muscle so that a portion of the vena cava is unroofed. Care should be taken to avoid lacerating perforating vessels when unroofing the vena cava. Encountering a perforating vein from the vena cava that cannot be controlled with monopolar electricity is unusual. However, large perforating vessels from the vena cava or aorta should be clipped. Dissection is continued up and down the vena cava. Small vessels and lymphatic channels are easily coagulated with monopolar electricity.

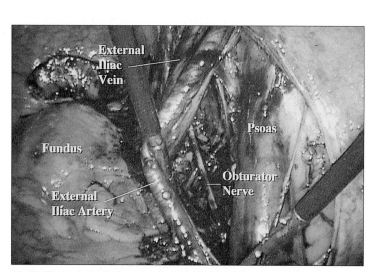

17.8 An adequate left pelvic lymphadenectomy can be performed despite the presence of the rectosigmoid on the left and the potential disadvantage of operating with scissors in the left hand.

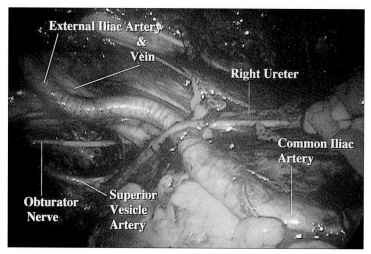

17.9 The right ureter can be seen as the only structure crossing the common iliac artery following a complete right lymphadenectomy and salpingo-oophorectomy.

17.10 The external iliac artery and vein can be retracted medially, separating these vessels from the psoas muscle. This facilitates access to the obturator space and allows a more thorough lymphadenectomy to be completed.

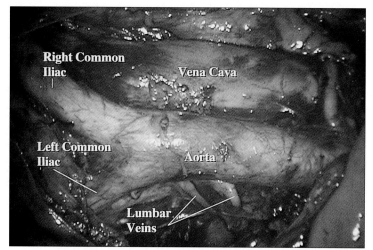

17.11 Following completion of a lower para-aortic lymphadenectomy, the aorta, vena cava, and proximal common iliac arteries are easily seen. Para-aortic lymphadenectomies below the inferior mesenteric artery are commonly utilized in patients with cervical and endometrial carcinoma. When performing a left para-aortic lymphadenectomy, the surgeon should be aware of the potential existence of large lumbar veins.

The nodal bundle is then transected, again with monopolar electricity, using a fulgurating technique. Once the nodal package is transected at one end, it is easy to peel the bundle off the vena cava toward the opposite end. Transection of the remaining end is again accomplished by monopolar electrocautery. The nodal tissue is extracted through the lower midline port. The operative field is irrigated and hemostasis is secured.

If the nodal tissue over the distal right common iliac artery is to be removed as well, this can be accomplished through the same peritoneal incision (**17.11**). The assistant uses his/her grasper to retract the ureter atraumatically in a caudad direction. This will provide exposure to the nodal tissue over this artery and beyond its bifurcation. The nodal dissection is then continued down the common iliac to the proximal internal and external iliac vessels.

LEFT-SIDED PARA-AORTIC LYMPHADENECTOMY

The surgeon, on the right side of the patient, performs this procedure using instruments placed through the lower midline and right lateral ports (**17.3**). The assistant holds the telescope and camera through the umbilical port. The camera is rotated so that the aorta and the vena cava are horizontal on the color monitor, with the patient's head to the left.

If the peritoneal incision has not already been made, an incision is made similar to that used for the right-side para-aortic lymphadenectomy. This incision over the aorta is extended in the cephalad direction as far as possible. The incision is extended in a caudad direction over the proximal left common iliac artery.

The surgeon dissects in the adventitial plane of the aorta in a cephalad and caudad direction. A key point on this side is to extend the arterial adventitial dissection as far as possible in both directions to allow ample room to safely perform the lymphadenectomy. Care should be taken to avoid injuring the inferior mesenteric artery. The more the aorta and left common iliac are 'cleaned off', the more space and visibility the surgeon will have!

Only after the adventitia over the aorta has been adequately dissected free should lateral dissection toward the left psoas muscle be carried out. The surgeon can safely dissect beneath the left ureter and mesentery of the rectosigmoid using this plane. This differs from the right-sided para-aortic lymphadenectomy, where lateral dissection is carried out after making the peritoneal incision but before dissecting the aortic adventitia.

Lateral dissection is continued until the psoas muscle and its tendon are identified. The assistant now places the grasper into the dissected space beneath the mesentery of the rectosigmoid, the ovarian vessels, and the left ureter. This retraction is paramount for adequate exposure, which is mandatory since the left-sided para-aortic lymph nodes are lateral to the aorta.

Once adequate exposure has been created, the surgeon grasps the nodal bundle near the bifurcation of the aorta and lifts it anteriorly. This frees the loose posterior attachments and assists in dissecting beneath the nodal chain. A window is created bluntly beneath the nodal chain. The dissection is extended in a cephalad direction using blunt and sharp dissection and electrocautery with the scissors as needed. The nodal chain is then transected at the cephalad end near the inferior mesenteric artery. The specimen is removed through the lower midline 12 mm port and the operative field is irrigated and inspected for hemostasis. Occasionally, large lumbar veins will be encountered on this side. The surgeon must be aware of their potential existence and exercise appropriate caution (**17.11**).

INFRARENAL PARA-AORTIC LYMPHADENECTOMY

This is the most difficult laparoscopic lymphadenectomy to perform and should be attempted only after ample experience is acquired. The transverse duodenum is separated from the vena cava and the aorta by blunt and sharp dissection. This dissection is continued in a cephalad direction, but lateral dissection is also accomplished by sweeping the laparoscopic instruments bluntly toward the psoas muscles. The assistant provides exposure by maintaining upward retraction on the transverse duodenum (**17.12**). It is helpful to place a fifth port in the mid to upper abdomen to assist in elevation of the duodenum, but after experience is gained this is usually not nec-

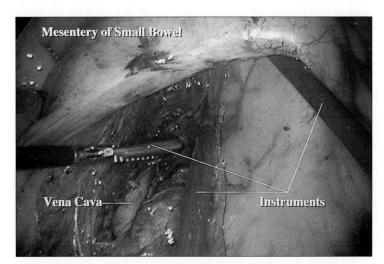

17.12 To perform an infrarenal para-aortic lymphadenectomy, the mesentery of the small bowel and third part of the duodenum must be mobilized and separated from the underlying aorta and vena cava. During this procedure, one laparoscopic instrument is needed to elevate the transverse duodenum. This allows the surgeon to operate with two instruments in a field with adequate exposure.

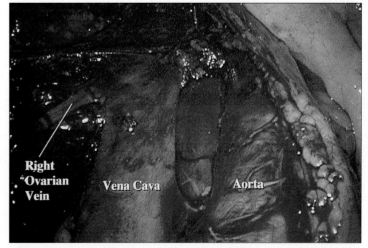

17.13 When dissecting para-aortic lymphatic tissue on the right side above the inferior mesenteric artery, care should be taken to avoid injuring the right ovarian vein and right ureter. If the surgeon is concerned about injuring the ovarian vein, a clip can be placed across the vein near its entry into the vena cava.

surgeon and assistant surgeon now face cephalad, with monitors moved toward the patient's head. As with the pelvic and lower para-aortic procedures, the surgeon stands on the contralateral side of the nodes to be removed; however, these higher nodes can be removed by the surgeon's positioning him/herself on either side of the patient or between the patient's legs.

After adequate cephalad exposure is obtained, the nodal dissection is begun. On the right, this was simply a matter of continuing the previously performed lymphadenectomy up to the origin of the ovarian vein, which may enter the vena cava distal to or very near the left renal vein (**17.13, 17.14, 17.15**). On the left, the surgeon is faced with the lateral location of the nodal chain, working around the inferior mesenteric artery and lumbar veins. It is extremely important to identify the left renal and ovarian veins as soon as possible (**17.14, 17.15**). They are often disguised in the endoabdominal fascia and could be easily damaged. Likewise, rapid identification of the right ovarian vein is important to prevent its transection during the removal of these high para-aortic nodes. Once these vessels are located, dissection in the adventitia of the aorta should be carried out. With generous use of monopolar electricity, annoying small bleeders will be minimized. The ovarian artery may need to be sacrificed, which can be done with bipolar or monopolar electricity, but this artery usually is not identified. The nodal bundle is transected near the left renal vein and the right ovarian vein as they enter the vena cava. The left-side dissection can be made easier by bluntly dissecting the nodal bundle from the left ovarian vein. The vein can then be retracted laterally, which keeps it and the left ureter out of harm's way. Once the nodal chain has been separated from its lateral attachment to the endoabdominal fascia and its medial attachments to the abdominal aorta, blunt dissection will easily separate the nodal chain from its posterior attachments. This also makes damage to any lumbar veins in this area less likely (**17.15**).

The peritoneum is not closed and no retroperitoneal drains are placed. The mesentery of the small bowel is repositioned over the para-aortic incision site at the end of the dissection. Patients undergoing laparoscopic surgery only are given a regular diet on the day of the procedure.

PITFALLS

Unfortunately, most physicians currently practicing gynecologic oncology have not developed their operative laparoscopic skills. This means that in many situations, novice laparoscopists will initially be performing lymphadenectomies. Early reports have demonstrated that the thoroughness of this procedure is compromised by inexperience and patient obesity. Depending on the patient's height and fat distribution, exposure to the para-aortic lymph nodes becomes difficult in patients who weigh 90 kg or greater. Even in lean patients, the thoroughness of the lymphadenectomy improves and complications are less likely to occur as the surgeon gains experience.

The laparotomy rate associated with complications during laparoscopic lymphadenectomy is reported to be in the range of 0–10%. These complications have been associated with the genitourinary, gastrointestinal, and vascular systems. Genitourinary complications likely to result in laparotomy include damage to ureter and bladder. The ureter is likely to be traumatized near the bifurcation of the common iliac artery during the pelvic lymphadenectomy, as is the lumbar ureter during para-aortic lymphadenectomy. Bladder lacerations occur during placement of the suprapubic port, or when dissecting in the perivesical space prior to removing the obturator nodes. Continuous bladder drainage and bluntly entering the perivesical space by retracting the obliterated umbilical artery medially will help avoid these complications.

Gastrointestinal complications likely to result in laparotomy are associated with bowel trauma and herniation. Enterotomy may occur during placement of trocars and ports, during 'packing' of the bowel into the upper abdomen, or during adhesiolysis. Care should be taken during all of these steps. Placement of ancillary ports under laparoscopic visualization, gentle manipulation of bowel with blunt instruments, and a good preoperative bowel preparation may

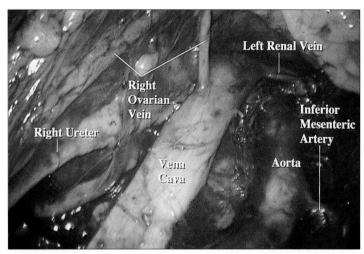

17.14 Following completion of an infrarenal lymphadenectomy, the ovarian veins, ureters, and left renal vein are easily identifiable. With anterior retraction on the transverse duodenum, the right ovarian vein can pull on the vena cava, causing elevation of the vena cava and separation from its underlying tissue and the adjacent aorta. This facilitates removal of lymphatic tissue between the vena cava and the aorta.

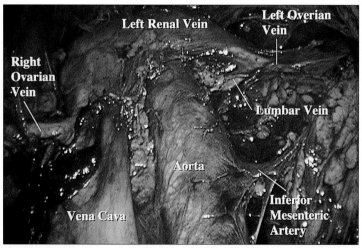

17.15 When dissecting left para-aortic infrarenal lymphatic tissue, extreme caution should be taken to avoid injuring the left ovarian vein, renal vein, and ureter. Lumbar veins are commonly present in this area and frequently will empty into the left ovarian vein.

assist in avoiding these complications. Bowel herniation is the most common laparoscopic gastrointestinal complication that results in laparotomy. This delayed complication occurs when small bowel herniates through the previous trocar sites (**17.16**). This can occur at both umbilical and nonumbilical sites and is more likely to occur at 12 mm sites than at 10 mm sites. It can be very difficult to close the fascia through small skin incisions; however, the incidence of herniation can be greatly reduced if fascia is closed. Extending the skin incision during closure, or use of one of the fascial closure devices currently available, will assist the surgeon with this onerous task.

Vascular injuries related to laparoscopic lymphadenectomy vary significantly. The majority will be a result of trocar injury to anterior abdominal wall vessels. The vessels most likely to be injured are the inferior epigastric, the superficial epigastric, and the obliterated umbilical artery. Visualization of the vessels during trocar placement, either directly with the laparoscope or via transillumination of the anterior abdominal wall, is difficult. A sound knowledge of the anatomy, lateral placement of the lateral ports, and a little luck will help the surgeon circumvent these common vascular injuries.

Injury to retroperitoneal vessels during laparoscopic lymphadenectomy is a major concern. Injury can occur with placement of the trocars; however, it is much more likely to occur during the operative procedure. Reported vascular complications associated with laparoscopic lymphadenectomy include injuries to the obturator vein, external iliac artery, a small vessel off the aorta, and the vena cava. Major vessels that could potentially be injured during this procedure include aberrant obturator veins, the obturator artery, the internal, external, and common iliac veins, the inferior mesenteric artery, the ovarian artery and vein, the lumbar veins, and the renal vein. It is likely that these yet-unreported complications will occur as the number of surgeons performing these procedures increases.

Injury related to non-specific vessels resulting in postoperative hematomas can also occur. Whether located in the retroperitoneum or in the anterior abdominal wall, the morbidity associated with hematomas can be significant (**17.17**). Obstruction of the ureter

and bowel as well as blood transfusion of the patient and infection of the hematoma are potential sequelae.

Complications of laparoscopic lymphadenectomy are in general the same as those reported following lymphadenectomies performed via laparotomy. Examples of miscellaneous complications associated with lymphadenectomy performed by either method include lymphedema, lymphocele, prolonged ileus, deep venous thrombosis, pulmonary embolus, and damage to the obturator nerve. Thus far, no deaths have been reported related to laparoscopic lymphadenectomy, and the major complication rate seems comparable to that of laparotomy.

CONCLUSION

Laparoscopic lymphadenectomy is in its infancy. The role that this technique will play in managing patients with pelvic malignancies is yet to be determined. Initial reports indicate that laparoscopic lymphadenectomy, both pelvic and para-aortic, is feasible, adequate, and safe. Utilization of this technique allows conversion of abdominal procedures to vaginal procedures for patients with cervical and endometrial cancer. Patients with early endometrial and ovarian malignancies who were incompletely surgically staged with their primary procedures may also avoid laparotomy by being staged laparoscopically.

It is imperative that the survival of patients with pelvic malignancies not be compromised by employing laparoscopic lymphadenectomy. Currently, survival data for patients with pelvic malignancies who have been managed with laparoscopy is lacking. The learning curve associated with this surgical procedure is significant and is unlikely to be overcome by the surgeon with no experience in abdominal pelvic and para-aortic lymphadenectomy, or by the experienced oncologic surgeon who performs this laparoscopic procedure only occasionally. Only the experienced, committed oncologic surgeon will master laparoscopic pelvic and para-aortic lymphadenectomy. Future clinical trials with experienced surgeons and long-term survival data will help determine the role of laparoscopic lymphadenectomy in oncology.

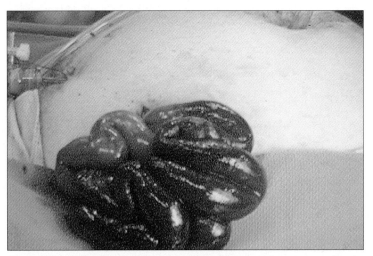

17.16 When small bowel herniates through a previous trocar site, it commonly compromises the vascular supply, resulting in necrotic bowel. These complications can often be managed through an incision over the herniation site. The herniated bowel can be inspected, resected, reanastomosed if necessary, and dropped back into the abdomen through the fascial defect.

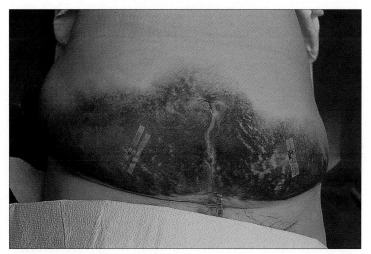

17.17 Injury to anterior abdominal wall vessels can result in significant blood loss. The inferior epigastric, superficial epigastric, and obliterated umbilical arteries can easily be injured; however, injury to nonspecific anterior abdominal wall vessels can result in significant blood loss, as demonstrated in this patient.

FURTHER READING

Boitke GM, Lurain JR, Burke JJ. A comparison of laparoscopic management of endometrial cancer with traditional laparotomy. *Gynecol Oncol* 1994; **52**:105

Burney TL, Campbell EC, Naslund MJ, Jacobs SC. Complications of staging laparoscopic pelvic lymphadenectomy. *Surg Lap Endosc* 1993; **3**:184–190

Childers JM, Brzechffa PR, Hatch KD, Surwit EA. Laparoscopic assisted surgical staging (LASS) of endometrial carcinoma. *Gynecol Oncol* 1993; **52**:33–38

Childers JM, Brzechffa PR, Surwit EA. Laparoscopy using the left upper quadrant as the primary trocar site. *Gynecol Oncol* 1993; **50**:221-225

Childers JM, Hatch KD, Surwit EA. Laparoscopic para-aortic lymphadenectomy in gynecologic malignancies. *Obstet Gynecol* 1993; **82**:741–747

Childers J, Hatch K, Surwit E. The role of laparoscopic lymphadenectomy in the management of cervical cancer. *Gyn Oncol* 1992; **47**:38–43

Childers JM, Spirtos NM, Brainard P, Surwit EA. Laparoscopic staging of the patient with incompletely staged early adenocarcinoma of the endometrium. *Obstet Gynecol* 1994; **83**:597–600

Dargent D. Laparoscopic surgery and gynecologic cancer. *Curr Opin Obstet Gynecol* 1993; **5**:294–300

Fowler JM, Carter J, Carlson J, Maslonkowski R, Byers L, Carlson L, Twiggs L. Lymph-node yield from laparoscopic lymphadenectomy in cervical cancer: A comparative study. *Gynecol Oncol* 1993; **51**:187–92

Kadar N. Laparoscopic vaginal hysterectomy: An operative technique and its evolution. *Gynaecol Endosc* 1994; **3**:109–122

Kavoussi LR, Sosa E, Chandhoke P, Chodak G, Clayman R, Hadley H, Loughlin KR, Ruckle H, Rukstalis D, Schuessler W, Segura J, Vancaille T, Winfield H. Complications of laparoscopic pelvic node dissection. *J Urol* 1993;**149**:322–325

Nezhat C, Burrell M, Nezhat F. Laparoscopic radical hysterectomy with para-aortic and pelvic node dissection. *Am J Obstet Gynecol* 1992; **166**:864–865

Querleu D. Laparoscopic para-aortic node sampling in gynecologic oncology: A preliminary experience. *Gynecol Oncol* 1993; **49**:24–29

Querleu D. Laparoscopically assisted radical vaginal hysterectomy. *Gynecol Oncol* 1993; **51**:248-54

Querleu D, LeBlanc E. Laparoscopic infrarenal para-aortic node dissection in the restaging of carcinomas of the ovary and fallopian tube. *Cancer* 1994; **73**:1467–71

Querleu D, LeBlanc E, Castelain B. Laparoscopic pelvic lymphadenectomy in the staging of early carcinoma of the cervix. *Am J Obstet Gynecol.* 1991; **164**:579–81

Vasquez JM, Demarque AM, Diamond MP. Vascular complications of laparoscopic surgery. *J Am Assoc Gynecol Laparoscop* 1994; **1**:163–67

COMPLICATIONS OF LAPAROSCOPY   18

Alan G Gordon and B Victor Lewis

INTRODUCTION

Laparoscopy carries a small but significant risk of complications. Many of these are relatively minor but some are major and may be life threatening. Most can be avoided by applying the basic principles of good surgical telchnique. It is fundamental that no surgeon should practice endoscopic surgery without adequate training which should include supervision by an expert during the early learning curve. Basic training should include an understanding of the principles of laser and electrosurgery, a knowledge of the instruments available and experience in recognizing the normal as well as the abnormal.

There are many training courses which provide didactic teaching using formal lectures, group discussion, practical laboratory sessions and videos of the common and not so common operations. The techniques of using a video screen to handle instruments, manipulate tissue and tie knots can be learnt on a training model. This is an excellent way to learn manual dexterity but there is no substitute for assisting an expert surgeon or of being assisted until the trainee is competent and confident to operate independently. Attendance at courses does not confer competence in endoscopic surgery. This can only be obtained by working with an expert.

Guidelines for safe endoscopic surgery have been published by several of the national and international societies in gynecologic endoscopy. A working party of the Royal College of Obstetricians and Gynecologists of London (RCOG) has recommended that laparoscopic operations be classified according to their complexity (**18.1**). Simple procedures can be performed by all gynecologists with appropriate training but more complicated operations are only suitable for surgeons with a special interest in endoscopy. Level 4 laparoscopic operations which include colposuspension, lymphadenectomy, and ablation of advanced endometriosis should only be performed by surgeons who spend a large proportion of their time doing endoscopic surgery. These are surgeons who may be nationally or internationally recognised for their expertise.

There have been several national and international surveys of the complication rates of laparoscopic and hysteroscopic surgery. The American Association of Gynecologic Laparoscopists (AAGL) has carried out surveys for over 20 years. National surveys have also been conducted in Australia and France.

INDUCTION OF THE PNEUMOPERITONEUM

EXTRAPERITONEAL GAS INSUFFLATION

It is usually simple to insert a Veress' needle to insufflate carbon dioxide (CO_2) into the peritoneal cavity (**18.2**). Failure may produce extraperitoneal emphysema. This may be suspected early by the feeling of crepitus below the site of insertion of the needle, a low flow rate or high gas pressure. The needle should be withdrawn and re-inserted through the same or another site. Alternatively the presence of emphysema may be diagnosed when the telescope is inserted by the typical 'spider web' appearance of the extraperitoneal tissues caused by the peritoneum being stripped off the underlying fascia. The telescope should be withdrawn and the gas expressed. The pneumoperitoneum should be reformed through another site or open laparoscopy performed.

The site of insertion of the needle may have to be modified if the patient is obese or the aspiration and sounding tests as described in Chapter 2 are suggestive of intra-abdominal adhesions. Alternative sites are the floor of the pouch of Douglas, the anterior axillary line in the 10th left interspace or suprapubically. If these sites are used care must be taken to avoid both the pleural cavity and the bladder.

PENETRATION OF A HOLLOW VISCUS

The Veress' needle may enter bowel, stomach or bladder. The aspiration test should allow early detection of gastrointestinal perforation but it is not foolproof. There may be a fecal smell from the proximal end of the needle, asymmetrical abdominal distension, belching or passage of flatus. The needle should be withdrawn and resited correctly. Laparoscopy should be performed and the bowel carefully inspected. A small hole usually seals spontaneously without leakage of bowel contents. Intravenous fluids and a broad spectrum antibiotic should be given and the patient observed for abdominal distension, guarding or tenderness. Laparotomy should be performed if there is any sign suggestive of peritonitis such as absent bowel sounds or rebound tenderness.

Classification of laparoscopic procedures by level of training
Level 1 Diagnostic laparoscopy
Level 2 Minor laparoscopic prccedures
Laparoscopic sterilization Needle aspiration of small cysts Ovarian biopsy Minor adhesiolysis not involving bowel Ventrosuspension Coagulation of endometriosis – revised AFS stage I
Level 3
Laser/coagulation of polycystic ovaries Laser/coagulation of endometriosis – revised AFS stages II and III Laparoscopic uterosacral nerve ablation Salpingostomy for infertility Salpingectomy/Salpingo-ophorectomy Adhesiolysis for moderate and severe adhesions Adhesiolysis involving bowel Laparoscopic ovarian cystectomy Laparoscopic/laser management of endometrioma Laparoscopically assisted vaginal/hysterectomy without significant associated pathology
Level 4 Extensive endoscopic procedures requiring subspecialist or advanced/tertiary level endoscopic skills
Myomectomy Laparoscopic surgery for revised AFS stage III and IV endometriosis Pelvic lymphadenectomy Pelvic sidewall/uretic dissection Dissection of an obliterated pouch of Douglas Laparoscopic incontinence surgical procedures

18.1 Classification of laparoscopic procedures by level of training.

The stomach may be damaged if an upper abdominal site is chosen or if the stomach is distended during induction of anesthesia or if anesthesia is maintained with a mask. It should be suspected if there is upper abdominal distension or increased tympanism. The stomach should be emptied by a naso-gastric tube and the pneumoperitoneum re-introduced. Treatment should be conservative provided there is no bleeding.

Bladder perforation may occur with a low insertion site of the Veress' needle or if the bladder is full. This event can be avoided by preliminary catheterization. If perforation has occurred, there may be pneumaturia but more often the injury is not recognized until the bladder is noted to be distended with gas at laparoscopy. Treatment is usually conservative.

BLOOD VESSEL INJURY

Insertion of the Veress' needle may damage omental or mesenteric vessels or any of the major retroperitoneal vessels. Injury to the major vessels can be avoided by lifting the abdominal wall and directing the needle correctly. Thin patients and children are at particular risk. It is impossible to ensure that the omentum is not in contact with the abdominal wall so its vessels are always at risk. The surgeon should take care not to insert the needle further than necessary.

The aspiration test should detect blood vessel damage. The needle should be re-sited and the pneumoperitoneum introduced. Careful inspection should reveal the extent of the injury. Minor bleeding may be controlled with coagulation or suture. Major bleeding or the development of a hematoma may be associated with dramatic collapse. This necessitates immediate laparotomy with the asistance of a vascular surgeon.

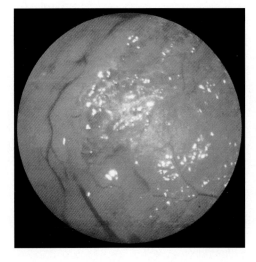

18.2 CO$_2$ gas in the extraperitoneal fat.

GAS EMBOLISM

Unrecognized intravascular insufflation of gas may lead to gas embolism or death. Routine use of the aspiration test should prevent this. The patient should be turned onto the left lateral position.

EFFECTS OF THE DISTENSION MEDIUM

Carbon dioxide is the most commonly used distension medium for operative laparoscopy. Gas embolism is uncommon because the gas is highly soluble in body fluids. A bolus of 400 ml produces no change in the ECG pattern. Circulatory changes return to normal within a few minutes.

Excessive absorbtion of CO$_2$ may produce cardiac arrhythmia. This may be prevented by endotacheal insufflation and positive pressure respiration and by using an automatic insufflator which cuts out if the intra-abdominal pressure rises.

Postoperative pain due to peritoneal irritation is common. Chest pain may be confused with coronary heart disease and may lead to the inappropriate use of anticoagulants. This may produce a wound hematoma or intraperitoneal bleeding.

Nitrous oxide (N$_2$O) has fewer side effects than CO$_2$ and is favored by some surgeons for diagnostic laparoscopy. Operative laparoscopy with N$_2$O is potentially dangerous if there has been inadvertent bowel perforation with escape of methane gas. The mixture of N$_2$O and methane may cause an explosion if high frequency electricity is used.

OTHER COMPLICATIONS

The Veress' needle may be inserted into the omentum and cause a pneumo-omentum. This should be suspected if the aspiration test is negative, the flow rate is low and the insufflating pressure high. There are typical blebs of gas within the omentum. The gas is quickly absorbed and no treatment is necessary.

Perforation of the uterine fundus is usually innocuous. The uterus should be inspected and any bleeding controlled with bipolar or thermocoagulation.

The liver or spleen may be punctured with a high insertion or if the organ is pathologically enlarged. It should be recognized by the routine tests. The needle should be withdrawn, resited and operation continued.

Gas from a correctly induced pneumoperitoneum may flow into the mediastinum and create a pneumomediastinum. Extensive interstitial emphysema may result in cardiac embarrassment.

A high insertion of the Veress' needle may produce a pneumothorax. This will produce difficulty in ventilating the patient, there will be mediastinal shift and increased tympanism over the affected area. The laparoscopy should be abandoned, the gas evacuated by a pleural tube if necessary and the patient kept under observation.

INSERTION OF TROCARS

The risks of trocar insertion are similar to those of Veress' needle insertion but the injury is likely to be more extensive. The primary trocar is nearly always inserted blindly and injury can only be prevented by careful application of the basic techniques of laparoscopy. Secondary trocars should only be inserted under direct vision.

INJURY TO A HOLLOW VISCUS

Injury to bowel, stomach or bladder may be avoided by careful attention to the technique of insertion of the trocars and use of the sounding test to map out a safe space (**18.3**).

The extent of the injury to bowel may vary from superficial serosal damage to complete penetration into the lumen. The viscus may slip off the trocar. alternatively the trocar can remain within the lumen or pass through a loop of bowel which becomes impaled on it. It is important at every laparoscopy to inspect the bowel in the axis of the primary trocar to ensure it has not been damaged. The eye or camera should be applied to the laparoscope immediately after insertion and the organs in line with the cannula inspected. The diagnosis of perforation is easy if the surgeon sees the mucosal folds of the bowel lumen. A through and through injury may be missed and only becomes apparent if there is fecal soiling or smell or the patient subsequently developes peritonitis.

When small bowel has been perforated the laparoscope should be left *in situ* while a minilaparotomy is performed and the bowel exteriorised and repaired. A large vertical incision is not usually necessary provided the site of the injury can be positively indentified and the surgeon is sure it is confined to a single perforation. Small bowel injuries can usually be closed with a simple purse-string suture. Intravenous antibiotics and intravenous fluids should be given until distension disappears and bowel sounds return to normal.

The most common site of injury to the large bowel is the transverse or descending colon. The classical treatment is to perform laparotomy to identify the hole because of the risk of contamination of the pelvis with feces. If the surgeon is expert and the injury is small, it may be permissible to repair the bowel by laparoscopic suturing provided that the principles of good management are not compromised. The defect should be closed in two layers in such a way as to avoid stricture formation. This should be followed by peritoneal lavage, abdominal drainage and the administration of antibiotics.

Laparotomy should be performed if the surgeon does not have sufficient skill to suture laparoscopically, if the injury is severe or if its extent cannot be defined. Transverse colostomy should be performed if there is significant fecal soiling but if the injury is small the hole may be repaired and the abdomen closed with drainage. Frequently the injury is not recognized at the time of surgery in which case the patient may present two or three days later with signs of peritonitis including abdominal distension, vomiting, rebound tenderness and pyrexia. A general surgeon should be consulted. The patient requires intravenous fluid and antibiotics, immediate laparotomy and meticulous examination of the whole of the intestine to determine the site and extent of the injury. A small injury may be treated by suturing or resection of the damaged area with end-to-end anastomosis and drainage. Larger injuries, especially if there has been delay in diagnosis, require exteriorization and temporary colostomy. The peritoneal cavity must be washed out with an antiseptic solution and the abdomen closed with drainage. It is important in all cases to enlist the help of a general surgeon and to ensure that documentation is complete and accurate because legal action may follow.

INJURY TO VESSELS IN THE ABDOMINAL WALL

Bleeding from the incision arely gives rise to concern and usually stops with firm pressure. Superficial bruising at the site of trocar insertion is common (**18.4**). The bruise may present an alarming appearance but always resolves in a few days. It is exceptional for superficial bruising to require incision and drainage.

Bleeding from injury to the deep inferior epigastric vessels is more serious. The vessels are at risk during insertion of the secondary trocars. Injury may be avoided by transillumination of the abdominal wall before insertion of the trocars but this is only appropriate in very thin patients. The vessels may be seen laparoscopically lying lateral to the obliterated umbilical arteries but frequently it is impossible to visualize them. The vessels may be avoided by inserting the trocars within the 'safety triangle' which is bounded by the obliterated umbilical arteries laterally, the roof of the bladder inferiorally and has its apex at the umbilicus or by inserting the trocars lateral to the rectus sheath taking care to angle them medially to avoid the external iliac vessels.

Injury to the deep inferior epigastric artery is characterized either by blood dripping, or even spurting, into the abdomen from the site of the secondary trocar. Alternatively an abdominal wall hematoma may develop with alarming speed and attain a considerable size.

The treatment is usually simple. The trocar and cannula should not be removed because they fix the position of the perforation and prevent the vessel from moving away thus making treatment more difficult. The easiest procedure is to remove the trocar from its slieve and insert a Foley catheter, inflate it and apply traction.

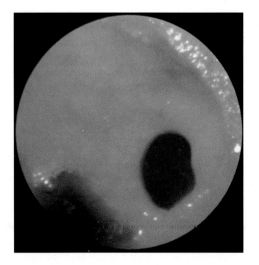

18.3 Perforation of stomach by trochar.

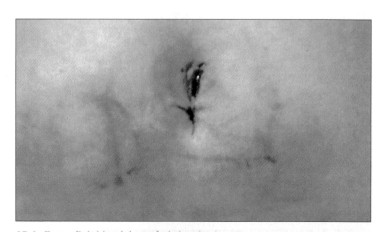

18.4 Superficial bruising of abdominal wall.

Alternatively the skin incision may be enlarged to 2 cm in length to expose the surface of the rectus sheath. A round-bodied needle can then be inserted through the full thickness of the abdominal wall from the sheath to the peritoneum under laparoscopic control. The needle point should be brought out again to the rectus sheath and the knot tied on the sheath. It may be necessary to insert two sutures, one above and one below the bleeding vessel. This is preferable to suturing on the skin which is painful and produces an unsightly scar. If these measures do not control the bleeding it may be necessary to enlarge the incision, locate the vessel and ligate it.

INJURY TO OMENTAL OR MESENTERIC VESSELS

Insertion of the primary trocar and cannula may injure omental or mesenteric vessels. Injury from insertion of the secondary instruments can only occur if they are not kept under constant visual control. The bleeding vessel can usually be grasped and ligated or coagulated with bipolar forceps but care should be taken not to coagulate too much mesentery in case there be ischemic damage to a loop of bowel or thermal injury to the bowel wall (**18.5**).

Injury by a Verress' needle to a mesenteric vessel my not be recognized at the time of injury because the telescope is directed into the pelvis or the bleeding is hidden behind loops of bowel. The patient may present 24 to 48 hours later with abdominal pain, palor and tachycardia. Laparotomy is now necessary. Occasionally a hematoma may develop which can be diagnosed by ultrasound. This may be treated by laparoscopic drainage or allowed to resorb if there is no associated pyrexia.

INJURY TO THE GREAT VESSELS.

The inferior vena cava and aorta are at risk from injury from the Veress' needle and the primary or secondary trocars if they are not inserted correctly. Any patient is at risk because the distance between the anterior abdominal wall and the great vessels is only one-third of the depth of the trunk (**18.6**). Predisposing factors include thin patients and blind insertion of the primary trocar. Injury can be avoided by elevating the abdominal wall and directing the trocar towards the pelvis at an angle to miss the sacral promontary. Laterally inserted secondary trocars should be directed medially under visual control to miss the external iliac vessels (**18.7**, **18.8**).

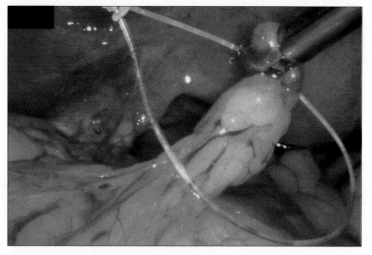

18.5 Ligation of vessel with endoloop.

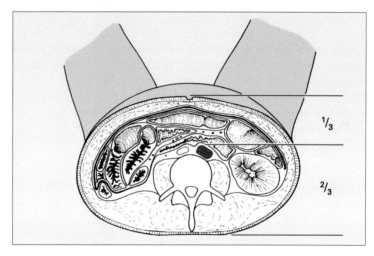

18.6 The distance from the abdominal wall to the great vessels is one third of the depth of the trunk.

These injuries are life-threatening. The first warning may come from the anesthetist who may detect a fall in blood pressure, the development of shock and possibly cardiac arrest. The surgeon may see blood welling into the pelvic cavity but, because the posterior abdominal wall peritoneum is loosely attached to the anterior surface of the aorta and inferior vena cava, a hematoma of up to 4 liters may develop without intraperitoneal spillage. If there is unexplained

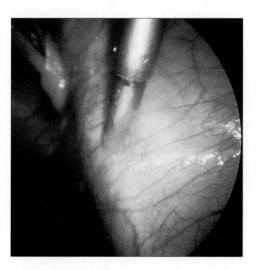

18.7 Danger of trauma to external iliac artery with secondary trocar even with retracting guard.

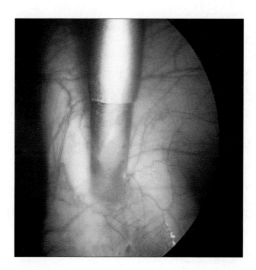

18.8 Danger of trauma to either artery or vein.

collapse, the patient must be rapidly resuscitated and an immediate search made for a cause (**18.9**).

A small leak from the inferior vena cava may not be immediately apparent. It may be temporarily controlled by the raised intra-abdominal pressure produced by the pneumoperitoneum and the lowered venous pressure resulting from the Trendelenburg position. As soon as the operation is complete and the abdominal and venous pressure return to normal, bleeding will recommence and the patient will become shocked.

Immediate resuscitation and laparotomy must be carried out and a vascular surgeon called. The bleeding point must be identified and pressure applied until skilled help arrives. Soft clamps should be placed above and below the injury and the vessel sutured with silk or vicryl to produce a water-tight seal.

BLEEDING FROM OTHER SOURCES

Bleeding frequently occurs during the dissection of ovarian cysts, myomectomy or the excision of an endometriotic cyst. The site of bleeding can usually be identified and controlled with bipolar coagulation, fulgaration or sutured using an endoloop ligature. Minor oozing may be controlled by the raised intra-abdominal pressure of the pneumoperitoneum or by lavage at 40° C. It is essential to examine all raw areas at the completion of surgery. The intra-abdominal pressure should be lowered to allow recognition of oozing points which may otherwise be missed.

THERMAL INJURIES

Burns from electrical current were one of the most common complications when monopolar tubal coagulation was the principle method of female sterilization. The incidence of burns was dramatically reduced by the introduction of bipolar and thermocoagulation. However, the vast increase in laparoscopic surgery both by gynecologists and surgeons who have not previously been aware of these complications has led to an increase in the incidence of electric burns.

Monopolar current passes into the patient's body from the electrode which may be forceps, a needle or probe. It then passes through the tissues to the return plate and thence to the generator. The current will usually take the path of least resistance which is often over the surface of bowel. It cannot pass through tissues which have been dessicated. This helps to determine its pathway. The effect depends on the power and power density which, in turn, depends on the area and duration of contact. If the area of contact is small and the power density high, such as at the tip of the

forceps, the tissues will be burnt. If the area of contact is large, as at the return plate, and the power density low, there will be no burn. However, if on its journey from the electrode to the return plate, there is small area of contact between two organs, there may be an inadvertent burn distant from the operation field.

Bipolar electrocoagulation removes some of these hazards. In this technique the current passes from one blade of the forceps through the intervening tissue to the other blade. There is thus less risk of distant burns but the risk of burning adjacent tissues by direct spread of heat remains.

Electrical safety must be maintained at all times. Electrosurgical units must be serviced at regular intervals. Defects in the insulation of forceps or scissors may produce burns on adjacent surfaces such as bowel when monopolar current is used. The insulation should be regularly checked.

SKIN BURNS

If the monitoring system is not properly earthed burns may occur at other sites such as ECG electrodes or points of contact with metal such as lithotomy poles. If ancillary instruments are not properly insulated there may be skin burns at the site of the secondary cannulae. Large areas of skin necrosis may result from an improperly applied or faulty return plate although modern electrosurgical generators will not allow current flow if the plate is misapplied.

BOWEL BURNS

The organs at most risk from accidental electrical burns are the large and small bowel. The injury may range from superficial serosal blanching to full thickness burns of the intestinal wall. It is reasonable to treat a minor superficial burn expectantly. Significant blanching indicates a more serious burn which, although it does not immediately produce a fecal fistula, may undergo avascular necrosis and result in delayed fistula formation. Clinically the patient may seem to be reasonably well for 48–72 hours or longer. Eventually she develops a fecal peritonitis characterised by the onset of insidious symptoms of malaise, sometimes low-grade pyrexia, abdominal discomfort and anorexia. Because the onset of symptoms is delayed the medical attendant may not be aware of the possibility of a bowel burn and may not recognise the signs of developing peritonitis. This leads to delay in readmission to hospital and the institution of appropriate treatment. Commonly these patients become very ill and eventually have laparotomy, colostomy, drainage and frequently prolonged ill health, Recourse to legal action is common.

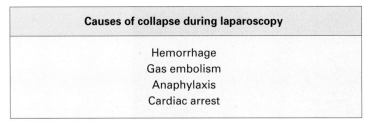

Causes of collapse during laparoscopy
Hemorrhage
Gas embolism
Anaphylaxis
Cardiac arrest

18.9 Causes of collapse during laparoscopy.

LASER BURNS

Carbon dioxide and Nd:YAG laser are commonly used at laparoscopy to treat endometriosis or to lyse adhesions. Accidental burns can occur distal to the target organ if no backstop is used in the case of CO_2 laser or the laser is fired inadvertently. The risk of burns is particulary high when treating deposits of endometriosis on bowel or on the peritoneum overlying the ureter or bladder.

No surgeon should use laser without special training and without observing all the rules of laser safety. These include the wearing of goggles by all members of the operating room staff, the posting of warning notices on the operating room doors and screening windows to prevent injury to passers by. Every institution should have a laser safety officer who must ensure all regulations are obeyed.

INJURIES FROM INSTRUMENTS

The commonest organ to be injured by scissors is the bowel. This is liable to occur during enterolysis for the sequelae of pelvic inflammatory disease (PID) or endometriosis when loops of bowel may be adherent to the uterus or each other. In this condition mechanical or hydro energy is the only form of energy which should be used. Laser and electrosurgery should be avoided because of the risk of thermal injury. Hydrodissection is the safest form of energy because the fluid will only pass along planes of cleavage and will not perforate the bowel.

The bowel may be cut or traumatized by traction with forceps. The injury may be immediately evident but can be missed. There may be no fecal soiling. If there is doubt, it is helpful to fill the pelvis with fluid and watch for bubbles from a fecal fistula.

Any patient known to have intestinal adhesions should have a preoperative bowel preparation. If this has been done then it is possible to effect primary suture of the tear either by laparoscopic suturing or by laparotomy. Otherwise it is wise to carry out colostomy for large bowel injury although small bowel may be sutured, antibiotics prescribed and the abdomen drained.

INJURIES TO THE URETER

Ureteric injuries are rare during diagnostic or minor laparoscopic surgery but are more common with advanced operations. There are three common sites for ureteric injury. The first is at the infundibulopelvic ligament where the ureter crosses the pelvic brim and the common iliac vessels. The ureter is at risk during dessication or stapling of the ovarian vessels during oophorectomy. The second is where the ureter passes deep to the ovarian fossa and may be damaged when operating on an ovary densely adherent to the pelvic sidewall as a result of endometriosis (**18.10**, **18.11**). The third is at the ureteric canal where the ureter passes under the uterine artery and may be damaged during laparoscopic hysterectomy either by burning or by the misapplication of staples. It is also

at risk at this site during uterine nerve ablation. It is essential at any operation to identify accurately the course of the ureter and to ensure no device or thermal energy is used in close proximity to it. At completion of the operation the ureter should be inspected again to ensure normal peristaltic movement is taking place.

The use of ureteric catheters is controversial. Some surgeons advocate the use of an ordinary catheter to identify the position of the ureter, some use an illuminated catheter to recognize it more easily but most rely on being able to identify the ureter by its peristaltic movement which is less obvious if it has a catheter in its lumen.

Ureteric injury may not be recognised immediately but the patient may return a few days later with a uretero-vaginal fistula or with urine draining into the peritoneal cavity causing abdominal distension, peritonitism and electrolyte imbalance. The diagnosis can be established by an intravenous pyelogram. A urologist should be consulted. These injuries can usually be treated by passing a double J-shaped catheter into the ureter following which spontaneous healing often occurs. Occasionally if a large length of ureter has been damaged or if it the injury is near the bladder insertion, it may be necessary to perform laparotomy and end-to-end anastomosis or ureteric implant.

INCISIONAL HERNIA

Incisional hernias containing omentum or loops of small bowel are well recognized as complications of advanced laparoscopic surgery. The laparoscopes in general use are 10–11 mm in diameter, the cannulae used to extract tissues are also 11 mm and the disposable cannulae to introduce stapling devices are 12 mm. Occasionally one of the abdominal incisions is enlarged to extract tissues too big to go through a cannula.

Any incision which is 7 mm or larger may lead to a Richter's hernia containing omentum or, rarely, bowel. All such incisions should be repaired in two layers – deep fascia and skin. It is not possible to suture the peritoneum of a laparoscopy without a special disposable J-needle (Rockets of London, Watford, UK) incision so it is always possible for a small amount of tissue to become incarcerated in the abdominal wall between the peritoneum and fascia. If this is recognized early it should be replaced but if it contains bowel and becomes obstructed, laparotomy, resection of the infarcted loop and end-to-end anastomosis may be needed.

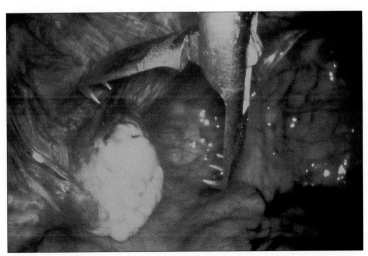

18.10 Grasping and mobilizing adherent ovary. The ureter lies on the lateral surface.

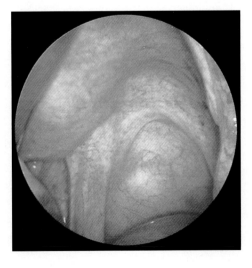

18.11 Oophrectomy in fully mobilized ovary.

COMPLICATIONS OF ANESTHESIA

The risks of anesthesia are the same as for any other form of surgery but may be compounded by the need for a steep Trendelenburg position and the influence of the pneumoperitoneum on cardiac function. An endotracheal tube and positive pressure respiration are essential for all but the simplest forms of laparoscopy. This should prevent regurgitation and inhalation of gastric contents and allows elimination of CO_2 from the circulation. The minimum necessary monitoring should be an ECG record and pulse oximetry.

OTHER COMPLICATIONS

INJURIES FROM THE OPERATING TABLE

The patient may be injured by any of the moving parts of the operating table. Injury can be caused to the nerves of the sacral plexus, the hip or sacro-iliac joints. Abduction of the arm may also produce a brachial plexus injury. Prolonged compression of the legs may lead to deep vein thrombosis. No part of the patient should be in contact with metallic parts of the table when electrical energy is being used.

It must always be remembered that the unconscious patient is not able to defend herself. It is the surgeon's responsibility to ensure that she is not at risk.

UTERUS

The uterus or cervix may be traumatized by the application and insertion of the cervical tenaculum, the hydropertubation cannula or a curette. The cervix should always be inspected at the completion of the operation and any bleeding controlled by pressure from sponge forceps. Suturing may occasionally be needed.

PELVIC INFLAMMATORY DISEASE

There is a small risk of producing or exacerbating PID by any procedure involving insufflation or surgery on the tubes. Postoperative PID is probably less common than with conventional surgery but still does occur occasionally

CONCLUSION

Most complications are avoidable. Careful assessment of the patient's needs, the facilities available and the surgeon's skill should enable the correct treatment to be offered. It is essential that the surgeon remains humble at all times. No operation which is too difficult should be attempted. It is never too late to change to laparotomy if the condition is demands it or if the surgeon's skill is insufficient. The alternative is disaster for the patient, well earned criticism for the surgeon and unjustifiable expense for the insurance company.

FURTHER READING

Baadsgaard SE, Bille S and Egeblad K. Major vascular injury during gynaecological endoscopy. *Acta Obstet Gynecol Scand*, 1989; **68**:283–285

Basil S, Nisolle M and Donnez J. Comlications of endoscopic surgery in gynaecology. *Gynaecological Endoscopy*, 1993; **2**:199-209

Chamberlain GVP, Orr CJB and Sharp F. Litigation – obstetrics and gynaecology. Proc 14th Study Group, Royal College of Obstetricians and Gynaecologists, London

Corfman RS, Diamond MP, DeCherney AH. Complications of laparoscopy and hysteroscopy. Blackwell Scientific Publications, Oxford, 1993

Gordon AG and Taylor PJ. Practical Laparoscopy, Blackwell Scientific Publications, Oxford, 1993

Howard FM. Breaking new ground or just digging a hole? *J Gynec Surg* 1992; **3**:143–155

Loffer FD and Pent D. Indications, contraindications and complications of laparoscopy. *Obstetrical and Gynecological Survey*, 1975; **30**: 407–427

Querleu D, Chevallier L, Chapron C and Bruhat MA. Complications of gynaecological laparoscopic surgery. A French multicentre study. Gynaec Endoscopy 1993; **2**:3–6

Report of RCOG Working Party on Training in Gynaecological Endoscopic Surgery, RCOG Press, London 1994

Soderstrom RM. Bowel injury litigation after laparoscopy. *J Amer Assoc Gynec Lap*. 1993; **1**:74–77

Sutton C and Diamond MP. Endoscopy for Gynaecologists. WB Saunders, London 1993

Yuspe A. Pneumoperitoneum,needle and trocar injuries in laparoscopy. *J Reprod Med*, 1990; **35**:485–490

INSTRUMENTS FOR DIAGNOSTIC AND OPERATIVE HYSTEROSCOPY

19

B Victor Lewis

INTRODUCTION

Hysteroscopy is a simple operation suitable for performing in the outpatient or office in the majority of patients. A simple hysteroscope consists of a telescope and a sheath (**19.1, 19.2**). The diameter of the telescope is usually 3.5 mm and the sheath 4 mm. The optical system in most rigid telescopes is a Hopkins rod lens system which gives a bright undistorted image as clear at the periphery of the field of view as at the centre. Telescopes have an angle of view of 0°12° or 30° depending on the preference of the surgeon. For simple diagnostic hysteroscopy a 0° or 12° telescope is probably the best because orientation within the uterine cavity is easier.

A flexible hysteroscope is preferred by some surgeons (**19.3**). This instrument is much more expensive than a simple rod lens telescope and produces a grainy view because of the fiberoptics. It has no advantage over the rigid telescopes except that it is easier to visualize the cornual orifice but this theoretical advantage is marginal.

DISTENSION MEDIA

The uterine cavity is a potential cavity only. In order to perform hysteroscopy the cavity must be distended using carbon dioxide gas or fluid. Gas must be insufflated from a hysteroflator which delivers a maximum flow of carbon dioxide of 100 mls per minute with a maximum pressure of 100 mmHg (**19.4, 19.5**). For simple diagnostic hysteroscopy the intrauterine pressure should not exceed 40 or 50 mmHg and the flow rate should not exceed 60 mls per minute. Deaths have occurred from carbon dioxide embolus when a high flow carbon dioxide source has been inadvertently used. Diagnostic hysteroscopy takes only a few minutes so the amount of carbon dioxide entering the abdominal cavity is only a a few hundred milliliters and is rapidly absorbed. Carbon dioxide diagnostic hysteroscopy is simple and gives a very good view particularly when the operation is performed in post-menopausal women or in the post-menstrual phase of the cycle. In the presence of blood, carbon dioxide causes bubbles which restricts the view.

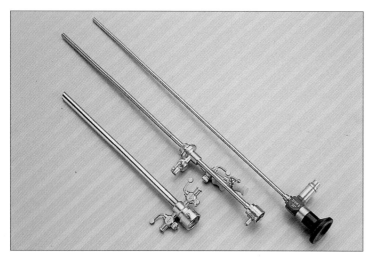

19.1 Diagnostic hysteroscope telescope with 30° lens with sheath showing inflow and outflow channels and channels for scissors or biopsy forceps.

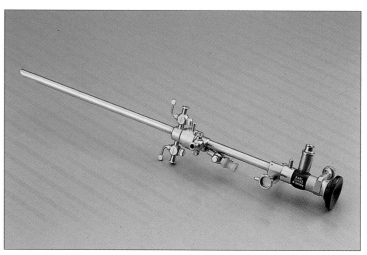

19.2 Hysteroscope assembled with sheath showing inflow and outflow channels and channel for biopsy forceps or scissors.

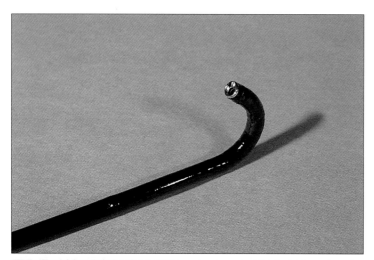

19.3 Tip of flexible hysteroscope.

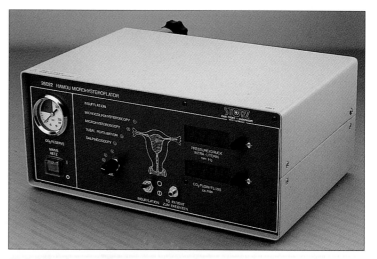

19.4 Microhysteroflator measuring intrauterine pressure and carbon dioxide flow rate.

The simplest method of distending the uterine cavity is with saline either injected with a 50 ml syringe or by gravity from an infusion bag elevated above the patient. Excess fluid escapes through the cervix around the sheath. This system is easy, cheap and gives a good view. Hyskon – a high molecular weight dextran, is popular in the United States but it is viscous and must be warmed prior to use. It has good optical qualities and allows an undistorted image even in the presence of blood. However, Hyskon is expensive and if it is allowed to dry it can block the stop-cocks on the inflow and outflow channels. Its other disadvantage is that it can cause acute anaphylactic reactions. If the diagnostic hysteroscopy is prolonged Hyskon enters the peritoneal cavity and is absorbed into the circulation where its hyperosmolar activity may lead to circulatory overload. It has been withdrawn from the market in the United Kingdom.

LIGHT SOURCE

Hysteroscopy should be performed with a high intensity light source. There is a tendency for cables to be mishandled and the fibers inside the cables can crack over a period of time which restricts transmission of light. For simple diagnostic hysteroscopy a low power light source of 150 watts is adequate but if a video camera is used a high intensity zenon or halogen light of at least 250 watts is essential.

THE MICROCOLPOHYSTEROSCOPE

A simple hysteroscope allows magnification of the image when the telescope is close to the object being viewed but panoramic hysteroscopy is at unit magnification. The microcolpohysteroscope has both a direct and an offset ocular which gives four levels of magnification (**19.6**). The telescope is 4 mm in diameter and 25 mm in length. The direct lens allows observation at unity or at a magnification x60 if the lens is in contact with the endometrium. The offset lens gives magnification x20 or x150. At high magnification the cellular structure of the endocervix and endometrium can be studied. The transformation zone can be identified when it is hidden within the endocervical cavity and cannot be seen with a simple colposcope. The columnar epithelium can be stained with Watermans blue dye and the squamous epithelium can be stained brown with Lugols iodine which produces a distinct border at the squamocolumnar junction. However, the interpretation of the visual findings is difficult and most observers find it technically difficult to use at higher magnification.

ANCILLARY INSTRUMENTS

A diagnostic sheath is made of stainless steel with a single inflow stop-cock for distension with fluid or gas. If ancillary instruments are used an operative sheath is needed which has two stop-cocks for inflow and outflow of the distension medium with a separate channel to permit the passage of ancillary instruments (**19.7**). These include a range of biopsy or grasping forceps, scissors and probes or laser fibers. The most commonly used instrument is a simple grasping forceps for biopsy under direct vision (**19.8**).

VIDEO SYSTEMS

Sophisticated cameras and video systems are available from a number of manufacturers. Light-weight two or three chip cameras produce superb images with minimal distortion (**19.9**). The image is displayed on a monitor and can be recorded on high quality videotape. Individual photographs can be made with a camera providing there is a high intensity light source or an external flash regulated by a computer. Today, permanent images can be obtained immediately with polaroid pictures which can be incorporated in the clinical notes. More sophisticated recorders allow slide photographs to be made of sufficiently high quality for projection.

RESECTOSCOPES

Most resectoscopes are modifications of cystoscopes and have an oval cross-sectional outline. The sheaths are wider than for diagnostic hysteroscopy, being about 7 mm in diameter with separate inflow and outflow channels for fluid distension. The working element is controlled by a proximal grip and may be either a ball, cylinder, cutting loop or knife. The working length of the instruments vary from 18–35 cm and the outer sheath diameter varies from 6.3 mm (19 Fr) to 9 mm (27 Fr). The metallic components are made from surgical stainless steel and the insulation is usually teflon.

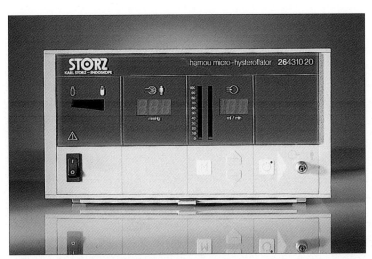

19.5 Electronic microhysteroflator.

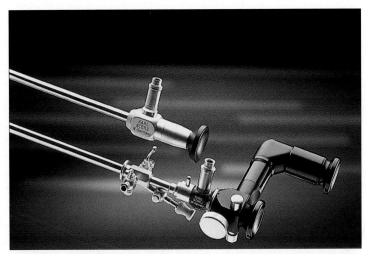

19.6 The microcolpohysteroscope with offset ocular which provides four magnifications.

There are two types of working mechanisms: the active and passive (**19.10**). The element of the active mechanism protrudes from the sheath at rest and requires the surgeon to withdraw it by traction on the trigger. In the passive mechanism the surgeon advances the element by pulling the trigger mechanism and return to the sheath is automatic when the pressure is relaxed (**19.11**). The pas-sive system is safer than the active system and is less likely to cause perforation of the uterus. The cutting loops vary in depth and diam-eter. Loops that are bent forward are used for resecting the fun-dus and cornua; loops that are bent backwards towards the surgeon are used to resect the endometrium on the uterine side walls. A 9 mm, resectoscope uses an 8 mm (24Fr) cutting loop

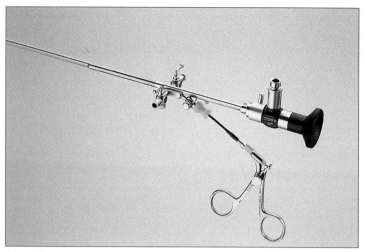

19.7 Hysteroscope with operating sheath and biopsy forceps in place.

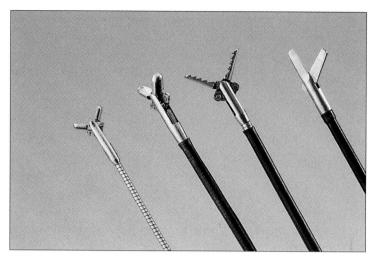

19.8 Range of grasping forceps, biopsy forceps and scissors.

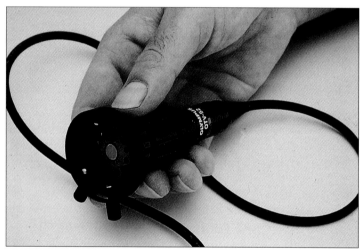

19.9 Chip camera for direct coupling to telescope eye-piece.

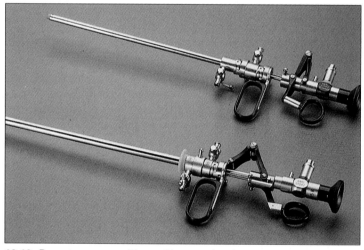

19.10 Resectoscopes with working mechanism.

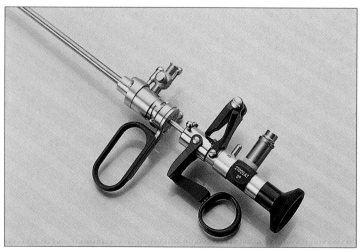

19.11 Resectoscope – close-up of working mechanism.

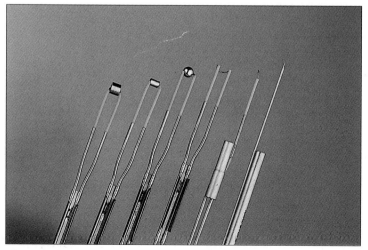

19.12 Rollerball, rollerbars, resectoscope loop and knife.

which is safe and efficient. Smaller loops may prolong the operating time and increase the risk of uterine perforation.

If the technique of electrocoagulation of the endometrium is used there is a wide range of ancillary instruments. The usual technique is to use a rollerbar as opposed to a metal ball but both come in large and small sizes (**19.12**, **19.13**). The larger bars or balls are more efficient in completing the operation in shorter time but they restrict the view of the surgeon, so for a normal size uterus the smaller device is preferable.

FLUID DISTENSION

If electro-resection or rollerball ablation is used a non-electrolytic solution such as 1.5% glycine is employed to distend the uterine cavity. Saline is suitable for laser ablation. Glycine can be infused by gravity from a 3 liter bag elevated 1 m above the patient. It is important to note that the volume of fluid in these bags can vary by 10% either way which may give rise to discrepancies when the fluid input and outflow are compared. Strict attention to the volume of fluid infused and collected is necessary in order to recognize intravasation of fluid into the circulation at an early stage because of the risk of pulmonary and cerebral edema and hyperamonemia.

An alternative but more expensive method of infusing fluid is to use an electronic pump (**19.14**, **19.15**). Several pumps are available which are pressure but not flow limited. When a fixed intra-uterine pressure of approximately 100 mmHg is set, the pump automatically turns itself off if this pressure is exceeded.

ELECTROSURGICAL UNIT

Solid state electrosurgical generators are used to deliver a pure cutting current, a pure coagulating current or a blended current. Most electrosurgical generators have a basic frequency of 475–750 KHz. In the cut mode the reference signal is amplified to produce a continuous output whereas in the coagulation or blend mode the reference signal is modulated through an electronic gate by an oscillator and an interrupted wave form is produced. The patient circuit consists of an active electrode which is usually the resectoscope loop or the rollerball. The current flows through the patient and returns to the generator via an electrode pad placed on the patient's thigh. The current density is highest under the resectoscope loop. Because the electrode is small it produces a concentration of current which generates heat. The modern generators have built in safety mechanisms that cut off the power if the dispersive electrode is not applied correctly (**19.16**). It is difficult to

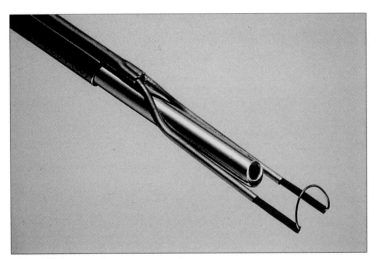

19.13 Close-up of resectoscope loop.

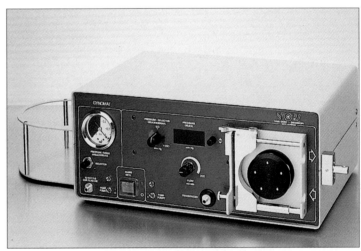

19.14 Electronic infusion pump – pressure controlled.

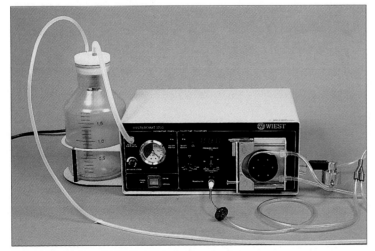

19.15 Hysteromat electronic infusion pump.

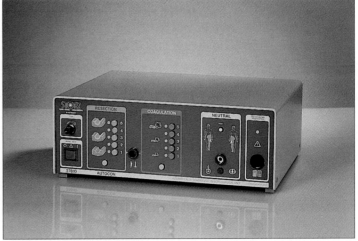

19.16 The electronic generator.

compare the power values for the different machines but it is usual to use a blend 100 watts cutting and 50 watts coagulating. If the power setting is too low the resected chips stick to the electrode but excessive tissue charring can occur if the power is too high.

The optimal setting for rollerball ablation varies but if the instrument is used in the pure cutting mode tissue is less likely to stick to the ball.

LASER

In laser ablation, Nd:YAG laser with a flexible quartz laser fiber is introduced into the uterine cavity through the operating channel of the multi channel hysteroscope. The Nd:YAG laser has a wavelength of 1.064 mu which destroys the tissue to the depth of 4–6mm only. Therefore, if this technique of ablation is used the patient should be pretreated with Danazol or GnRH agonists to thin the endometrium before surgery.

DIAGNOSTIC HYSTEROSCOPY 20

B Victor Lewis

INTRODUCTION

The traditional method of investigating women with irregular menstrual bleeding by dilatation and curettage is diagnostically inaccurate and therapeutically ineffective. The operation should be replaced by diagnostic hysteroscopy and directed biopsy. In the majority of women hysteroscopy is an out-patient or office procedure which can be performed without anesthesia. Preliminary counselling and explanation is essential and the patient must be accompanied by a relative or friend. The examination couch should be comfortable and the lithotomy poles should be angled forward at an angle of 45° so the patient's hips are not hyperflexed. A good light source must be available and ideally there should be facilities for permanent recording of the findings. A video system is excellent for teaching and also to demonstrate to the patient any pathology that is discovered. Out-patient hysteroscopy is not suitable for nervous patients and may not be suitable for nulliparous or post-menopausal women with a stenosed cervix. With patience, office hysteroscopy can be performed in most women but some patients require a para-cervical block or an injection of local anesthetic into the cervix. No attempt should be made to pass the hysteroscope until the anesthetic is fully effective which takes 3–5 minutes.

In post-menopausal women some authorities recommend a short course of estrogen tablets because this softens the cervix and allows a small dilator to pass through the endocervical canal. Although it is unlikely a short course of estrogen will cause endometrial hyperplasia, this treatment is not popular because of the potential risk.

Hysteroscopy should be preceded by a bimanual examination to determine whether the body of the uterus is anteverted or retroverted. A single tooth tenaculum is first attached to the anterior lip of the cervix which allows traction on the cervix while a fine uterine sound is passed to measure the uterine length and to determine the angle of the cervical canal. It may be necessary to pass several dilators of increasing size but they should not be passed too deeply into the uterus because they cause bleeding which obscures the view. In most women cervical dilatation is neither desirable or necessary. If possible hysteroscopy should be performed in the immediate post-menstrual phase of the menstrual cycle when the endometrium is thin and there is minimal bleeding. This is not always easy to arrange particularly in women with irregular menstrual cycles or intermenstrual bleeding and in these women blood can be washed away with saline. The rigid hysteroscope is passed through the endocervical canal under direct vision. If carbon dioxide gas is used at a flow rate of 40 ml per minute and a pressure of 50 mmHg, the gas bubble at the end of the telescope distends the endocervical canal and allows atraumatic passage of the hysteroscope into the uterine cavity (**20.1**). Sometimes it is helpful to pass the hysteroscope through the cervix at a magnification of x20 if the Hamou telescope is being used (**20.2**).

When the telescope enters the uterine cavity a panoramic view of the uterus at unit magnification is seen (**20.3**). The main causes of poor vision are carbon dioxide gas bubbles, blood in the uterine cavity or inadequate illumination. Because the telescope is only 4 mm in diameter a high powered light source is essential particularly if a video camera is used. Gas bubbles usually disperse with time as the carbon dioxide leaks around the cervix or escapes through the tubal ostia. If blood obscures the view it should be washed away with a continuous flow of a small volume of normal saline.

In the post-menstrual phase of the cycle the endometrium is flat and atrophic. A similar picture occurs in a post-menopausal woman but the endometrium is even whiter. The cornual orifices are easily seen if the telescope is angulated or rotated depending on whether the lens is 0° or 30°. As the telescope is advanced towards the ostia a magnified picture appears. As the gas pressure rises the cornual orifice opens and then shuts as the pressure falls when carbon dioxide leaks into the abdomen (**20.4**, **20.5**). The fundus of the uterus is convex into the uterine cavity with each cornu recessed. This appearance can produce an artefact suggesting a bicornuate uterus but it is normal. In a true bicorunate uterus the septum can extend almost to the endocervical canal and if the telescope is passed to one side of the septum the diagnosis can be missed.

In a pre-menstrual woman the endometrium is more vascular and edematous and may be indented with the tip of the telescope but this manoeuver can make the endometrium bleed. If the end of the telescope is placed close to the endometrium the openings of glands can be seen. After a panoramic view of the endometrium is obtained a directed biopsy should be taken from the endometrium. Alternatively if there is no focal lesion the telescope can be removed and a biopsy obtained by curettage or aspiration.

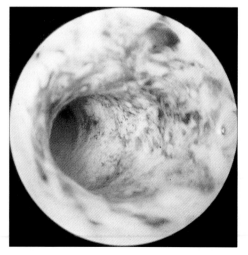

20.1 Endocervical canal.

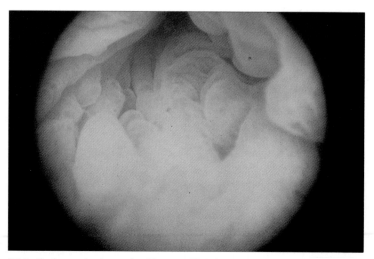

20.2 Endocervical canal x 20 magnification.

PATHOLOGIC FINDINGS

MUCOUS OR ENDOMETRIAL POLYPS

Just before menstruation the endometrium is thick and has a polypoid appearance that can be mistakenly thought to be abnormal. The timing of hysteroscopy is therefore essential and should be carefully recorded. A true adenoma may be associated with endometrial hyperplasia and is polypoidal in shape but hardly ever exceeds the size of a grape and is usually no larger than a pea. Histopathologic examination of a biopsy will show endometrial glands and stroma which respond to ovarian hormones. Most mucous polyps are multiple and tend to recur unless the underlying hormonal dysfunction is corrected (**20.6**). A single endometrial polyp may be symptomless but if the tip becomes necrotic and ulcerated it will cause bleeding. A mucous polyp can also cause dysmenorrhea. Blind curettage is likely to miss the endometrial polyp and it is best removed with a biopsy forceps under direct hysteroscopic vision.

FIBROID POLYPS

Fibroids are the commonest of all pelvic tumors and are composed of muscle fibers with connective tissue. They tend to be spherical in shape surrounded by compressed normal myometrium which produces a pseudocapsule. The presence of a filling defect may be apparent on a hysterosalpingogram but hysteroscopy is necessary to determine its nature (**20.7**). Sub-mucous fibroid polyps are relatively avascular with a white appearance which distinguishes them from endometrial polyps on hysteroscopy (**20.8, 20.9**). They are often associated with endometrial hyperplasia, adenomyosis or cancer of the corpus uteri. Dual pathology should always be considered. A sub-mucous fibroid polyp is usually small but may cause heavy periods and spasmodic dysmenorrhea. Small fibroids can easily be seen and identified with the hysteroscope but paradoxically a large fibroid filling the uterine cavity may be missed because the telescope slips between one side of the fibroid and the endometrium. This possibility should always be considered. If fibroids are seen, their number and position should be recorded. It is important to examine the fibroid from all angles by rotating the telescope so a pedicle can be seen or an assessment can be made as to what proportion of the fibroid is intramural. The length of the uterine cavity is also important when a decision has to be made as to whether a fibroid is suitable for transcervical resection or laser ablation. Fibroids with a narrow pedicle are easily removed by cut-

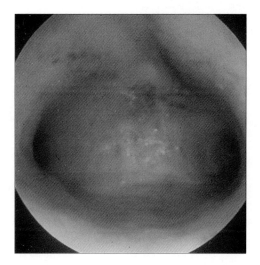

20.3 Panoramic view of the uterus.

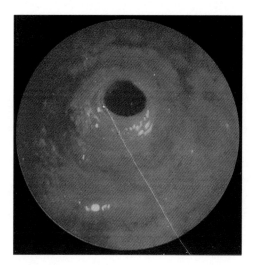

20.4 Magnified view of tubal ostium (opened).

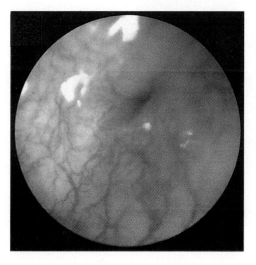

20.5 Magnified view of tubal ostium (closed).

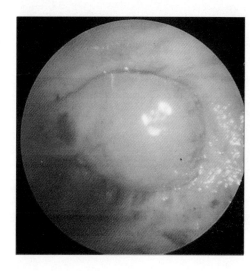

20.6 Endometrial polyp.

ting the pedicle and, if it cannot be extracted with polyp forceps, it can be left *in situ* to be expelled spontaneously. A fibroid that is mainly intramural can be resected in two separate operations but great care must be taken not to perforate the uterus.

INTRAUTERINE CONTRACEPTIVE DEVICES

It is common for an intrauterine device to be misplaced usually because the tail wraps itself around one arm of the coil and is withdrawn into the uterus. It is easy to see the coil with a hysteroscope and remove it with grasping forceps (**20.10**). More difficulty occurs if the coil is fractured and only a small segment is left in the uterine cavity. The hysteroscope is very useful under these circumstances because blind exploration of the uterine cavity may not retrieve all the fragments. If the coil has perforated the wall of the uterus, hysteroscopy may need to be combined with laparoscopy to locate the device and remove it, either through the hysteroscope or the laparoscope depending on the depth of perforation.

RETAINED PRODUCTIONS OF CONCEPTION

Pregnancy is a contraindication to hysteroscopy and the patient's last menstrual period should always be recorded. Retained products of conception after an incomplete miscarriage are best removed by blind suction curettage but if a woman continues to bleed after an evacuation and ultrasound scans suggest there are retained products, hysteroscopy is useful in identifying a placental or fetal remnant (**20.11**, **20.12**).

ENDOMETRIAL CANCER

Most endometrial cancer occurs in post-menopausal women and presents with bleeding. Hysteroscopy not only allows the diagnosis to be confirmed and a directed punch biopsy to be obtained for histologic confirmation, but it also delineates the limits of the tumor and enables the surgeon to decide if the cancer is invading the endocervical canal. This decision is important because it influences therapy. One of the difficulties with endometrial cancer is that it bleeds and the view into the uterine cavity may be obscured. Also

women with polypoid carcinoma may have a thin uterine wall where the tumor invades the myometrium and it is easy to perforate the uterus with the rigid telescope unless it is inserted very gently, under direct vision.

It is possible to distinguish endometrial adenomatous hyperplasia (**20.13**) and carcinoma on hysteroscopic appearances but the differentiation can be difficult. The final diagnosis must always rest on histology and a biopsy is essential.

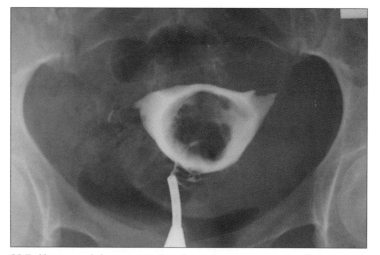

20.7 Hysterosalpingogram showing a large intrauterine filling defect.

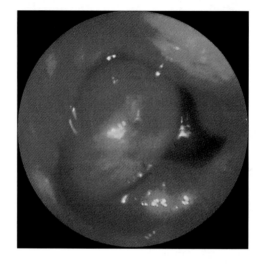

20.8 Endometrial polyp.

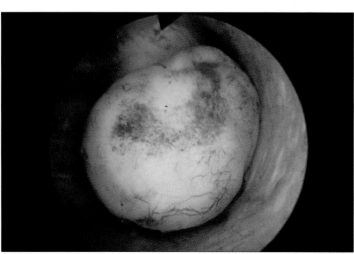

20.9 Submucous fibroid polyp on narrow pedicle.

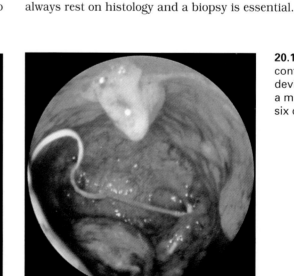

20.10 Intrauterine contraceptive device. There is also a missed abortion at six o'clock.

CONGENITAL ABNORMALITIES OF THE UTERUS AND INTRAUTERINE SYNECHIAE

A bicornuate uterus with a septum is easily seen (**20.14**) and most can be cut with scissors, electrosurgical cutting current or Nd:YAG laser. This operation should be combined with laparoscopy to ensure the fundus of the uterus is not divided. Single soft synechiae can usually be broken down with the bevelled edge of the telescope but thicker synechiae need cutting with microscissors or laser.

CATHETERIZATION OF THE FALLOPIAN TUBE

A fine catheter can sometimes be inserted into the cornual orifice of the fallopian tube for a few millimeters (**20.15**). If there is proximal cornual block with a thin septum, catheterisation of the tube using a fine catheter with a curved end and a concentric guide wire can overcome the block which can be confirmed by injecting a radio-opaque dye through the catheter (**20.16**).

In vitro fertilization or GIFT has been attempted by implanting four cell embryos into the fallopian tube through a catheter passed into the cornu through a hysteroscope. The results of this are poor.

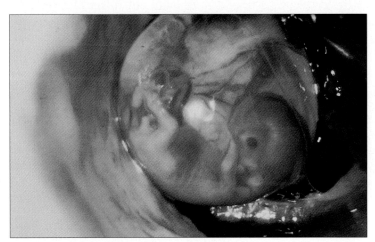

20.11 Incomplete abortion.

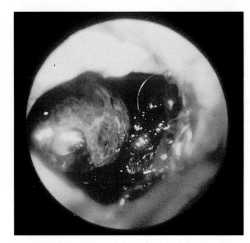

20.12 Retained products of conception.

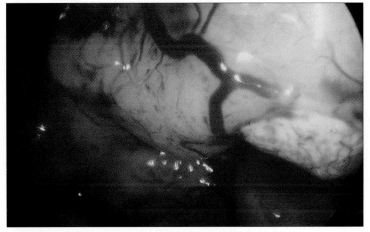

20.13 Polypoid surface of endometrial hyperplasia.

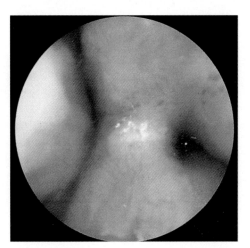

20.14 Uterine septum looking into left horn.

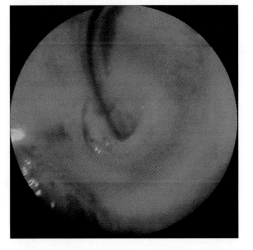

20.15
Catheterization of the fallopian tube.

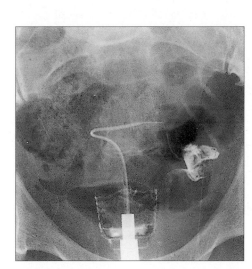

20.16
Catheterization of fallopian tube using fine catheter with guide wire. Radio-opaque dyes enter the peritoneal cavity.

MICROHYSTEROSCOPY

The Hamou modification of the standard hysteroscope allows magnified images to be obtained with the offset occular. In the contact mode the end of the telescope touches or is very close to the endometrium and the openings of individual mucous glands and even the cellular structure can be seen. Adenomyosis sometimes gives rise to an appearance which is diagnostic but the classical appearance is not always present and the diagnosis can be notoriously difficult. Hysteroscopic techniques have been described for deep biopsy of the myometrium to confirm adenomyosis, but usually the diagnosis is made in retrospect by the pathologists examining a uterus removed by hysterectomy.

CONCLUSION

Hysteroscopy is a simple inexpensive diagnostic technique which should be a standard method of investigating women with abnormal uterine bleeding. It is particularly valuable to investigate postmenopausal bleeding to exclude endometrial cancer.

Some anxiety has been expressed about the possibility of disseminating cancer cells into the abdominal cavity by flushing the cells through the fallopian tubes. However, this is unlikely and laparoscopy or laparotomy after hysteroscopy in women with endometrial cancer do not show viable endometrial cancer cells in washings from the Pouch of Douglas.

Hysteroscopy can be performed in the out-patient clinic or office in most women and is relatively free from complications. The greatest danger is perforation of the uterus which can always be avoided with good technique if the telescope is inserted through the cervical canal under direct vision without force.

FURTHER READING

Gordon AG, Taylor PJ. Practical Laparoscopy. Blackwell Scientific Publications, Oxford, 1993

Hamou J. Microhysteroscopy. *J Repro Med.* 1981; **26**:375–382

Hill NCW, Broadbent JAM, Braumann R, *et al.* Local anesthesia and cervical dilatation for out-patient hysteroscopy. *J Obstet Gynecol* 1992; **12**: 33–37

Lewis BV. Hysteroscopy in clinical practice. *J Obstet Gynecol* 1988; **9**: 47–55

Lewis BV. Hysteroscopy for the investigation of abnormal uterine bleeding. *Br J Obs Gynae* 1990; **97**: 283–284

Taylor PJ and Hamou JE. Hysteroscopy. *J Repro Med* 1984; **28**: 359–389

STERILIZATION 21

Jan Brundin

INTRODUCTION

The development of rigid and flexible hysteroscopes in the last few decades has made possible accurate visualization of the uterine cavity. Ultrasound-guided transcervical cannulation of the fallopian tube has gained an increasing importance. Cannulation may be of value for sterilization, gamete intrafallopian transfer (GIFT) or to overcome cornual obstruction.

Before the introduction of ultrasound, blind methods were used to occlude the uterine tube (**21.1**). These methods were hazardous and toxic and resulted in failures. None of these methods are now approved.

The situation is different when it comes to hysteroscopic sterilization. Electrocoagulation with a probe introduced through the cornua is dangerous and may cause bowel damage or lead to extrauterine pregnancies.

More success has been achieved with mechanical devices inserted at hysteroscopy (**21.2**). In recent years a great number of studies on various mechanical devices have been published. Today, only three of them are in current medical use. These are the hydrogelic P-block, the silicon rubber plug – the Ovabloc, and the Hamou plug.

THE P-BLOCK

The efficacy of the hydrogelic P-block has been tested during almost 20,000 cycles, i.e 1665 women years (**21.3**). During this time 35 pregnancies have occurred due to expulsion of one or both P-blocks. Thus, the Pearl index of the P-block method is 3 but with the P-block *in situ* it is 0. The method is comparatively popular and the continuation rate is 99%. Approximately 50% of the women who became pregnant after expulsion of one or both P-blocks returned after pregnancy to have new plugs inserted. The complication rate is very low. It should also be emphasized that after 2.5 years of continuous P-block use, no patient became pregnant. This is probably due to the surrounding tissue growing into the hydrogelic compound and anchoring the device. No pregnancy has occurred with the P-block in position over 12 years of observation.

The P-block is applied under local anesthesia and bilateral insertion takes 4 to 7 minutes and can be completed as an out-patient procedure (**21.4–21.9**). P-blocks may also be inserted blindly using transvaginal or abdominal-guided ultrasound with varying success.

The position of the P-blocks is easily checked either by transvaginal or transabdominal ultrasound.

Methods used for human transcervical sterilization	
Blind methods	
Silver nitrate	Froriep 1849
	Neuwirth *et al.*1974
Electrocoagulation	Kocks 1878
	Prudnikoff 1912
	Dickinson 1916
	Hyams 1934
	Sheares 1934
Commercial gum with admixtures of dust, chalk, marble, polyvinyl-pyrolidone, urethane, quinine	Rakshit 1968, 1972
Quinacrine	Zipper, Stachetti & Medel 1970
	Zipper & Insunza 1972
Methylcyanoacrylate (MCA) FEMCEPT-device/MC	Stevenson 1976 Neuwirth, Richart, Stevenson, Bolduc, Zinser, Baur, Cohen, Eldering & Argueta-Rivas 1980
Paraformaldehyde/Vagister	Dafoe 1976
Phenol-mucilage-glycerine-mixture	Research group of Tubal Occlusion by Drugs, Zhongshan China, 1979

21.1 Blind methods used for transcervical sterilization.

Methods used for human transcervical sterilization	
Hysteroscopic methods	
Tissue destruction: Electrocoagulation	Israngkun *et al.* 1976 Quinones *et al.* 1976 Darabi *et al.* 1978
Mechanical devices: Hosseinian's uterotubal junction device UTJD	Hosseinian, Lucero & Kim 1976
The hydrogelic P-block	Brundin 1980, 1982, 1987
The silicone rubber plug – Ovablock	Erb 1976, Reed & Erb 1979, Erb 1982, Demaeyer 1982
The Hamou nylon plug	Hamou & Taylor 1991
Sugimoto's silicone rubber ITCD	Sugimoto 1978
Uterotubal ceramic plugs (few tests in humans)	Craft 1976
The Popp claw device (not tested in humans)	Popp 1980
Metal alloy (not tested in humans)	Richart, Neuwirth, Nuwayser & Fenoglio 1978
Portos silicone plugs (not tested in humans)	Porto 1974

21.2 Hysteroscopic methods used for transcervical sterilization.

The hydrogelic P-block	
Observation months by May 12th 1992	19984
Woman years	1665
Average months/woman	48
Standard deviation (months)	33
Number of pregnancies	35
Pearl index (pregnancies in 100 woman years)	3
Pearl index (when no rejection takes place)	0
Continuation rate – without pregnancy	99%
Continuation rate – in spite of pregnancy	48%
Complications causing withdrawal of P-blocks:	
Perforation with sequelae	0
Perforation without sequelae	2
Bleeding	1

21.3 The hydogenic P-block.

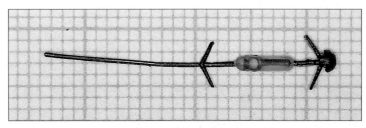

21.4 P-block Mark 9 in non-hydrated state on mm scale background.

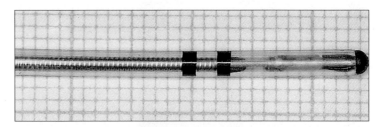

21.5 P-block Mark 9 loaded into the insertion catheter.

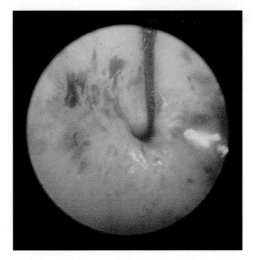

21.7 Indicator thread of a P-block protruding through a tubal orifice into the uterine cavity.

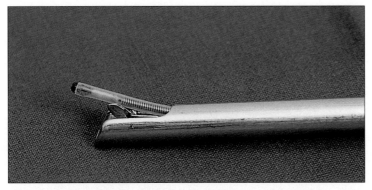

21.6 Distal end of hysteroscope with Albarran bridge and end of the loaded P-block insertion catheter.

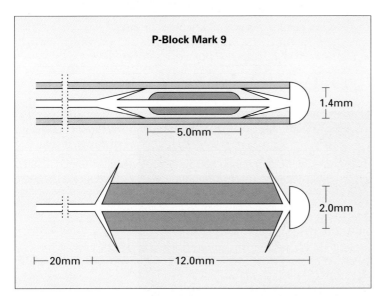

P-Block Mark 9

1.4mm
5.0mm
2.0mm
20mm
12.0mm

21.8 Schematic drawing of a P-block. Loaded into the insertion catheter in non-hydrated state (upper diagram). P-block after hydralization due to accumulation of body fluids (lower diagram).

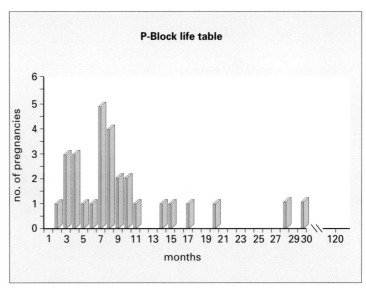

21.9 P-block life table after 10 years of experience showing number of pregnancies over time.

THE SILICON RUBBER PLUG – THE OVABLOC

The Ovabloc was developed by Robert Erb in Philadephia in the 1970's. A catheter is pressed into the uterine tubal ostium under hysteroscopic control (**21.10**) and silicon rubber is injected by a pump (**21.11**) to occlude the tubal lumen as far as the ampulla. Stannous octoate is added immediately before injection as a catalyst. The plug solidifies within about 90 seconds. The Ovabloc thus

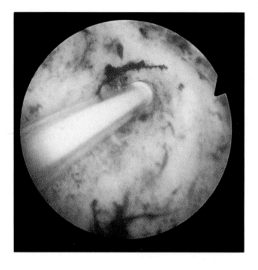

21.10 Intrauterine picture of insertion catheter placement at tubal uterine os.

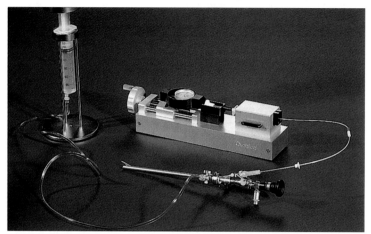

21.11 Injection pump used for silicone rubber injection into the oviduct.

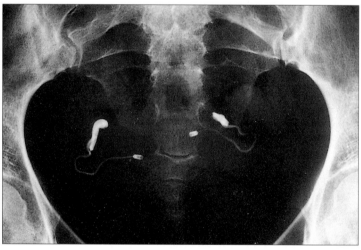

21.13 X-ray picture of a pair of Ovablocs in situ.

Ovabloc intratubal device clinical trials – phase I and III			
Start of study	Reed 1978	De Maeyer 1978	Loffer 1981
Women months of use*	14.309	8.040	12%
Method failure	10**	2***	11%
Pearl index	0.84	0.30	0%
Life table index	0.84	0.30	0%

* These are calculated from the moment the patient relies on Ovabloc alone for contraception, i.e. after the 3-month follow-up visit

** One pregnancy was ectopic

*** all pregnancies were ectopic

21.12 Ovabloc clinical trial results.

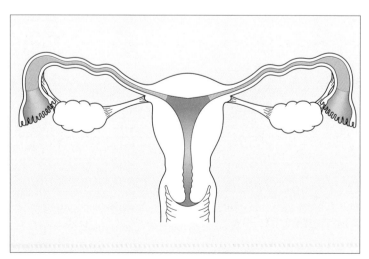

21.14 Ovabloc in situ.

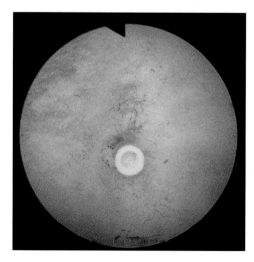

21.15 Intrauterine picture of uterine tip of device in situ.

becomes moulded in place. The procedure has been performed in several thousand patients (**21.12**) and is an alternative to laparoscopic sterilization. An experienced hysteroscopist needs to perform the operation. The efficacy of the method is excellent and very few pregnancies have occurred. The size and shape of the Ovabloc can be seen on a plain X-ray picture (**21.13**) of the abdominal cavity by addition of silver to the silicon rubber. The method must be considered as a permanent sterilization. Even if the isthmic part of the plug can be extracted through the uterus, the remaining plug in the ampulla may not be expelled into the abdominal cavity (**21.12, 21.14, 21.15**).

THE HAMOU PLUG

The Hamou plug is made of nylon and resembles the early versions of the P-block (**21.16**). The Hamou plug has an extraction sling protruding from the tubal orifice into the uterine cavity instead of a plane indicator thread hanging down into the uterus. The mode of action of the Hamou plug is debatable. It is so thin that it can not occlude the tubal lumen. The main contraindication to the Hamou plug is menorrhagia. Of 237 successful insertions, 27 required a local anesthetic and 16 a general anesthetic. The remainder were inserted without an anesthetic. With the plug in place, there were eight pregnancies in 13,252 cycles. In seven patients from whom the plugs were removed, four pregnancies occurred (**21.17**).

MODERN HYSTEROSCOPIC SURGERY

During the last few years, hysteroscopic surgery has advanced. Hysteroscopic resection of the endometrium and Nd:YAG laser ablation instead of hysterectomy for functional bleeding cannot guarantee sterility even though most of the endometrium is destroyed. If sterility is essential, the application of P-blocks at the end of the resection is worth considering.

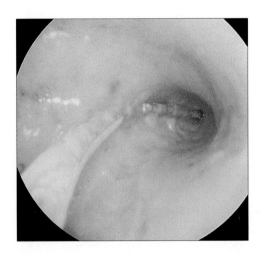

21.16 The Hamou plug for intratubal sterilization.

The Hamou plug	
257 insertions from March 1982 to July1, 1988	n= 257
Contraindications to intrauterine devices	159
Metrorrhagia	109
Infections	21
Others	29
Contraindications to oral contraception	182
Metabolic disorders	114
Vascular disorders	27
Others	41
Results	
Bilateral insertion at 1st attempt	222
Bilateral insertion at 2nd attempt	15
Insertion under local anesthesia	27
Insertion under general anesthesia	16
Insertion failure	14
Spontaneous expulsion	11
Number of cycles without other contraception	13.252
Pregnancies	8
Elective removal	7
Pregnancies	4

21.17 The Hamou plug – results. Reprinted from Hysteroscopy and Microcolpohysteroscopy. Hamou J and Taylor PJ. Appelton and Lange, Conn., USA 1991, pp201–210.

FURTHER READING

Brundin J. Intratubal devices. In: *Biodegradables and delivery systems for contraception. Progress in contraceptive delivery systems series* 1980 Eds: Hafez ESE, Vanos WAA. MTP Press, Lancaster, England. pp123–137

Brundin J. Observations on the mode of action of an intratubal device, the P–block. *Am J Gynecol*, 1987; 156; **4**:997–100

Cohen MR, Dmowski WP. Modern hysteroscopy: diagnostic and therapeutic potential. In: Hysteroscopic Sterilization 1974. Eds: JJ Sciarra, JC Butler and JJ Speidel. Intercontinental Medical Books, New York. pp9–44

Dafoe CA. Transcervical tubal occlusion. In: Advances in Female Sterilization Techniques 1976. Eds: JJ Sciarra, W Drogemueller and JJ Speidel 1976. Harper & Row, Hagerstown pp225–229

Loffer FD. Hysteroscopic sterilization with the use of formed–in–place silicone plugs. *Am. J Obstet Gynecol* 1984; **149**:261–270

Richart RM, Neuwirth RS, Nielsen PA *et al.* The effectiveness of the FEM-CEPT method and preliminary experience with radiopaque MCA to enhance clinical acceptability. In: PARFR series on fertility regulation 1983. Eds: Zatuchni GI, Shelton JD, Goldsmith A, Sciarra JJ. Harper & Row, Philadelphia. pp212–218

Quinones R, Aznar RR, Alvarado DA. Tubal electrocauterization under hysteroscopic control. *Contraception* 1973; **7**:3

HYSTEROSCOPY IN INFERTILITY AND REPEATED PREGNANCY LOSS

22

Patrick J Taylor and Jacques E Hamou

INTRODUCTION

Infertility, the inability to conceive a pregnancy after 12-months of unprotected intercourse, affects approximately one couple in six. Of the identifiable causes of infertility, tubal abnormalities account for 26%, other lesions of the genital tract including lesions of the uterine cavity contribute only 4%. It is in the diagnosis and management of these lesions that hysteroscopy may play a part.

Habitual abortion is strictly defined as the occurrence of three or more consecutive spontaneous abortions. The term 'recurrent spontaneous abortion' describes two or more spontaneous abortions. It has been estimated that habitual abortion affects 1% of the population. Lesions of the uterus are said to account for 15–25% of cases. In these patients hysteroscopy can be invaluable.

The instruments used and the techniques for performing hysteroscopy have been described in chapters 19 and 20. Details of the various operative procedures are also provided elsewhere.

It is the purpose of this chapter to describe briefly the preliminary investigations that should be performed for the infertile couple or those suffering from habitual abortion prior to recourse to hysteroscopy. The complementary roles of hysterosalpingography (HSG) and hysteroscopy will be discussed. The findings and their significance, with respect to the presenting symptom and the indications for office hysteroscopy and hysteroscopy combined with laparoscopy, will be described in some detail. Information about therapeutic maneuvers and the outcome of such interventions will be provided.

PRELIMINARY INVESTIGATIONS

Whether the complaint is one of infertility or habitual abortion, a complete history should be taken from, and an examination performed on, both partners. Historical clues, suggesting the presence of a uterine lesion may be elicited. Heavy menstrual flow may be related to uterine malformations or the presence of fibromyomata. Intermenstrual spotting might suggest that the patient harbors endometrial polyps. Diminution or cessation of menstruation, especially if following curettage, should raise the suspicion that the uterus may contain adhesions.

It is wise to ascertain the woman's hemoglobin level and degree of immunity to rubella. Genital tract specimens should be sent for bacteriologic culture. At this point the further investigation of infertility and habitual abortion differ.

In cases of infertility the occurrence or, otherwise, of ovulation should be noted. A history of a regular menstruation indicates ovulation in 91–97% of women. If further confirmation is required, a single measurement of progesterone in the mid-luteal phase will suffice. Values greater than 16mmol/L are diagnostic. Conversely, a history of amenorrhea is indicative of anovulation or the presence of uterine adhesions. At the same time two semen samples should be analyzed. The post-coital test is of little predictive value. By these simple methods, those ovulatory patients with normospermic partners can be identified. The investigation of anovulatory or amennorheic patients (except those in whom uterine adhesions are suspected) and male factor infertility will not be discussed here.

If the complaint is one of habitual abortion, blood samples should be taken from the female partner to assess the level of T_4, thyroid–stimulating hormone and prolactin. Abnormalities of thyroid or prolactin metabolism will require treatment. Luteal–phase insufficiency should next be excluded by appropriately timed endometrial biopsies or measurement of serum progesterone values. Following these simple investigations a group of euthyroid, normoprolactinemic women who have no evidence of luteal–phase insufficiency will have been identified.

At this stage, the lower genital tract and fallopian tubes of both groups of patients (infertile and aborting) should be evaluated. Investigations of the anatomy of the genital tract can be carried out by HSG, hysteroscopy and laparoscopy. The next section will describe the relative places of HSG and hysteroscopy in the evaluation of the uterine cavity.

INVESTIGATION OF THE UTERINE CAVITY BY HYSTEROSALPINOGOGRAPHY AND HYSTEROSCOPY

It has been argued that hysteroscopy can replace HSG. Purely from the perspective of evaluation of the fallopian tubes in infertile patients, HSG is a valuable preliminary screening test. It will identify cornual occlusion with reasonable accuracy. Salpingitis isthimica nodosa can be diagnosed by this means. Distal tubal occlusion and the endotubal architecture will be delineated. The prior knowledge that the presence of tubal disease is to be anticipated will permit scheduling of the operating room for an operative, rather than purely diagnostic, laparoscopy. Therefore, HSG should be the preliminary investigation in cases of infertility.

The sensitivity of HSG in detecting intrauterine lesions is 95%, and the specificity 79%. It would seem reasonable to use HSG also to screen for intrauterine lesions. If such lesions are detected radiographically, hysteroscopy is warranted. The prevalence of such hysteroscopically detected lesions is about 10%. If HSG is normal with respect to the fallopian tubes, conventional wisdom suggests that laparoscopy should be delayed for 6 months, except in women with very suggestive histories or older than 35 years. Only those who do not conceive during this waiting period will require laparoscopy.

Should hysteroscopy be used in a similar fashion if HSG has revealed an apparently normal uterine cavity? If the sensitivity (95%) and specificity (79%) of the test, and the prevalence of lesions in the study population (10%) are known, it is possible to calculate the likelihood that hysteroscopy will identify lesions in patients with normal HSGs. This calculation indicates that a normal HSG will be corrected by hysteroscopy in only 1% of cases. It is probably unnecessary to perform hysteroscopy in such patients, except when the HSG has suggested cornual occlusion. This approach is shown schematically in **22.1**.

The situation is rather different in cases of habitual abortion, and is dependent on the availability of an ambulatory hysteroscopy facility. If no such facility is available, HSG is once again adequate to exclude patients with a normal uterus, and to permit scheduling of the operating room for definitive hysteroscopic corrective procedures for those in whom an abnormality is detected. If outpatient facilities for hysteroscopy are available, the use of smaller diameter hysteroscopes and carbon dioxide, as the distension medium, is the preliminary investigation of choice. This method is usually less uncomfortable than HSG and, whereas HSG may serve to identify a 'filling defect', only direct visualization will provide an immediate- and accurate diagnosis. If lesions are identified, minor ones can be dealt with immediately. The operating room can be scheduled for the performance of more extensive procedures. This approach is shown in **22.2**.

FINDINGS AND THEIR SIGNIFICANCE

Lesions of the uterine cavity may be found in women suffering from infertility or habitual abortion. There may be a place for hysteroscopy immediately preceding an *in vitro* fertilization attempt. This section will describe the lesions, consider their significance in both infertility and habitual abortion, and discuss the potential usefulness of hysteroscopy as an adjunct to assisted reproduction.

Lesions

Intrauterine lesions occur with varying frequency in infertile women and those who habitually abort. This issue will be discussed when the significance of the lesion is considered. Suffice to say at this point that the most frequently noted are polyps, fibromyomata, adhesions and congenital malformations. Less commonly seen are endometritis and bony fragments.

1. Polyps. These are overgrowths of the endometrium and may be single or multiple, pedunculated **(22.3a,b)** or sessile **(22.4)**. Polyps are covered with endometrium and are easily recognizable. The pedunculated type can be overdiagnosed because strips of endometrium can be dislodged owing to cervical dilatation which gives a very similar appearance. In addition to uterine polyps small polypoid lesions may be noted in the first few millimeters of the fallopian tube.

2. Fibromyomata. Subserous fibromyomata cannot be visualized hysteroscopically nor can intramural fibroids, although the distortion of the uterine cavity produced by such lesions may be readily appreciated. Hysteroscopy comes into its own in the evaluation of submucous lesions. They may be pedunculated **(22.5)** or sessile, **(22.6)** and occupy space within the uterine cavity **(22.7)**. They can vary in size from a few millimetres to several centimetres in diameter. The endometrium over their surface is usually thin and lighter in color than the surrounding healthy endometrium. They may be covered with large surface blood vessels. The endometrium surrounding the lesion may contain areas of endometrial hyperplasia. When touched gently with the tip of the hysteroscope they are typically firm in consistency.

3. Adhesions. The presence of adhesions, the eponymous Asherman's Syndrome, was in fact first described by Fritsch in 1894. Adhesions may be found in association with amenorrhea, hypomenorrhea or eumenorrhea. Previous uterine trauma is an almost invariable antecedent. Histologically three types can be identified: endometrial, muscular and fibrous. Endometrial adhesions are very fragile. Muscular adhesions are more dense and covered by pale endometrium. Fibrous adhesions are poorly vascularized **(22.8)**, devoid of an endometrial covering, and of the three types are by far the strongest. Adhesions may lie centrally, that is crossing the uterine cavity and anchored at two poles or marginally. These latter tend to project like shelves from the lateral walls or fundus of the uterus. Very dense adhesions can severely distort and even obliterate the uterine cavity. They obscure the landmarks and interfere with orientation. Often the fibrosis extends into the myometrium. Hysteroscopic dissection of such lesions carries a high risk of uterine perforation.

4. Congenital malformations. Major malformations of the Müllerian system may represent failure of fusion of the Müllerian ducts with the formation of bicornuate or didelphic uteri or failure of development of one duct which results in the presence of a unicornuate organ. In these cases hysteroscopy offers little, unless information about the configuration of the uterine cavity or cavities is required in the same way that information may be required about the normal uterus. If the Müllerian ducts fuse but the central septum fails to break down a septate or subseptate uterus will result. The appearance is typical. The septum is often paler than the surrounding endometrium, appearing as a partition between the two uterine cavities each of which is seen as a dark orifice at least while the endoscope is at the level of the internal os **(22.9)**. As each cavity is entered in turn the single tubal ostium will be identified laterally and the pale septum medially.

22.1 Investigation of female infertility.

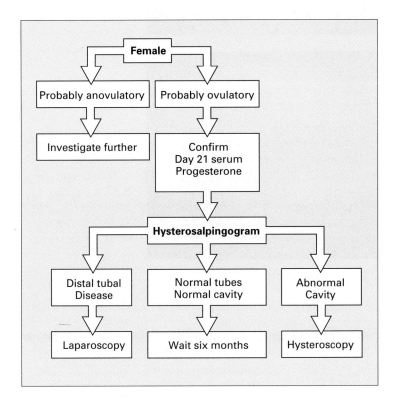

5. Endometritis – hysteroscopy is contraindicated. If it is clinically obvious that there is acute infection of the lower genital tract. A surprising number of cases of both active and chronic endometritis can be identified in asymptomatic patients. Those familiar with cervicitis observed colposcopically will have no difficulty in recognizing the hysteroscopic appearance of endometritis. There is congestion of the endometrium and the glandular orifices are white giving the endometrial surface a speckled appearance (**22.10**). The lesions may be generalized or may exist in small isolated islands.

6. Bony fragments. Whether bony fragments which can be detected in the uterus represent osseous tissue which has been retained following an abortion or true osseous metaplasia is unclear. The lesion furtunately is rare. The hysteroscopic appearances are typical. Lamellae of yellowish white osseous tissue which may be fan shaped or discoid, are clearly noted deeply embedded in the surrounding mucosa. (**22.11**).

Significance of the findings

1. Infertility. Since physicians began to investigate infertility there has been an understandable, but regrettable tendency to assign causation arbitrarily. Simply because a lesion is detected in an infertile patient is insufficient reason to assume that it is the cause. It should be an absolute requirement that any putative cause of infertility be demonstrated unequivocally to occur more frequently in an infertile than a fertile population.

22.12 compares the findings in two similar groups of patients in whom dextran or carbon dioxide was used as the distension medium. The rate at which lesions were observed was considerably lower in the carbon dioxide group, at least with respect to polyps and adhesions. It was concluded that forcible cervical dilation, necessary for the performance of dextran hysteroscopy, may have dislodged strips of endometrium which were misinterpreted as being either adhesions or polyps. It will be noted that fibroids and septa, the appearances of which are unmistakable, occurred with similar frequency in both groups.

Both of these studies were performed in an attempt to answer the question, 'do polyps adhesions or fibroids occur more frequently in infertile or at least potentially fertile (previous tubal ligation) populations?' In no case was this found to be so. It is unlikely therefore that the finding of polyps, adhesions or fibroids in normally menstruating women has uncovered a cause of infertility. In those patients who harbor adhesions of sufficient severity to cause amenorrhea or severe hypomenorrhea it is that the lesions are causative.

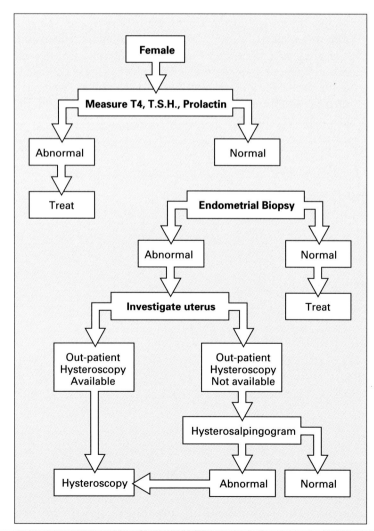

22.2 Investigation of habitual abortion.

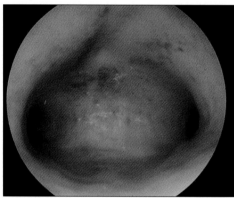
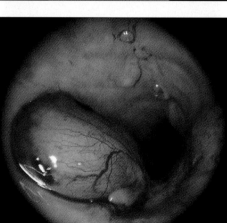

22.3a,b Normal uterine cavity (upper figure) and a mucous polyp (lower figure).

Septa do not cause infertility. The role of endometritis is unclear, and will be discussed when the potential role of hysteroscopy prior to *in vitro* fertilization (IVF) is considered.

Very few cases of intrauterine bone have been described. As such, prevalence studies are impossible. If such lesions are detected it is not unreasonable to assume that they may act like natural intrauterine contraceptive devices and treat them accordingly.

HABITUAL ABORTION

The prediction, made in the late 1930's that after three conceptions a woman had a 73% of losing a subsequent pregnancy was clearly incorrect. Follow-up studies of these patients show that 53–68% of such women will carry a subsequent pregnancy. This spontaneous cure rate must always be considered when claiming that any ther-

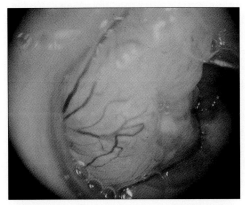

22.4 Polyps. A sessile mucous polyp. No obvious pedicle is visible. The color is very similar to that of the surrounding endometrium.

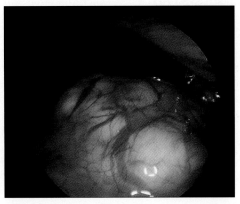

22.5 Fibroids. A pedunculated, sub-mucous fibromyoma. Note the pedicle at 2 o'clock and the prominent blood vessels.

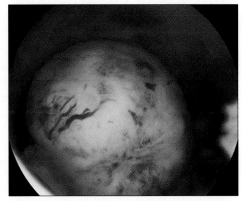

22.6 Fibroids. A large sessile submucous myoma.

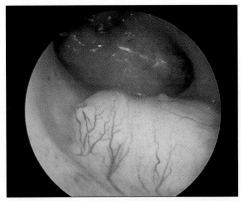

22.7 Fibroids. A submucous myoma which is distorting the uterine cavity.

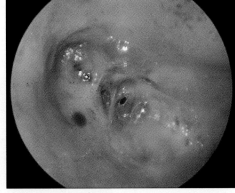

22.8 Adhesions. Very dense adhesions which have practically obliterated the upper part of the uterine cavity. Note their pale color.

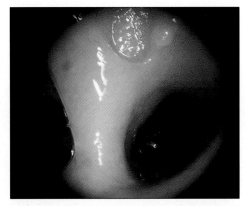

22.9 Septum. A uterine septum. The two uterine cornua are seen as dark areas on either side of the septum.

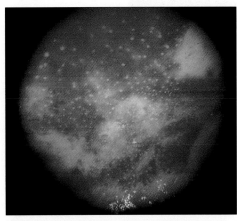

22.10 Acute endometriosis. Note the yellow, punctuate foci. This appearance is similar to that of acute cervicitis when observed colposcopically.

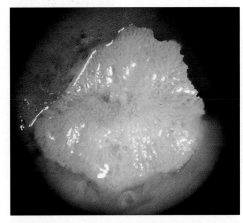

22.11 Bony metaplasia. Osseous metaplasia. The bone is clearly visible and is deeply embedded in the endometrium.

apeutic maneuver has overcome tendency to abort. The abortion rate in women with a bicornuate uterus is 33.8%, 34.6% in women with a single uterine horn and 22% in women with a uterine septum. Of these lesions only the septum can be managed hysteroscopically. As many as 41% of women with fibroids may abort. It is possible that adhesions have an association with habitual abortion, but whether they represent a cause of abortion or the effect of repeated curettage is unclear.

HYSTEROSCOPY AS AN ADJUNCT TO ASSISTED REPRODUCTIVE TECHNOLOGY

There may be a role for hysteroscopy either in the assessment of the uterine cavity prior to attempted IVF and embryo transfer, or one of its variants, gamete intrafallopian transfer (GIFT), zygote intrafallopian transfer (ZIFT), pronuclear stage intrafallopian transfer (PROST) or in permitting access to the tubal ostium to allow the placement of gametes or pre-embryos.

Despite excellent rates of oocyte recovery, fertilization and embryo replacement the successful pregnancy rate following IVF or one of its variants is disappointingly low. While embryonic causes may represent the majority of reasons for this lack of success it is not unreasonable to postulate that abnormalities of the uterine cavity may be contributory. It is recommended that obvious polyps, fibroids or septa should be dealt with hysteroscopically prior to an *in vitro* attempt. These lesions may predispose to the clinically recognizable abortion of a very precious pregnancy. It is less clear

whether the identification and treatment of more subtle uterine disorder can improve the success rate by reducing the rate of very early embryonic loss. This subject will be discussed in greater detail in chapter 28.

Access to the fallopian tubes can be achieved either laparoscopically or through the cervix. There is increasing interest in the placement of gametes or pre-embryos directly within the tubes. The earliest approach was GIFT used as a treatment for unexplained infertility. Variations on this technique have included ZIFT and PROST. Originally, return of the gametes (GIFT) or pre-embryos (ZIFT and PROST) was performed laparoscopically. As oocytes can be collected ultrasonographically their return to the tube either with spermatozoa or as pre-embryos is much less traumatic if effected by the transcervical route. Hysteroscopic tubal canalization **(22.13)** and GIFT, ZIFT or PROST have been described. In addition this technique can be used to perform direct intratubal insemination. Although in these circumstances it is probable that direct intrauterine insemination is equally effective (or equally lacking in efficacy) it is probable that rapid developments in ultrasonography will provide transcervical access to the tubes with greater ease than by hysteroscopy. Furthermore it must be remarked that while there are a large number of publications apparently demonstrating the superiority of GIFT over IVF for the treatment of unexplained infertility only two prospective randomized studies exist. Neither has demonstrated one technique to be superior to the other. Both lacked sufficient numbers of subjects to possess the statistical power to make this conclusion unequivocally.

Hysteroscopic findings in groups of infertile patients compared by the distension medium used			
Distension medium Group and findings	Primary infertility (n=493)	Secondary infertility (n=344)	Reversal (n=155)
Dextran 70			
Normal	350 (71%)	188 (55%)	104 (67%)
Adhesions	74 (15%)	103 (30%)	28 (18%)
Polyps	59 (12%)	40 (12%)	19 (12%)
Fibroids	6 (1%)	7 (2%)	2 (1%)
Septa	4 (0.8%)	6 (2%)	2 (1%)
Total abnormalities	143 (29%)	6 (41%)	51 (33%)
CO$_2$	(n=160)	(n=118)	(n=57)
Normal	153 (95.6%)	105 (89%)	54 (94.7%)
Adhesions	4 (2.5%)	5 (4.2%)	1 (1.75%)
Polyps	2 (1.25%)	0	0 (1.75%)
Fibroids	1 (0.62%)	0	1 (1.75%)
Septa	0	8 (6.8%)	1 (1.75%)
Total abnormalities	7 (4.4%)	13 (11%)	3 (5.3%)

22.12 Hysteroscopic findings in groups of infertile patients compared by the distension medium used. (Reproduced from Taylor PJ, Lewinthal D, Leader A, Pattinson HA. A comparison of dextran 70 with CO$_2$ medium for hysteroscopy in patients with infertility or requesting reversal of a prior tubal sterilization. *Fertil Steril* 1987; **47**:861 with permission.

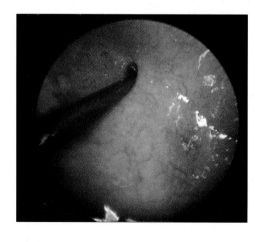

22.13 Tubal catheterization. Hysteroscopic placement of an intra tubal catheter.

HYSTEROSCOPIC MANAGEMENT OF INTRA-UTERINE LESIONS

Hysteroscopy now offers the opportunity to deal transcervically with polyps, adhesions, fibroids and septa. It must be re-iterated that in cases of infertility it is prudent to remove such lesions. The removal of polyps is probably of no therapeutic significance for either infertile or aborting patients but most patients will be puzzled, to say the least, if the physician leaves *in situ* what at least to their minds, is a cause for their troubles. Fibroids and septa should where possible be dealt with as prophylaxis against abortion in the infertile and as a possibly curative measure in cases of habitual abortion. Removal of dense adhesions may be of help to infertile and aborting women alike. This section will describe briefly the setting and techniques of hysteroscopic management.

SETTING

Diagnostic hysteroscopy may be performed as an out-patient procedure under no or local anesthesia. In other circumstances day care admission, general anesthesia, with or without concomitant laparoscopy, may be required. Those patients who have undergone hysterosalpinogography as the initial screening procedure for infertility in whom an intrauterine lesion is suspected should undergo combined laparoscopy and hysteroscopy.

If the uterine cavity is normal hysteroscopy will add little except in cases of apparent cornual occlusion. These patients should undergo laparoscopy which will permit evaluation of the distal tubes and any peri-adnexal lesions. In some of these patients chromopertubation may demonstrate cornual patency. If the cornua are still apparently occluded hysteroscopically guided selective perhydrotubation may clarify the situation. Attempts can be made at this time, if occlusion is still demonstrated, to perform cannulation and dilatation of the proximal tube (**22.14**, **22.15**). The intrapelvic architecture can be assessed and in addition major hysteroscopic procedures can be monitored laparoscopically in an endeavour to reduce the likelihood of uterine perforation.

If outpatient hysteroscopy is performed in place of hysterosalpingography in cases of habitual abortion, some minor lesions can be dealt with immediately. More significant lesions will require to be dealt with under general anesthesia.

TECHNIQUES

Whether hysteroscopic surgery is performed under local or general anesthesia as just described, will be dependant in part on the setting in which the diagnostic hysteroscopy is being performed and in part the feasibility of the operative procedure. This section will consider those operations which can be performed using local and those which require general anaesthesia.

Procedures Which Can Be Performed Using Local Anesthesia

Polyps or small pedunculated fibroids of less than 1 cm in diameter can be dealt with at the time of the diagnostic evaluation. If the Hamou microcolpohysteroscope is used the 6.5 mm operative

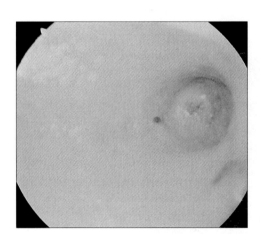

22.14 Proximal tubal occlusion. A thin membrane can be seen narrowing, and possible occluding the tubal ostium.

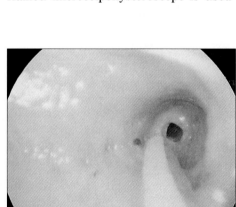

22.15 Proximal tubal occlusion. A catheter has been introduced and has dilated the tubal ostium. The catheter is clearly shown.

sheath will accommodate a 5 Fr electrode. The power is set at 15 watts and the tip of the electrode buried in the base of the pedicle. Once the current is applied the pedicle will be seen to blanch **(22.16)**. Burying the tip reduces the amount of smoke. Once coagulated the pedicle is electroresected using cutting current. The polyp or fibroid can be left in the uterine cavity as they will invariably be expelled spontaneously.

Polyps or myomata of between one to two centimetres in diameter will require resection with the resectoscope loop. While small lesions can be treated using carbon dioxide as the distension medium use of the diathermy loop requires the use of glycine or sorbitol.

Less dense adhesions can be ruptured by simple pressure with the tip of the hysteroscope. Even denser adhesions can be dealt with by the technique of target abrasion **(22.17)**. The tip of the Hamou instrument is set at an angle of 30°. The area of least vas-cularization is identified and the hysteroscope used like a chisel to chip it away. The procedure is repeated at the other pole. Myofibrous adhesions may bleed slightly whereas fibrous adhesions are invariably avascular. They may be more resistant to target abrasion. This technique can be successful in up to 85 % of cases.

Procedures Which Require General Anesthesia

All of the techniques just described can also be performed under general anesthesia if the setting requires it. The apprehensive patient may also require general anesthesia for minor procedures. It is possible that as more experience is gained some of the techniques to be described will move to the local anesthetic domain. This shift is already occurring with endometrial ablation. Presently, however, the excision of septa, very dense adhesions, and larger fibroids require a general anesthetic.

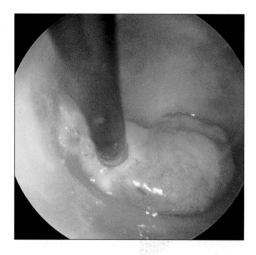

22.16 Electrocautery of a small polyp. The blanced area at the base of the polyp, following the first application of the current, is clearly noted.

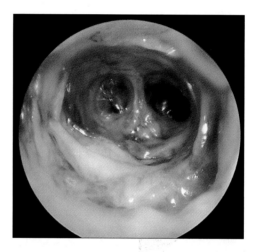

22.17 Adhesiolysis. The same uterus as shown in **22.8**. Adhesiolysis by target abrasion has almost been completed.

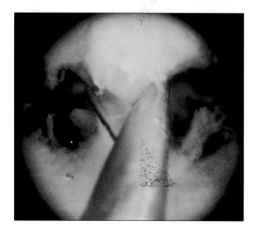

22.18 Excision of a septum. Scissors about to be closed on the lower edge of a uterine septum.

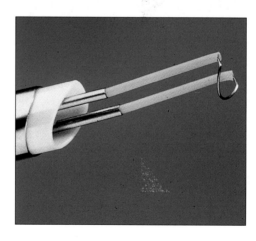

22.19 The resectoscope. The working element of the resectoscope.

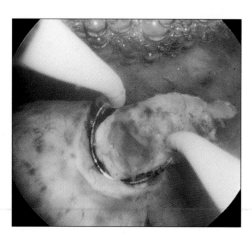

22.20 Resection of a fibroid.

Septa. In the first place the exact configuration of the uterus can only be determined laparoscopically. This alone requires a general anesthetic. Once it has thus been determined that the deformity is not didelphic or bicornuate, resection of the septum can be performed with scissors (**22.17**), the resectoscope (**22.18**) or the laser. The complete details of the technique have been described elsewhere. The principles of resection include identification of both tubal orifices and continuing the incision until there is a small amount of bleeding. The septum itself is avascular. Bleeding indicates that the upper limit of the septum has been reached. Postoperatively an intrauterine device should be inserted and high dose estrogen, to which a progestational agent is added in the latter days, prescribed for 20 days. Follow-up hysteroscopy should be performed following the withdrawal bleeding. The intrauterine device can be removed at this time. If any adhesions have formed despite the adjunctive therapy they can easily be broken down.

Dense Adhesions. If more than half of the uterine cavity is obliterated or the adhesions are known to have been present for more than two years target abrasion will be ineffective. Attempts to deal with them hysteroscopically may be monitored laparoscopically or by using ultrasound. The risk of uterine perforation is high. The adhesions may be removed with scissors, electroresection or with the Nd:Yag Laser. A useful technique is to introduce a dilator directed towards each uterine corner. The hysteroscope is used to identify each tubal ostium. The adhesions have now been converted into an acquired septum which can be dealt with in a fashion similar to that which is used to deal with a congenital septum. Postoperative adjunctive therapy and follow up hysteroscopy are useful.

Larger myomata. Pre-treatment with a progestational agent will thin the endometrium over the lesion and facilitate dissection. Removal is best effected with the resectoscope loop (**22.19, 22.20**). If it is necessary to leave residual intramural tumor to avoid uterine perforation, a repeat procedure two to three months later may be needed. Often the intra-mural portion will have become extruded into the cavity. If myoma exist in more than one uterine wall only one wall should be treated. Delaying resection of the other lesions for two or three months will reduce the likelihood that two opposing raw areas will become adherent. Because of the recognized trophic effect of estrogens, postoperative hormone therapy is contraindicated. A second look hysteroscopy should be performed six weeks after the final resection. Any adhesions which may have formed can be identified and dealt with easily.

OUTCOME

While it is clearly possible to deal with polyps, septa, adhesions and myomata hysteroscopically it is important to consider the effects upon reproductive outcome of such procedures. It is unlikely that removing any but the largest polyps exerts any influence other than on the patient's state of mind.

DeCherney in 1986 resected septa in 105 women complaining of habitual abortion. Resection was successfully performed in 72. One uterine perforation occurred. There were 58 successful deliveries. Daly in1989 achieved a pregnancy rate of 92%, 80% of these pregnancies were viable and 73% went to term. Only 18% were lost in the first trimester of those patients with a history of recurrent first trimester abortions. While these figures are impressive it must be realized that the abortion rate in women with intact septa is 22%. It would not be impossible to design a prospective randomized study of treatment versus no treatment in such patients. The results might be interesting.

Adhesiolysis was performed in 39 women who had dense adhesions. Twenty pregnancies occurred of which 15 delivered successfully (38%). Other authors have reported live birth rates of 26, 23 and 16%. In these patients the prevalence of third stage complications was high. The situation with fibroids is discouraging. Fibroids tend to occur in older women and age alone may be contributory. Only 20% term pregnancies were achieved in a group of women who underwent hysteroscopic resection of their fibroids.

CONCLUSION

Hysteroscopy is coming of age in the diagnosis and management of intrauterine lesions in patients suffering from infertility or habitual abortion. The desire to attribute causality and cure must be kept in mind constantly. It is improbable that polyps cause reproductive difficulties or that their removal is curative. Septa do not cause infertility but appear to be associated with habitual abortion. Hysteroscopic resection of these lesions may improve the pregnancy rate but absolute confirmation will require a properly conducted clinical trial.

The role of fibroids is unclear as a cause of infertility. They may contribute to habitual abortion. Results of hysteroscopic resection of submucous fibroids are disappointing. Dense adhesions cause infertility and can be identified in cases of habitual abortion. Reasonable success attends their removal.

Nevertheless just as the role of laparoscopy has evolved and become refined so will that of the hysteroscope in infertility and habitual abortion.

FURTHER READING

Gomel V, Taylor PJ, Yuzpe AA, Rioux JE. Laparoscopy and Hysteroscopy in Gynaecologic Practice 1986. Chicago. Year Book Medical Publishers

Hamou JE. (Translated by Taylor PJ) Hysteroscopy and Microcolpohysteroscopy Text and Atlas 1991. Conn., USA, Appleton and Lange

HYSTEROSCOPIC ELECTROSURGERY 23

Robert S Neuwirth

INTRODUCTION

Hysteroscopic electrosurgery began early in the modern era of hysteroscopy, in 1970, for tubal cauterization. The search to find a method of transcervical tubal sterilization had been a factor in accelerating the refinement of the equipment and practice of hysteroscopy between 1950 and 1965. The final piece of technology to be developed was a safe, reliable uterine distension system. In rapid sequence the CO_2 system introduced by Lindemann, the 32% dextran system developed by Edstrom and Fernstrom, and the 5% dextrose and water system advocated by Quinones were refined and applied to tubal sterilization by electrocautery. While the safety and effectiveness of electrocautery of the isthmic segment of the fallopian tubes fell short of general clinical acceptance, hysteroscopy and electrosurgery survived and evolved into very useful techniques.

The first major report on hysteroscopic electrosurgery was by Neuwirth and Amin in 1976 who used a modified resectoscope. Other series were reported but the hysteroscopic laser ablation techniques pioneered initially by Goldrath overshadowed DeCherney's report of resectoscopic ablation of the endometrium. By 1990 it was evident that hysteroscopic laser was useful for endometrial ablation and some hysteroscopic myomectomies, but that hysteroscopic electrosurgical ablation and myomectomy were less expensive, less hazardous, more widely applicable and equally effective. Indeed, the recognition of thermal surgery as a technology which could be produced by cryosurgical, electrosurgical, laser, and direct heating methods is the current state of the art.

To elaborate more fully on hysteroscopic electrosurgery we will review the principles of electrosurgery, and its application to the resectoscope. Finally, hysteroscopic electrosurgical cutting and coagulation procedures will be discussed.

The basic principle of electrosurgery is the passage of a high frequency current through the body. Historically, diathermy for deep heat treatment was produced by a high frequency generator delivering short wave electrical current to the body via two wide area electrodes or paddles in contact with an area of skin covered with electrolyte paste. The generator had positive and negative electrodes and the body tissues acted as a leaky capacitor resisting the flow of electrons. This resistance to flow produced mild internal heating which improved blood flow to deep tissues such as joints or the abdominal cavity. Unipolar electrosurgical currents were formed when one of the electrodes was reduced in contact surface area to the point that the power density per square millimeter was high enough to produce tissue temperatures which would coagulate protein or destroy tissues by vaporization at the point of contact. No electrolyte paste was used at the active electrode in order to raise resistance to electron flow.

Two wave forms were identified which had different electron-flow characteristics. The cutting current was a continuous sine wave which produced a less penetrating heat but a higher contact temperature which caused the tissue to divide with minimal depth of penetration of heat (**23.1**). The coagulation current was a intermittent sine wave which produced deeper penetration of the heat from resistance to the electron flow and tended to produce a lower temperature but wider penetration of the heat leading to tissue coagulation and destruction and at times charring (**23.2**). One wave form was good for incision. The other was preferable for hemostasis by coagulation. The surface area of the active electrode and the time of activation were important in determining the temperature of the tissue at the contact point for any given power output.

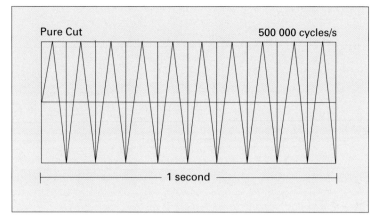

23.1 Pure cutting (From Sutton C and Diamond MP. Endoscopic Surgery for Gynaecologists. WB Saunders, London, 1993, with permission).

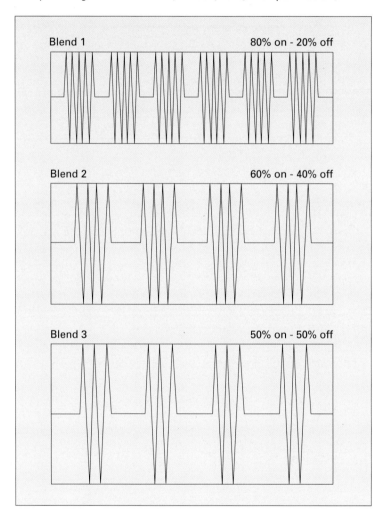

23.2 Blended wave forms (From Sutton C and Diamond MP. Endoscopic Surgery for Gynaecologists. WB Saunders, London, 1993, with permission).

Bipolar electrosurgery resulted from making both paddles of the early diathermy machine small in surface area. They were incorporated into the same surgical instrument, such as coagulation forceps, in which each area of the forceps is electrically isolated and one is positive and the other negative. Current flow is from one tip to the other through tissue held in between the tips. This causes the tissue to heat and become coagulated. The power output limit of bipolar generators is lower than the unipolar or diathermy generators because the electrodes are in close proximity.

The equipment for electrosurgery consists of the generator, the connecting wires and the electrodes. In hysteroscopic electrosurgery

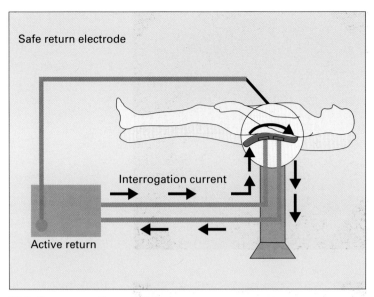

23.3 Contact quality monitor.

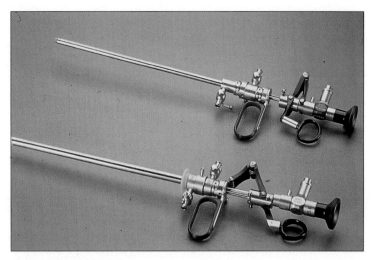

23.4 Resectoscopes.

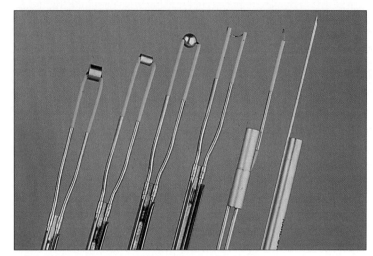

23.5 Electrodes – loop, rollerball, rollerbar and knife.

the electrodes are usually incorporated into the resectoscope as a loop, rollerball, or rollerbar. Other electrodes are available such as a needle or knife. The generators have outlets for the active and ground electrode wires for unipolar surgery and the positive and negative contacts for the bipolar systems. The controls include power output, usually calibrated in maximal watt output against a standard resistance ranging from zero to 400 watts. The output may also be calibrated from zero to 100 which usually means % of the maximal output. Wave forms are usually options which include pure cutting, pure coagulation and blended. The blended options refer to the output wave which may be one quarter, one half or three quarters cutting mixed with coagulation wave forms. This produces more or less coagulation component to the electrosurgical current in use.

The ground electrode in unipolar electrosurgery is a broad plate on which an electrolytic material is coated to improve current flow and lower resistance so as to prevent the temperatures of the tissue in contact from rising to the point of injury. The most advanced electrosurgical generator models have circuit controls to detect an incomplete circuit of the electrosurgical high frequency current. Essentially these generators are equipped with an ammeter on the output and input sides of the generator which monitor the current flow. If the differences between current flow to the patient significantly exceeds the current flow returning to the generator it will shut down to avoid a burn from deviant high frequency current escaping the circuit such as through an ECG lead (**23.3**).

The leads must be heavily insulated and care must be used when the generator is on and the leads not connected to the active and ground electrodes. Accidental burns can occur if the generator is activated and the leads of the electrodes are in contact with the patient so that a complete or deviant circuit occurs.

The electrodes in hysteroscopic electrosurgery are predominantly those used in the resectoscope. The resectoscope consists of the endoscope and fiberoptic light bundles, sheaths for distension fluid, and the electrodes which are mounted on the working element (**23.4**). The endoscopes are standard hysteroscopic models and have an offset objective lens. The sheaths are electrically insulated and consist of two channels for continuous flow irrigation. The electrode may be a loop, rollerball or rollerbar (**23.5**). The electrodes are back loaded into the working element and into a contact point where the current flows and which is fully insulated. The endoscope fits into the working element which, in turn, is inserted into the inner irrigation channel. The electrodes have guide elements which align the electrode with the endoscope and permit movement backwards and forwards. The electrode motion is controlled by a pistol or trigger grip system operated by a spring. This enables careful electrode motion under direct illumination and visual control from the endoscope within an insulated set of sheaths which direct the flow of the non- electrolytic distension medium. It is safer if the electrode has a passive action so that it is within the sheath at rest. The electrode is extended by finger pressure on the spring and should only be activated as it returns to the resting position.

The operating conditions needed for proper use of the resectoscope include high intensity lighting, an undistorted image, and effective distension of the uterine cavity. The resectoscope image is produced by a rigid lens system with a field of view of about 70°, and an infinity focus lens which gives normal size images at roughly 4 cm between the objective lens and the object. The angle of view may be between 12° to 30° and permits viewing of the electrode during its full excursion. The image becomes enlarged as the lens approaches the object. Consequently the manipulation of the resectoscope requires movement of both the electrode and the whole resectoscope in order to keep the image magnification relatively stable during an electrosurgical maneuver.

The light is transmitted by fibroptic cable which gives an even intensity of light in the operating field. Light intensity is limited with the 150 watt incandescent bulb light source and is in the yellow range. The higher power halogen light sources provide light in the blue range with a greater intensity. Television and photographic documentation require a halogen light and/or a flash generator. A video camera attached to the resectoscope must be orientated to the vertical and horizontal axis as landmarks in the uterus are few and disorientation is easy with potentially serious consequences.

The uterine distension needed for electrosurgery is very important. Carbon dioxide is not acceptable because of smoke and inadequate lens washing of blood and debris during the course of surgery. Liquids must be non-electrolytic as the presence of ionic material will defocus the electrosurgical impact on the tissue making cutting and coagulation unpredictable and hazardous. There are two groups of non-electrolytic fluids, the high viscosity, such as 32% dextran 70 (Hyskon) or the low viscosity such as 3% sorbital, 1.5% glycine, or 5% dextrose in water. Pure water is hazardous because it will cause intravascular hemolysis if it enters the circulation. 'Hyskon' can only be used with a non-continuous flow system due to its viscosity. Its lack of miscibility in blood permits surgery even in the presence of bleeding. Its disadvantages include allergic reactions and the need to clean the instruments carefully and promptly after use to avoid sticking of valves and tubing. The absorption of 'Hyskon' into the vascular system should be limited to 400 ml or less because it is hyperosmotic and draws into the vascular compartment 8 ml of serum for every millilitre of 'Hyskon' absorbed. Careful fluid balance measurements are essential. It does not cause caramelization on electrodes although coagulated tissue will adhere to electrodes whether high or low viscosity fluid is used.

Low-viscosity fluids require a continuous flow resectoscope to achieve an adequate intrauterine pressure without intravasation of the distension medium. The fluid enters the uterus via one channel of the resectoscope and exits via the second, connected to a negative pressure pump. Flow should be controlled by the surgeon at the outlet valve of the resectoscope. As the intrauterine pressure needed to distend the uterus and control venous and arterial bleeding is between 80 and 150 mm Hg, a bag of solution can be placed 1–2 m above the patient so that the force of gravity will provide the desired pressure. The rate or flow should be controlled by the surgeon to give clear vision. Ideally, if there is no bleeding or leakage of fluid from the uterus the flow can be reduced. This prevents fluid overload and pulmonary edema. In practice a fluid balance must always be maintained and if the fluid deficit is over 2 litres the procedure should be terminated immediately. Serum electrolyte levels should also be monitored.

The applications of hysteroscopic electrosurgery are limited to cutting and coagulating. Original work to coagulate the interstitial fallopian tube for sterilization failed because it did not occlude the uterine cornua in 20% of cases and there was a high ectopic pregnancy rate.

Subsequent work has been directed at endometrial ablation and resection of submucous fibroids. Endometrial ablation has been performed by electrocoagulation and electroresection.

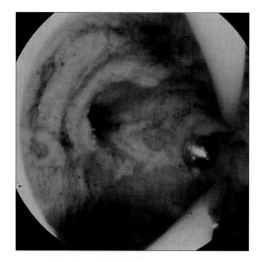

23.6 Coagulation of right cornu.

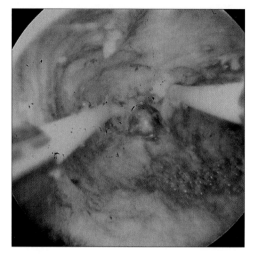

23.7 Complete endometrial coagulation.

Electrocoagulation usually employs a rollerball or rollerbar electrode at a power of 50 to 75 watts. It is preferable to begin at 12 o'clock on the anterior uterine wall because bubbles of water vapor accumulate there making this sector more difficult to coagulate due to loss of clear vision. The fundus and cornual areas are treated by lateral motion of the extended electrode, care being taken in the cornual region not to hold the electrode at any point for more than one or two seconds because the myometrium is thin at this point and perforation may occur (**23.6**). The speed of motion of the electrode is determined by the surgeon. The degree of white coagulation, charring and vertical grooves from desiccation of the endometrium determine the appropriate speed (**23.7**). We perform the operation under general anesthesia and give prophylactic antibiotics.

Surgeons in training would be wise to test these effects in hysterectomy specimens before treating patients. This gives insight into the relationship between the power setting, contact pressure and rate of movement of the rollerball electrode.

Preoperative and postoperative endometrial suppression with Depo Provera, danazol, or gonadotrophin releasing hormone (GnRH) agonists should improve the success of ablation. The patient may have bloody or clear discharge for two or three months following the operation. Clinical assessment is best after three months when about 90% of patients will have oligo- or amenorrhoea. About 10% of patients will have persistent heavy bleeding and may seek hys-

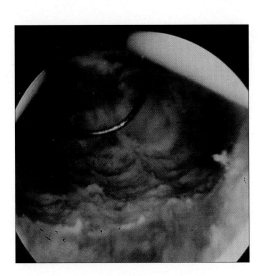

23.8 Loop resection of posterior wall.

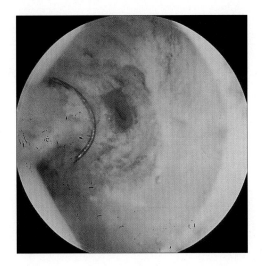

23.9 Loop resection completed.

terectomy or repeat ablation. It is not always possible to repeat the ablation because of scar tissue. Hysterography or transvaginal ultrasound will show the size of the uterine cavity.

Endometrial ablation is indicated in patients with dysfunctional uterine bleeding who would otherwise be offered hysterectomy. Endometrial cancer and hyperplasia should be excluded by a preliminary biopsy and a normal cervical smear obtained. The uterine cavity should not measure more than 14 cm. Patients should be warned of the possibility of laparoscopy or laparotomy should perforation, hemorrhage or visceral injury occur. Complications from rollerball ablation are rare. None of our cases have required emergency laparotomy or transfusion. One patient required intravenous antibiotic therapy postoperatively.

Long-term follow-up for six years has shown an 85% chance of avoiding repeat ablation and hysterectomy. Longer-term follow-up has not yet been published.

Experience with electroresection is similar. The majority of the ablations in the USA have been performed by electrocoagulation. In electroresection a loop is used with a cutting or blended current to excise the endometrium and the superficial myometrium (**23.8, 23,9**). It tends to be more bloody and the tissue fragments may obscure the field much as in a resectoscopic myomectomy. It gives pathologic information which may include fragments of small myomata or adenomyosis. It is a most useful technique when combined with a submucous myomectomy in a patient with menorrhagia.

Hysteroscopic myomectomy is useful for patients with a submucous myoma who are infertile or who are experiencing menorrhagia and desire to maintain their fertility. Resectoscopic surgery in patients with submucous myomas was first described 20 years ago. Since that time it has become clear that normal menstruation and childbirth with vaginal delivery are possible following this technique.

Office hysteroscopy and transvaginal ultrasongraphy are essential if fibroids are suspected. The size of the uterine cavity can be measured and the number and position of the fibroids estimated. If two fibroids are seen opposite each other the resection should be performed in two stages to prevent formation of synechiae.

Fibroids with a large intramural component are unfavorable for a single-stage operation. If the intramural component is less than 50% the procedure may be performed under general anesthesia with concomiment laparoscopy.

Larger lesions are more prone to heavy bleeding and uterine perforation is relatively easy. Our transfusion rate is about 3% and the emergency laparotomy rate nearly 1% in this group. The operation is performed with a 90° loop using pure cutting current. The lesions are resected down to the normal myometrium. The morcellated fragments of myoma may be removed with ovum forceps or a suction curette.

The pedicle of a pedunculated fibroid may be cut with the resectoscope, and then removed through a dilated or incised cervix. If cervical incision is performed the cut is made at 6 o'clock as far as the internal os. Care must be taken not to perform an accidental colpotomy. When the fibroid has been removed the cervix should be repaired and hysteroscopy performed to evaluate the endometrial cavity. An intrauterine balloon is sometimes needed postoperatively for several hours to tamponade bleeding until clot forms.

Patients with fibroids should be treated for at least three weeks pre-operatively with GnRH agonists.

Control of bleeding is usually good. Fertility has been restored or preserved in most patients. Longer-term follow-up for 8 years shows that 20% of these patients require further surgery.

FURTHER READING

Neuwirth RS, Amin H. Excision of submucous fibroids with hysteroscopic control. *Am J Obstet Gynecol* 1976; **126**: 95

Goldrath MH, Fuller T, Segal S. Laser photovaporization of endometrium for the treatment of menorrhagia. *Am J Obstet Gynecol* 1981; **140**:14

DeCherney AH, Polan ML. Hysteroscopic management of intrauterine lesions and intractable uterine bleeding. *Obstet Gynecol* 1983; **61**: 392

Derman SG, Rehnstrom J, and Neuwirth, RS. The long-term effectiveness of hysteroscopic treatment of menorrhagia and leiomyomas. *Obstet Gynecol* 1991; **591**:1991

ENDOMETRIAL RESECTION

24

Adam L Magos

INTRODUCTION

Transcervical resection of the endometrium (TCRE) is one of the hysteroscopic techniques for ablating the endometrium in women with abnormal dysfunctional uterine bleeding, typically menorrhagia. In contrast to the other methods such as laser ablation or rollerball coagulation, it is the only one which provides an operative specimen for histologic examination as the endometrium is physically cut away from the myometrium rather than being destroyed *in situ*. The resectoscope also provides a fast and efficient way to remove small to medium sized submucous fibroids which are often found in such patients, although the instrument should not be used to treat deeper myomas because of the risk of uterine perforation.

PATIENT SELECTION

The ideal case for endometrial resection is a woman over 35 years of age whose primary complaint is of regular, heavy periods, possibly with pain during menstruation. She would have tried medical treatment without success, have no wish for further pregnancies, and is now prepared to undergo hysterectomy (as an alternative). Clinical examination and investigations such as ultrasound, hysteroscopy and endometrial biopsy may suggest that she is suffering from dysfunctional uterine bleeding, but equally, she may have fibroids, although her uterus should not be larger than the equivalent of a 12 weeks' gestation, and none of her fibroids should be greater than 5 cm in diameter. There should be no evidence of other gynecologic pathology such as endometriosis or prolapse, and she should understand that surgery cannot guarantee either amenorrhea or sterility. Finally, she should be aware that there is scanty information about the long-term outcome of surgery, particularly in terms of treatment failure and possible risks such as uterine malignancy. Adequate counselling is of paramount importance with TCRE as with any new form of treatment.

PREOPERATIVE ASSESSMENT

History, clinical examination and basic blood tests are all that are required in many cases, additional investigations being reserved for special indications. Although endometrial resection provides excellent specimens for histologic testing, much better than with dilatation and curettage, it is preferable to exclude before surgery a diagnosis of endometrial atypia by endometrial biopsy in women aged over 45 years who are at a higher risk of endometrial carcinoma. Similarly, any history of irregular bleeding such as intermenstrual or postcoital bleeding should be investigated fully by cervical cytology, hysteroscopy and endometrial biopsy. Ideally any assessment of the uterine cavity should include hysteroscopy to ensure that small lesions are not missed.

Women with bulky uteri suggestive of fibroids should also be investigated by hysteroscopy, this being the optimal means of judging the degree of intra-cavity extension of the myoma. This should be combined with pelvic ultrasound to determine the number and size of deeper fibroids. Ultrasound is also useful to ensure the absence of ovarian pathology which is particularly important with hysteroscopic surgery as the ovaries will not be visualized as they would be at hysterectomy.

ENDOMETRIAL PREPARATION

Endometrial resection is also most easily performed when the endometrium is thin although it is not as critical with TCRE as with other ablative techniques such as laser ablation or rollerball coagulation, where the depth of tissue effect is limited to 4–5 mm. This can be ensured by operating on women immediately after menstruation, performing suction curettage prior to surgery, or preparing the endometrium hormonally with agents such as LHRH agonists, danazol, progestogens or the combined contraceptive pill. It has been shown that prior treatment with danazol, for instance, produces an atrophic endometrium measuring 1–2 mm in depth irrespective of the phase of the menstrual cycle. There are other advantages as well to hormonal pre-treatment such as correction of anemia secondary to menorrhagia, reduction in the size of intrauterine fibroids facilitating their hysteroscopic excision, and a change in the consistency of the endometrium making it firmer and less fluffy and thus less likely to block the small outflow holes on the resectoscope sheath. All this adds up to an easier and faster operation and a reduced risk of fluid overload. Against these advantages must be placed the cost of pretreatment and side-effects which can be severe enough to warrant stopping medication in some cases.

EQUIPMENT

Conceptually, TCRE shares many similarities with endoscopic prostatectomy (TURP) and the instrumentation for the hysteroscopic procedure has essentially been adapted from the equipment used by urologists. Apart from the resectoscope itself with its cutting loops, other essential equipment for TCRE include a fluid uterine distension/irrigation system, an electrosurgical generator, light source and cable, and ideally a video camera and monitor.

RESECTOSCOPE

A continuous flow resectoscope is used by most physicians for performing TCRE as it gives optimal control of uterine distension and irrigation, and thus vision. It is a relatively simple instrument made up of five parts, including the endoscope, handle mechanism, an inner inflow and outer outflow sheath, and a cutting loop (**24.1, 24.2**).

Endoscope
The optical part of the resectoscope is available in a number of sizes and angles of view, but a 4 mm diameter telescope with a 30° fore-oblique lens is the most popular. Narrower optics are available, but the field of view is then unnecessarily limited and orientation becomes more difficult. Similarly, lenses at 0°, 12° and 15° are also manufactured but a shallower angulation means that the cornual areas are less easily viewed. Whichever size or angle of endoscope is chosen, it can also be used for diagnostic hysteroscopy when fitted with the appropriate sheathing system.

Handle Mechanism
The handle-mechanism of resectoscopes can be of two types: active or passive (**24.3**). 'Active' and 'passive' refer to the action required to make a cut with the electrode when it is moving towards the sheathing system, and this depends on the properties of the spring mechanism which is part of the handle. With an active resectoscope, the cutting loop is forced outside the sheathing system at

rest by the spring, and a cut is therefore made by actively pulling the cutting loop towards the sheath. Conversely, a passive handle mechanism maintains the electrode within the sheathing system, and cutting is achieved by pushing the loop outside and then allowing the spring to pull the loop into the sheath while making the cut.

A passive type of handle mechanism with the cutting electrode totally housed within the inflow and outflow sheaths in the resting position is to be recommended for hysteroscopic surgery for several reasons: it is easier to insert the resectoscope into the uterine cavity when the loop is not protruding, the view of the cavity is not obscured by the loop, and of most importance, accidental trauma to the uterine walls is virtually impossible when the cutting loop is shielded within the sheaths even if the electrode is unintentionally activated. It is evident from this discussion that for reasons of safety, the activated electrode should only be pushed outside the body of the resectoscope immediately prior to a cut being made.

Continuous Flow Sheaths

As with the size of the telescope, the in- and out-flow sheaths also come in a variety of sizes ranging from 21–28 Fr gauge. The narrow Hallez type resectoscope (Karl Storz, Tuttlingen, Germany) was the first designed specifically for gynecologic use, and in particular for the excision of small, submucous fibroids. While it may be an ideal instrument for this type of procedure, the view afforded by its narrow optic combined with the fragility of its small, round cutting loop means that it is not suited to more extensive procedures such as TCRE. Instead, a larger 26–27 Fr gauge sheathing system is to be recommended as it can house a 4 mm endoscope and larger, sturdier cutting loops, but without necessitating excessive cervical dilatation.

A recent adaptation of the urologic resectoscope for intrauterine use is the siting of irrigating perforations around the entire circumference of the tip of the outer outflow sheath. This has the advantage that bubbles produced during surgery from heating of the irrigating fluid is aspirated from the uterine cavity even when operating on the anterior wall with the resectoscope rotated 180°.

Cutting Loop

Cutting loops are available in a number of dimensions and wire diameters depending on the size of the sheathing system used. With the usual 26 Fr gauge outer sheath (diameter approximately 9 mm) used for endometrial resection, the cutting loop measures 24 Fr (diameter approximately 8 mm), which therefore produces a 4–5 mm deep furrow during surgery. This is ideal for TCRE where the aim of surgery is to undercut the basal layer of endometrium by 2–3 mm, as this size of cutting loop inherently resects 2–3 mm of hormonally thinned endometrium together with 2–3 mm of underlying myometrium per cut. The use of smaller loops means that surgery takes longer as the resection has to be repeated until the endometrium is sufficiently undercut, while larger loops may lead to inadvertent opening of the deep branches of the uterine artery, as well as increase the risk of uterine perforation.

While a standard loop is used to resect the body of the uterine cavity, a slightly forward-angled loop, made by bending the wire electrode 15-20° off the perpendicular, makes treatment of the fundus and ostial areas technically easier (**24.4**). Alternatively, a rollerball can be utilised to coagulate the ostial areas where the myometrium is known to be relatively thin and thus at greater risk of perforation by the cutting loop.

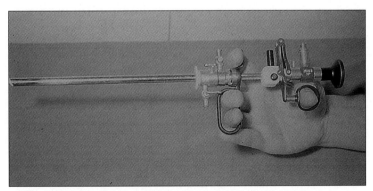

24.1 A typical resectoscope used for hysteroscopic surgery including endometrial resection.

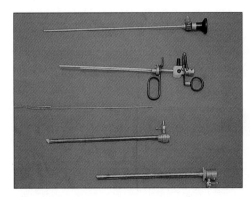

24.2 The five components of a resectoscope (from top to bottom: telescope, handle mechanism, cutting electrode, inner inflow sheath and outer outflow sheath.

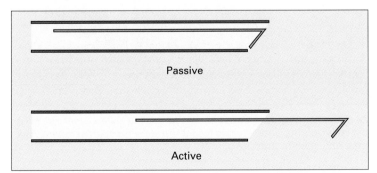

24.3 Diagrammatic representation of a passive and active resectoscope. At rest, the electrode is situated within the sheaths in the case of a passive handle mechanism, and outside the sheath with an active one.

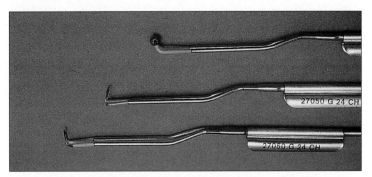

24.4 Cutting and coagulating electrodes used for endometrial ablation. The cutting loop at the top has been bent forward for resection of the uterine fundus and ostial areas; the loop in the middle is the standard loop which is used for treating the rest of the cavity; and the rollerball at the bottom is used for electro-coagulation of the endometrium and for additional hemostasis.

UTERINE DISTENSION AND IRRIGATION

The uterine cavity is a potential space which has to be distended to obtain a panoramic view for surgery. While a gas such as CO_2 is suitable for diagnostic procedures, electrosurgery is associated with bleeding and the production of smoke, and for these reasons a liquid medium must be used to keep the operative field clear. As a further consideration, the use of electricity for TCRE means that the solution must be electrolyte-free to avoid dissipation of the current and possible electrical burns distant from the operative site. Several near isotonic sterile solutions are available, including 1.5% glycine, 5% dextrose, and sorbitol or sorbitol/mannitol mixes. Whichever distension fluid is used, it must be remembered that they do not contain electrolytes such as sodium, and over-absorption is therefore associated not only with fluid overload but also hemodilution including hyponatremia.

The thick muscle wall of the uterus makes it a relatively non-compliant organ to distend, and in contrast to the thin-walled bladder, higher pressures of 60–120 mmHg are required to obtain an adequate operative view of the entire cavity. Such distension pressures can be achieved using gravity by elevating the bags or bottles containing the irrigating fluid to a sufficient height above the patient. Although such a system is simple and cheap, adjustment of the distension pressure relies on altering the height of the supporting poles which can be both inconvenient and insensitive. Use of a sphygmomanometer cuff around bags of fluid is a possible alternative, but suffers from the progressive drop in distension pressure as the bag gradually empties.

Most convenient is the use of a purpose-built pressure pump such as the Hamou Hysteromat (Karl Storz, Tuttlingen, Germany) **(24.5)**. This is a constant pressure, variable-flow pump which monitors the intrauterine pressure throughout surgery and allows fine control over intrauterine pressure and flow rate of the distending fluid **(24.6)**. The maximum distension pressure is generally set at 80–100 mmHg but can be adjusted easily to the minimum which produces adequate uterine distension as defined by a complete view

of the uterine fundus and ostial areas. The maximum flow-rate is not so critical but is often preset at 250 ml/minute.

An alternative design of pump, one which produces a constant flow of irrigant at a variable pressure, should not be used for hysteroscopic surgery as very high intrauterine pressures can be produced with resultant excessive fluid absorption.

The outflow circuit of the resectoscope can be connected to any standard suction unit, remembering that the intrauterine pressure and hence the degree of distension is a balance between the inflow and outflow pressures. Generally, only minimal suction needs to be applied to maintain a clear view of the uterine cavity and remove any debris, especially if the endometrium has been pretreated. A suction pump is conveniently built into the Hamou Hysteromat.

ELECTROSURGICAL GENERATOR

Any modern solid-state electrosurgical generator can be used for endometrial resection which provides safe monopolar cutting, coagulating and blended currents for surgery, although specialised generators are also available. As the output characteristics of electrosurgical generators vary depending on the manufacturer and the model, it is impossible to generalize as to the ideal power settings. Instead, as with uterine distension, the minimum power should be applied which produces the desired tissue effect, that is easy resection of the endometrium and myometrium with minimal drag and charring. Using such settings a loop electrode can be used for 10–15 procedures before failing.

Use of a blended cutting current, that is a mixture of cutting and coagulation, has a number of theoretical advantages compared with a pure cutting current: small vessels are coagulated while being cut, and this may have a beneficial effect on intraoperative fluid absorption and postoperative bleeding, and any unresected endometrium may be destroyed by the deeper penetration of the coagulating waveform. Whether theory translates into practice remains to be proven.

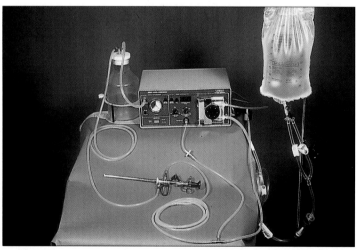

24.5 The Hamou Hysteromat pump used to distend and irrigate the uterine cavity with low viscosity fluids during hysteroscopic surgery showing how the inflow and outflow circuits are connected.

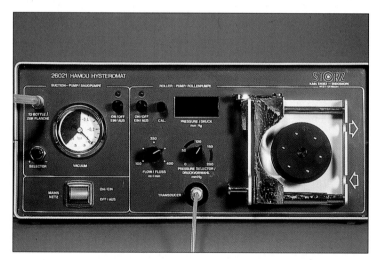

24.6 Close-up of the front panel of the Hamou Hysteromat showing the roller-pump, and controls for intrauterine pressure, irrigant flow rate, and suction pressure.

Finally, a rollerball may occasionally be used to ablate the endometrium of the uterine fundus or for hemostasis at the end of surgery. The desired tissue effect for these two indications is coagulation, and for this reason a coagulating current is, at least in theory, the waveform of choice. Some gynecologists, however, prefer to use a cutting current for rollerball ablation. Whichever type of current is utilized, surgery has to be performed slowly enough to allow sufficient contact time between the electrode and tissue for full thickness coagulation.

ILLUMINATION AND VIDEO MONITORING

The importance of adequate illumination during surgery hardly needs to be emphasized. The use of a relatively narrow optic means that the cold-light fountain should have an output of at least 250 watts, particularly if surgery is to be performed under video monitoring using a chip camera. This is to be recommended on several counts: superior comfort of the operator, interest of the theater staff (and patient if TCRE is performed under local or regional anesthesia), and to facilitate teaching and supervision.

PRINCIPLES OF RESECTOSCOPIC SURGERY

Two basic principles regarding the use of the resectoscope and electrosurgery must be understood for its effective and safe use. Firstly, it is the cutting current applied to the loop which 'cuts' not the loop itself; the wire loop is merely an electrode transmitting the cutting current on to the target tissue and will not resect the endometrium unless the generator is activated. Secondly, with rare exceptions, cuts should only be made by moving the activated cutting loop towards the resectoscope sheath and not away; if this rule is adhered to, uterine perforation becomes a virtual impossibility unless repeated cuts are made in the same place deep into the myometrium.

ANESTHESIA

Hysteroscopic surgical procedures can be performed not only under general or regional anesthesia, but also under local anesthesia supplemented by light sedation/anxiolysis. This is possible because of the relatively poor sensory innervation of the uterine cavity for stimuli such as heat and cutting, the modalities utilized for endometrial resection. As there appears to be advantages with local anesthesia in terms of faster patient recovery and reduced nausea, thus making it ideal for out-patient or day-case surgery, it is our routine practice to offer patients a choice of anesthesia. There are also cases for whom general anesthesia is contraindicated on medical grounds but who can now be offered surgery.

Our technique consists of premedicating with a hypnotic (temazepam, 20 mg orally) and an long-acting analgesic (diclofenac, 100 mg rectally) one hour before surgery. In the operating theater intra-venous access is established and an opiate analgesic (fentanyl 50mg iv) followed five minutes later by an anxiolytic (midazolam 2 mg iv) are slowly injected. The patient is continuously monitored (pulse, ECG, BP, sPaO$_2$) throughout the sedation process and thereafter during surgery. A dilute solution of a local anesthetic (1% lignocaine with 1:200,000 adrenaline) is injected paracervically (10 ml), intracervically (10 ml) and after cervical dilatation, into the myometrium (20 ml) via an injection needle fitted to the resectoscope **(24.7, 24.8)**. The intrauterine injections are placed all over the cavity but primarily into the fundus and ostial areas which are spared by the paracervical block. Small supplemental doses of midazolam and fentanyl can be given during surgery as symptomatically required, but it is unusual to exceed 8 mg of the former and 100 mcg of the latter in total.

Patients are 'street fit' within hours of their surgery, nausea is unusual, and postoperative pain is generally slight and easily treated with non-opiate oral analgesics.

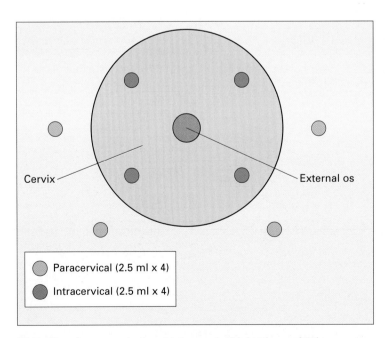

24.7 Site of paracervical and intracervical injections of 1% lignocaine and 1:200,000 adrenaline injected prior to cervical dilatation in patients undergoing hysteroscopic surgery under local anesthesia.

Cervix — External os

- ● Paracervical (2.5 ml x 4)
- ● Intracervical (2.5 ml x 4)

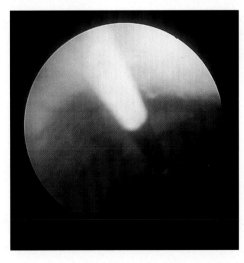

24.8 Hysteroscopic view of the needle used to inject local anesthetic into the myometrium prior to endometrial resection. Several injections are made all over the uterine cavity to achieve total anesthesia. A similar technique is used for focal lesions except the anesthetic is only injected around the target lesion.

SURGERY

The position of the patient, operative personnel, and equipment in our theater is shown in **24.9–24.11**. To the right of the surgeon are the scrub nurse, a cut-down D&C tray containing only the essential instruments for hysteroscopic surgery (e.g. Sims speculum, volsellum, uterine sound, Hegar dilators sizes 3-10, resectoscope, polyp forceps, non-toothed forceps, drapes, etc.), and the pump and fluids for uterine distension and irrigation. To the left are electrosurgical generator, light source, and video system, the latter in such a position as to be comfortably visible to the surgeon, scrub nurse and patient if appropriate. A tall plastic bucket is placed immediately at the foot of the operating table to collect any transcervical leakage of the irrigant, and the two foot-pedals controlling the surgical generator are positioned on either side of the bucket, the right one being for cutting and the left for coagulation. This is preferable to keeping the pedals next to each other and risking inadvertent activation of the wrong current circuit.

The patient's legs are placed in lithotomy poles, and she is washed and draped as for any vaginal gynecologic procedure. Bimanual examination is performed to check the uterine position and size; the bladder is only catheterized if it is full and palpation is difficult or if laparoscopy is to be carried out simultaneously. A

Sims speculum is placed into the vagina, and the anterior lip of the cervix grasped with a volsellum before sounding the uterus and dilating the cervix sufficiently to admit the resectoscope (10 mm in case of a 26–27 Fr gauge outer sheath). The operating table is also given a slight Trendelenburg tilt, partly to avoid the vaginal speculum from falling out, but mostly to encourage the bowel to slide off the uterus and thereby reduce the risk of serious bowel trauma in case of uterine perforation. The resectoscope and accessories are meanwhile assembled by the scrub nurse.

Before starting the resection it is important to ensure that all the air has been drained out of the inflow irrigation tubing and the wire lead to the electrosurgical generator is not in contact with the patient, to avoid air embolism and capacitance burns respectively. Beginners may find laparoscopic monitoring of the procedure by a colleague reassuring to provide early warning of impending (or actual) uterine perforation. Laparoscopy can also be valuable if resection is to be combined with resection of a relatively large and deep fibroid. Laparoscopy, however, adds to the invasiveness of the procedure and is unnecessary under normal circumstances. Conversely, if laparoscopic sterilization is planned, it should be performed before the start of TCRE to prevent transtubal fluid loss of the uterine irrigant and thereby reduce the risk of fluid overload.

24.9 Diagram of the position of the operating personnel, patient and equipment for hysteroscopic surgery.

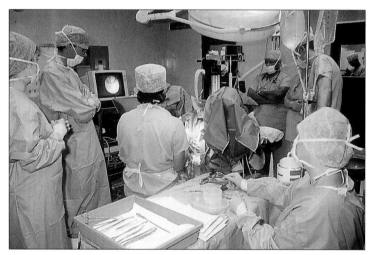

24.10 Picture of the operating theatre viewed from the foot of the operating table.

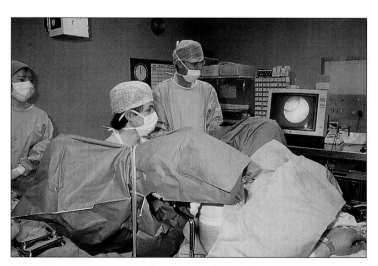

24.11 Picture of the operating theatre viewed from the head of the operating table.

Inspection of the Uterine Cavity

When all is ready, the tip of the resectoscope is inserted into the external cervical os, and the irrigation and suction systems opened. The resectoscope can then be guided into the uterine cavity under direct vision making allowance for the angulation of view of the fore-oblique optic. Once inside the uterus, the cavity must be inspected carefully, particularly if preoperative diagnostic hysteroscopy had not been carried out, and any abnormality noted. Focal lesions such as benign polyps and submuscous fibroids are relatively common in women with menorrhagia and do not contra-indicate surgery. Similarly, the presence of a septate or bicornuate uterus merely means that the resection technique has to be adapted in the mid-line. On the other hand, the finding of areas suspicious of endometrial malignancy is an absolute contra-indication to TCRE, and surgery should be aborted and biopsies taken, this being easily carried out with the resecting loop itself.

Excision of Focal Lesions

Any polyps or submucous fibroids which are primarily intracavity are best excised at the start of surgery before the endometrium is resected, especially if they obscure the upper part of the uterine cavity. This is a simple procedure unless the lesion is very large, and it is best to remove the resected tissue and send it for histo-logic examination separate from the rest of the chippings. The resection proper can then be started in a 'clean' cavity.

Uterine Fundus

It is best to begin the resection in the fundus and ostial areas before proceeding to the remainder of the cavity (**24.12a,b**). There are two reasons for this which are inter-related. This is the most awkward area to treat and is therefore best resected before vision becomes restricted by chippings from the body of the uterus. Because of the angles involved between the resectoscope and tissue surface, it is easier the perform this part of the surgery with a cutting loop which has been bent forward slightly (**24.13**), using a scooping action across the fundus, and taking shallow shavings around the tubal ostia until myometrial fibers are identified. Most care has to be taken while doing the latter as the underlying myometrium can be as thin as 4 mm making perforation a hazard if too deep a cut is made.

An alternative approach to treating the top of the uterine cavity involves using a rollerball to coagulate the endometrium (**24.14, 24.15**). This is technically easier than resection especially for the beginner. There is probably less risk of perforation, although this has been recorded with the rollerball. It is important to keep the ball moving and not to 'over coagulate' the ostia by treating one area for too long.

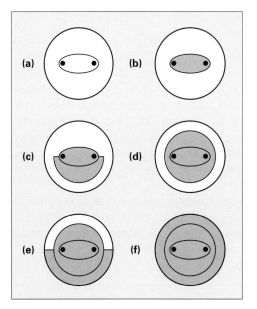

24.12 Diagram of the operating sequence used to perform TCRE. The fundus and ostial areas are treated first followed by the upper part of the posterior wall, the upper part of the anterior wall, the lower part of the posterior wall and finally the lower part of the anterior wall.

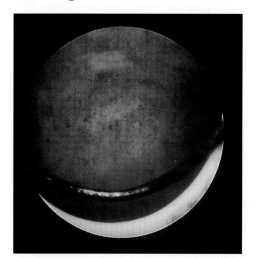

24.13 View through the resectoscope at the start of TCRE showing the forward-angled cutting loop which projects out of the sheath even when the handle mechanism is fully drawn in.

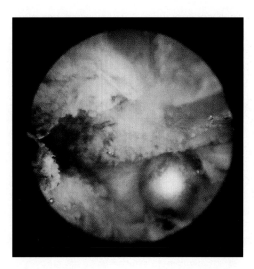

24.14 Rollerball coagulation of the right tubal ostium as an alternative to resection.

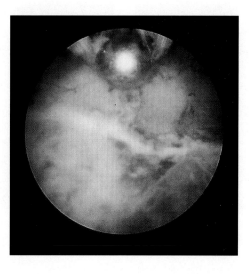

24.15 Rollerball coagulation of the uterine fundus.

Uterine Body

Once the fundus and tubal ostia have been treated, resection of the main bulk of the endometrium can continue towards the cervical canal in a systematic fashion (**24.12c–f, 24.16, 24.17**). As the resected chips tend to fall onto and cover the posterior uterine wall, it is logical to treat this area early before it becomes obscured. Therefore the posterior wall is resected first, and surgery is continued by gradually rotating the resectoscope clockwise (or anticlockwise) so as to leave no area untreated. The anterior wall is treated last (**24.18**). If the cutting loop is fully extended at the start of each cut, the chips will measure approximately 2.5 x 0.8 x 0.5 cm; it is relatively easy to push these pieces of tissue away from the area being resected and towards the fundus, which of course has already been treated. Surgery can then be continued until the cervical canal is reached without having to remove the resectoscope (**24.19**).

An alternative method used by some surgeons is to make full length cuts of the endometrium from the fundus to the cervix by not only moving the cutting loop into the sheathing system, but also slowly withdrawing the resectoscope itself from the uterine cavity as the cut is being made. This produces long pieces of resected tissue which are difficult to manipulate within the cavity because of their size, so it is usual to remove each chip immediately it has been cut. This has the advantage that the uterine cavity remains free of debris during surgery, but has the disadvantage that the resectoscope has to be removed with each cut which both slows down surgery and encourages bleeding.

As TCRE relies primarily on the full-thickness excision of the endometrium, the adequacy of surgery depends on visualizing the circumferential myometrial fibers. In practice, because of the undulating character of the basal layer of the endometrium, the endometrium has to be under-cut by about 2–3 mm to have a good chance of achieving this. Deeper resection is potentially dangerous as larger vessels are opened resulting in increased fluid absorption and greater risk of haemorrhage.

Uterine Isthmus and Cervical Canal

Surgery can be continued to 1 cm or so above the uterine isthmus (viz. partial TCRE) or into the endocervical canal (viz. total TCRE). This distinction is not made with other ablative techniques where treatment universally extends over the entire endometrial lining. In theory, excision around the isthmic region and upper endocervical canal may lead to cervical stenosis and hence the development of hematometra if any functional endometrium is left behind; while this complication can develop following surgery, hematometra tend to be fundal resulting from fibrosis in the upper uterine cavity rather than a cervical obstruction. Conversely, the menstrual results of partial TCRE are inferior to the more extensive procedure and it gives no chance of amenorrhea. Most of our patients request and undergo total TCRE.

Resection of the lower part of the uterus / upper part of the cervix has to be performed gently. The cuts must not be too deep especially laterally where the descending branches of the uterine artery are located (**24.20**). Rollerball coagulation is an alternative technique as for the fundus and ostial areas, but care has to be taken not to over-treat as this can be followed some time afterwards by sloughing and hemorrhage.

Once the resection is deemed complete, the resectoscope is withdrawn from the uterus and the endometrial/myometrial chips are removed from the cavity using a flushing curette connected to a bag of normal saline. It can be difficult to remove all the debris as is evident when the resectoscope is re-inserted to check for any untreated areas of endometrium (**24.21, 24.22**). A final look inside the uterus also gives the chance to coagulate bleeding vessels, made more obvious if the distension pressure is reduced. All the operative specimen is routinely sent for histologic examination (**24.23**).

Special Situations

Apart from the presence of polyps and fibroids, there are two other special situations worthy of comment. If hysteroscopy reveals a double cavity suggestive of either a septate or bicornuate uterus, the middle portion of the uterus should be treated by rollerball coagulation as resection may lead to perforation if the uterus is in reality bicornuate. Alternatively, laparoscopy can be performed to check the contour of the uterine fundus and distinguish between the two anomalies; if the diagnosis is then one of a septate uterus, the septum can be excised hysteroscopically prior to resection, although this is by no means essential.

Care also has to be taken in women who have had lower segment Caesarean deliveries. The anterior wall of the uterus may be thin in the isthmic area, and indeed it is not unusual to see a fibrous indentation under the scar. Resection should therefore be extremely shallow, or once again, gentle coagulation with a rollerball can be used instead.

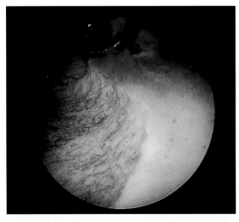

24.16 Resection of the posterior wall of the uterus.

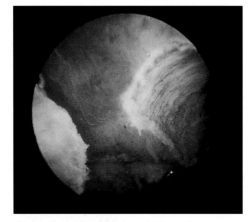

24.17 Resection of the anterior wall of the uterus.

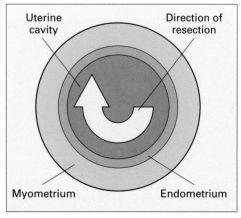

24.18 Systematic resection of the endometrium can be achieved by gradually rotating the resectoscope in a clockwise (or anticlockwise) direction after each cut.

OPERATIVE COMPLICATIONS

With the appropriate choice of patients and correct technique, TCRE is a safe operation. Serious complications are rare but nonetheless one has to be aware of what can potentially go wrong so that corrective action is taken as quickly as possible. Fluid overload, uterine perforation and hemorrhage are at least in theory the three major operative risks.

The volume of irrigant absorbed by the patient during surgery depends on a number of factors, of which the duration of surgery and the intrauterine distension pressure are the two most influential. To minimize the risk of fluid over-load, TCRE should be performed as quickly as possible, remembering that the operative time will be prolonged when treating a patient with a large uterine cavity, fibroids or thick endometrium. Over distension of the uterine cavity should also be avoided, which in practice means working at the lowest pressure which provides a complete view of the uterine fundus. It is essential to monitor fluid balance throughout surgery by comparing the in- and outflow volumes of the uterine irrigant; if the deficit exceeds 2000 ml, it is our practice to stop surgery, give an i.v. diuretic, catheterize the patient, and check her serum electrolytes.

The uterus can be perforated at the time of cervical dilatation, resection or at the end of surgery when the chippings are being removed. Of these, perforation caused when the resectoscope is being activated is the most serious as it can be associated with major intra-abdominal trauma to bowel, the urinary tract or major vessels. This type of perforation is most likely to occur as a result of inexperience, particularly when treating the ostial areas of the uterus. The perforation may be obvious, either because extrauterine structures can be seen, or as is the case more often, because of a sudden and rapid absorption of fluid by the patient. In either event, surgery should be stopped immediately, and laparoscopy or laparotomy performed to assess the extent of any injury inside the abdomen. Save in exceptional circumstances, trauma to vital structures should be managed by laparotomy with appropriate surgical assistance.

Intraoperative hemorrhage is an unusual complication of TCRE provided resection is not carried too deeply into the myometrium. The area most at risk of major vascular trauma is the isthmic/cervical regions, where the endometrium is naturally thin even without hormonal treatment, and the arterial supply runs relatively close to the surface. Hemorrhage can usually be controlled by

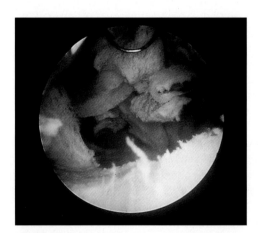

24.19 View of the uterine cavity when the body of the uterus has been resected showing the chippings which have yet to be removed.

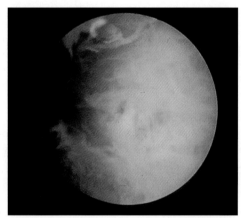

24.20 Resection of the uterine isthmus and endocervical canal should be done carefully by making shallow cuts only.

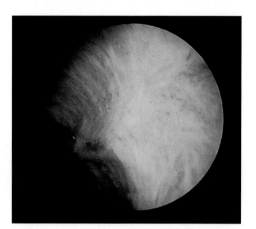

24.21 A small island of endometrium which was missed during the initial resection but which is obvious once the resected chippings have been removed and the cavity is checked at the end of surgery.

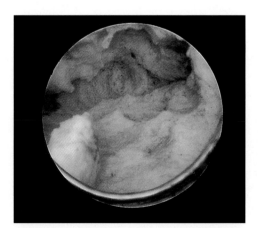

24.22 The appearance of the uterine cavity at the end of surgery with the pale fibers of the myometrium easily visible all over.

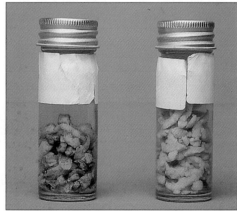

24.23 On the left, a typical specimen pot of resected endometrium which is sent for histologic evaluation. For comparison, on the right, is a similar pot of prostate chippings obtained at TURP.

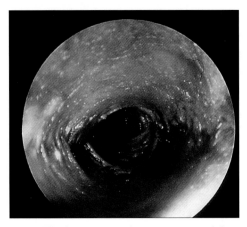

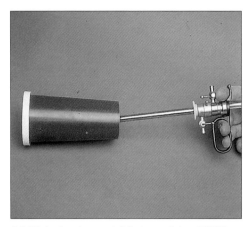

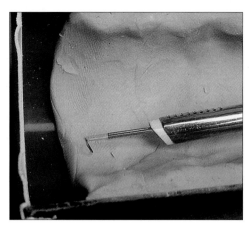

24.24 The hysteroscopic appearance of the uterine cavity 12 months after TCRE: the uterine cavity is narrow and fibrotic, the tubal ostia are rarely seen, and it is difficult to find any normal endometrium.

24.25 A simple model for practising TCRE consisting of a plastic beaker with a 1 cm hole in its base and a plasticine lining.

24.26 The plasticine lining can be resected without using an electrosurgical generator.

electrocoagulation using the cutting loop itself or a rollerball, or alternatively, balloon tamponade can be achieved using a standard bladder catheter. Hysterectomy may be the only solution if these measures fail.

RECOVERY AND MENSTRUAL RESULTS

TCRE is similar to other endoscopic procedures in that it can be performed as a day case in most patients, with minimal postoperative discomfort and fast recovery. Being a newer technique than laser ablation, data regarding the efficacy of endometrial resection are less complete. However, the series which have been published suggest that the menstrual results are comparable in terms of rates of amenorrhea, menstrual improvement, and failure rates. Our most recent analysis of over 450 patients show that the cumulative success rate, defined as avoidance of further treatment, is over 80% after four years, while the chance of undergoing hysterectomy during that period is 13%.

This improvement in menstruation is probably related to the extensive intra-uterine shrinkage and fibrosis which develops after surgery. Hysteroscopy even only three months after TCRE typically shows a small, contracted and tubular cavity, the fundus and ostial areas being obscured by scar tissue (**24.24**). Endometrium becomes difficult to distinguish visually, but biopsy of the cavity can reveal endometrial deposits even on those women who have become amenorrheic.

LONGER-TERM COMPLICATIONS

Treatment failure occurs in some patients either because of a return of their original complaint, menorrhagia, or because of the development of new symptoms, the commonest of which is dysmenorrhea. Pelvic pain may be associated with the development of a hematometra, but sometimes no obvious explanation can be found. In cases of recurrent menorrhagia or hematometra, surgery can be repeated as an alternative to hysterectomy; when pelvic pain is the sole abnormality, hysterectomy may be the only choice of therapy.

Pregnancies have been recorded following TCRE, women generally opting for early termination. Whether any of the ablative techniques will influence the risks of endometrial carcinoma in years to come remains to be shown.

CONCLUSION

TCRE can be an effective and relatively atraumatic solution to the common complaint of menorrhagia. It has several advantages compared with the other ablative techniques in terms of cost, speed of surgery, ability to deal easily with submucous fibroids, and the availability of an operative specimen for histologic examination. Endometrial resection is inherently a more difficult procedure to learn (**24.25, 24.26**) but the versatility of the instrument means it is well worth the effort.

FURTHER READING

Baumann R, Magos AL, Kay JDS, Turnbull AC. Absorption of glycine irrigating solution during transcervical resection of the endometrium. *BMJ* 1990; **300**: 304-5

Brooks PG, Serden SP, Davos I. Hormonal inhibition of the endometrium for resectoscopic endometrial ablation. *Am J Obstet Gynec* 1991; **164**: 1601-8

DeCherney A, Polan ML. Hysteroscopic management of intrauterine lesions and intractable uterine bleeding. *Obstetrics and Gynecology* 1983; **61**: 392-7

Lockwood GM, Baumann R, Turnbull AC, Magos AL. Extensive hysteroscopic surgery under local anaesthesia. *Gynaecological Endoscopy* 1992; **1**: 15-21

Magos AL, Baumann R, Lockwood GM, Turnbull AC. Experience with the first 250 endometrial resections for menorrhagia. *Lancet* 1991; **337**: 1074-8

ENDOMETRIAL LASER ABLATION 25

Ray Garry

INTRODUCTION

Dysfunctional uterine bleeding (DUB) frequently fails to respond to medical therapy and is one of the most common indications for hysterectomy. More than 50% of the 700,000 plus hysterectomies performed each year in the United States are performed for DUB. Many patients and their doctors are, however, unhappy about this and would prefer a less invasive approach which retains the structurally normal and healthy uterus and removes only the bleeding endometrium. Many local destructive agents and modalities had been used unsuccessfully until Goldrath described the hysteroscopic use of the Nd:YAG laser to ablate the endometrium in 1981. Later this same modality has been shown to be effective in treating uterine polyps, submucous fibroids and intrauterine septae.

The early attempts at treatment were unsuccessful because the endometrium has amazing powers of regeneration. It is shed at the end of each menstrual cycle and rapidly replaces itself. The endometrium is repaired from the glands situated in the pars basalis deep in the zone of the endometrium retained when the more superficial layers are shed at menstruation **(25.1)**. Any successful attempt to prevent the rapid regrowth of endometrium after trauma must effectively and completely remove these basal glands. Techniques which simply remove the superficial endometrium are certain to fail.

EQUIPMENT FOR ENDOMETRIAL LASER ABLATION

ND:YAG LASER

The Nd:YAG laser wavelength of 1064nm is particularly suitable for endometrial laser ablation (ELA) because of three properties laser energy of that wavelength possesses:

1. Nd-YAG laser energy can be readily directed down a flexible quartz fiber from the laser generating equipment through an endoscope to virtually any cavity in the body. The laser can be situated a convenient distance from the patient and directed via an operating hysteroscope into the uterine cavity.
2. Nd:YAG laser energy is not absorbed when passed through water and clear fluid. It can therefore be used therapeutically inside the uterine cavity distended with fluids. Laser energy is not conducted by electrolyte containing solutions and so any optically clear fluid can be used.
3. Nd:YAG produces a clinical effect mainly by coagulating tissue protein. When applied to the surface of a tissue such as the endometrium it penetrates to a depth of 5–6 mm. This is deeper than the CO_2 laser or the argon and KTP laser wavelengths can penetrate **(25.2)**. This greater depth of penetration ensures a greater probability of destroying endometrium to a depth adequate to remove all the basal glands and so make this the most suitable of the available medical wavelengths. The energy is delivered directly from the end of the quartz fiber – the so called 'bare-fiber' system. Contact tips are neither necessary nor useful in this situation which, if they are cooled with gas, can be dangerous in the uterine cavity because of the risk of embolus.

Lasers are inefficient energy machines with a low conversion rate from electrical power input to laser energy output. Most of the energy is lost as heat so it is important the laser is adequately cooled. Air cooled devices are more convenient than water cooled devices. The effect of the laser on tissue is dependant on the power density of the laser energy at the fiber tip and the time the laser is held in contact with the tissue. Thus, the higher the power of the laser the more rapidly the fiber can be moved to produce a consistent effect. The minimum power required for reasonable treatment time is 60 watts delivered to tissue and as there is some loss of energy down the fiber a higher power is needed. I prefer to use a 100 watt laser set to deliver 80 watts to the endometrial surface **(25.3)**.

QUARTZ FIBER

The Nd:YAG laser energy is directed through a quartz fiber which is usually 600μ in diameter, although wider fibers of 800, 1000 or even 1200μ are available. The wider fibers ablate larger areas of tissue at any moment in time but because the power must be spread over a wide area the fiber must be moved slowly to produce the desired effect. I prefer the standard 600μ diameter fiber. The long quartz fiber is directed down one of the channels of a suitable operating hysteroscope **(25.4)**.

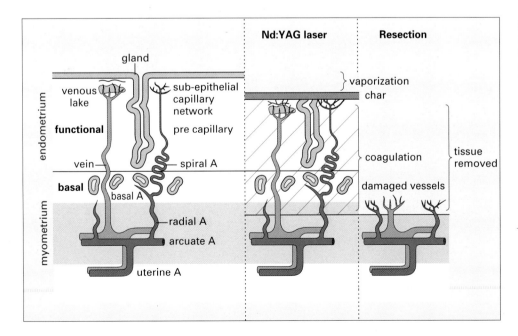

25.1 A diagrammatic representation of the endometrium. This shows the location of the basal glands and how they can be removed either by ablative or excisional techniques.

OPERATING HYSTEROSCOPE

The early hysteroscopes used for ELA were ill designed. Goldrath originally used a hysteroscope without a channel for the outflow of fluid from the cavity of the uterus. The way in which he obtained drainage was to over dilate the cervix to allow the distension fluid to escape in the space between the hysteroscope and the cervix. Continuous clear vision is an essential prerequisite for safe hysteroscopic surgery. This can only be maintained by ensuring all bubbles and particles produced during surgery are continuously flushed out of the cavity. It is essential to ensure that the hysteroscope employed for any operative procedure is a specifically designed continuous flow instrument with separate channels for fluid inflow and outflow. I favor the operating hysteroscope designed by Michael Baggish (Bryan Corp. MA, USA) with three or now five parallel individual channels **(25.5)**. Other companies such as Olympus and Storz have also produced continuous flow designs.

UTERINE DISTENSION SYSTEMS

Distension Media

The uterine cavity is only a potential space and must be distended with fluid and gas under pressure to ensure adequate visualization of the endometrial surface. Gaseous distension media such as CO2 can be used but most surgeons prefer fluid distension for operative hysteroscopy. When electrosurgical power is used inside the uterus it is essential to use non-electrolyte containing fluids such as glycine. If excess volumes of glycine are absorbed during hysteroscopic surgery there is the risk of fluid overload but there are also a risk of the 'TUR' syndrome with the possibility of dilutional hyponatremia, cardiac failure, metabolic disturbances, and cerebral edema, coma and, rarely, death. The Nd:YAG laser wavelength works equally well in all clear fluids and so the simplest, safest and cheapest solution should be chosen. I prefer the crystalloid normal saline for uterine distension during ELA.

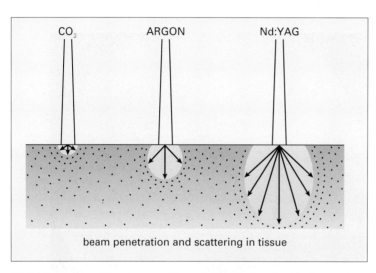

25.2 Diagrammatic representation of the relative depth of penetration of three different laser wavelengths.

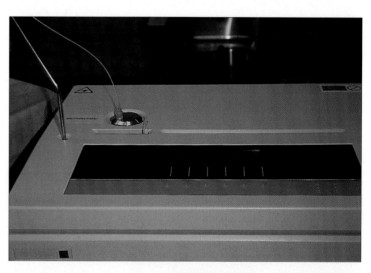

25. 3 The control panel of an SLT CL 100 watt Nd:YAG laser.

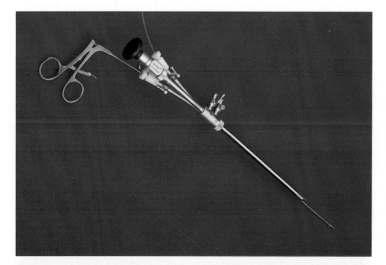

25.4 A Baggish operating hysteroscope with quartz laser fiber down one channel and semi-rigid forceps down the other.

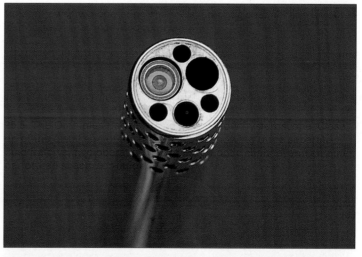

25.5 The Omniplus Baggish Continuous-Flow hysteroscope. Close up of the distal end of the hysteroscope showing three separate fluid inflows, two operating channels, an optic channel and an outer perforated sheath for fluid return.

Infusion Pumps

The distension fluid must be forced into the uterine cavity under pressure. This pressure can be obtained by gravity and suspending the infusion bag above the patient. The infusion pressure is proportional to the height of the bag above the patient and flow rates can be altered by adjusting the height. Fluid can also be forced into the cavity with simple rotary pumps (**25.6**). These are more easily controllable than gravity feed and are capable of producing a constant flow of fluid into the uterine cavity irrespective of the intrauterine pressure.

ELA and, indeed, any form of intrauterine surgery inevitably disrupts the subendometrial blood vessels (**25.7**). Bleeding from these vessels will quickly cloud the distension fluid and impair vision. The uterus is a thick walled muscular structure and if the cervix and the hysteroscope fit tightly with each other a closed circuit distension system can be produced. Increasing the pressure in the cavity will then tamponade the vessels and stop the bleeding. In my personal series of 1000 ELAs performed with such a closed circuit no case was abandoned because of bleeding and a clear view was maintained throughout the procedure.

Excessive absorption of the distension fluid is one of the most important potential complications of ELA. If the intrauterine pressure is maintained within acceptable limits, fluid usually stays in the uterine cavity and is not absorbed. This effect can be demonstrated by taking a hysterogram at the completion of an ELA operation. **25.8** shows an x-ray taken with the intrauterine pressure set at 75mm/Hg. The important point is that at this pressure the radio-opaque medium is confined inside the uterine cavity. Uncontrolled elevation of intrauterine pressure will force fluid from the uterine cavity into the open vessels. This effect can be demonstrated by deliberately raising the intrauterine pressure to 150mm/Hg and observing the free flow of medium into the whole of the pelvic venous system (**25.9**). This 'high pressure' fluid absorption occurs commonly when simple constant flow pumps are used. The outflow channel frequently becomes blocked with small particles and if the rate of flow remains constant the pressure inside the cavity will rise. The treatment of this problem is to recognise the block and reverse flush the outflow channel to clear it.

Low intrauterine pressure results in bleeding into the cavity but no risk of excess fluid absorption. High intrauterine pressure results in blood vessel tamponade and no bleeding into the cavity but may force fluid into the patient's circulation. The optimum fluid distension system would titrate the intrauterine pressure against the patient's blood pressure so that there is neither bleeding from the vessels nor fluid infusion into them (**25.10**).

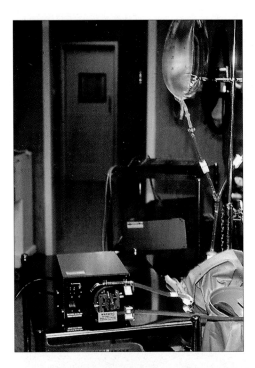

25. 6 A simple roller pump (constant flow) which will infuse fluid at a constant rate no matter what the outflow channel conditions.

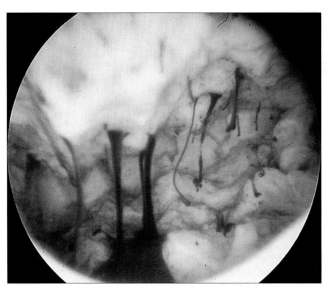

25.7 Intrauterine bleeding. Bleeding from the disrupted endometrial capillaries inevitably follows ablation when the intrauterine pressure is too low.

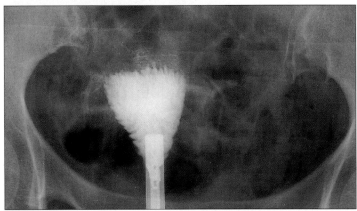

25. 8 A hysterosalpingogram taken at the end of an ELA procedure with the IUP at 75mm/Hg. Note the radio-opaque dye is confined to the uterine cavity.

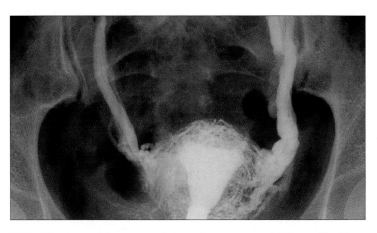

25.9 A hysterosalpingogram taken at a pressure of 150mm/Hg. The dye is forced into the uterine circulation with the production of a dramatic pelvic venogram.

To ensure this I therefore prefer to use pressure controlled uterine infusion pumps such as that designed by Hamou **(25.11)** (Stortz, Tuttlingen Germany) or the one I am helping to develop with W.O.M (Berlin, Germany) which, in addition to controlling the infusion pressure, also measures the volume of fluid infused and collected and calculates the quantity of fluid absorbed **(25.12)**. The dramatic reduction in fluid absorption produced by substituting a pressure-controlled pump for a simple pump is shown in **25.13**. The maximum intrauterine pressure should equal the mean arterial pressure of the patient. In a healthy woman this should be 80–100mm/Hg. 'High pressure' absorption can be avoided by controlling the intrauterine pressure and ensuring the outflow channel remains patent throughout the procedure.

In a few cases, even with good control of the intrauterine pressure, excess fluid absorption may still occur. Such cases are not associated with increased intrauterine pressure and indeed the intrauterine pressure may fall. We have demonstrated this is due to ablating too deeply into the myometrium and inadvertently entering major large calibre uterine vessels. This can be demonstrated by taking an HSG during such 'low-pressure' absorption **(25.14)**. This type of absorption may be avoided by good technique and ensuring the level of destruction is confined to the endometrium and the superficial myometrium.

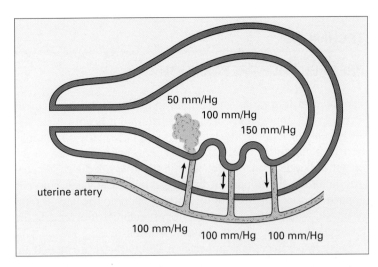

25.10 Diagram of IUP titration against arterial pressure. If the IUP is too low bleeding will occur into the uterine cavity obscuring vision. If the IUP is too high the net flow will be in the opposite direction and fluid will be forced into the patient's circulation. With the correct IUP the forces will be in equilibrium and there will be neither bleeding nor absorption.

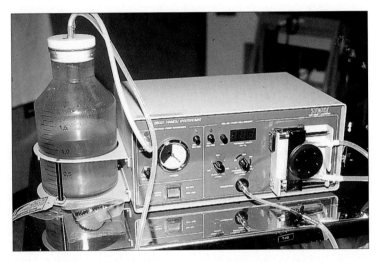

25.11 A Hamou Hysteromat – a pressure-controlled roller pump with facilities to monitor IUP and restrict the IUP to a pre-set maximum.

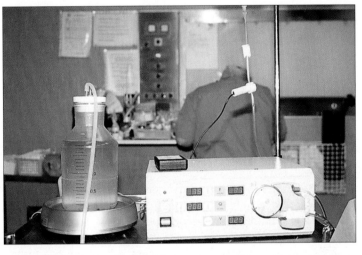

25.12 WOM Infusion System. A prototype system which controls IUP and calculates fluid absorption.

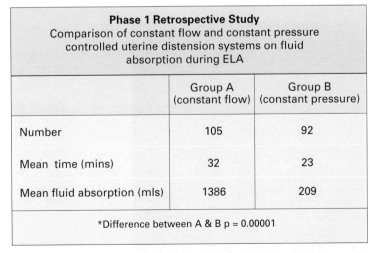

Phase 1 Retrospective Study Comparison of constant flow and constant pressure controlled uterine distension systems on fluid absorption during ELA		
	Group A (constant flow)	Group B (constant pressure)
Number	105	92
Mean time (mins)	32	23
Mean fluid absorption (mls)	1386	209
*Difference between A & B p = 0.00001		

25.13 A table demonstrating the effects of controlling IUP on fluid absorption during ELA.

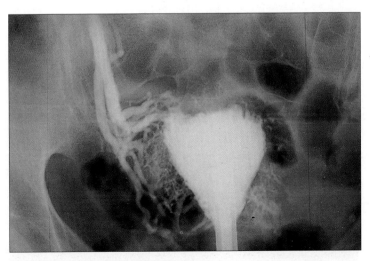

25.14 Hysterosalpingogram of 'low pressure' absorption taken after ablation had been taken too deeply producing a fistula between the cavity and major caliber vessels deep in the myometrium.

TECHNIQUE

PREOPERATIVE PREPARATION

The endometrium varies considerably in thickness during the menstrual cycle. Immediately after menstruation it is only a few layers of cells thick but by the late secretory phase of the cycle it may be 10–12 mm thick. If Nd:YAG laser energy is applied early in the menstrual cycle it will destroy the full thickness of the endometrium including the important basal glands. If the same power is applied for the same time to the endometrium in the late secretory phase, it will only destroy the upper endometrium leaving the basal glands intact. This is clinically worthless.

It is always necessary to perform ELA early in the menstrual cycle or pretreat the endometrium so that it is thin at the time of treatment. Danazol has long been regarded as the 'gold standard' for endometrial thinning and is usually given in a dose of 600–800 mgs daily for 4–8 weeks prior to ELA. Recent studies have indicated that GnRH agonists such as goserelin ('Zoladex', Zeneca Cheshire, UK) are at least as effective in causing endometrial thinning and are associated with shorter operating times, less operative complications and is better tolerated by patients. Goserelin is particularly indicated when the length of the uterine cavity is greater than 8 cms and/or when the uterus contains submucous fibroids.

ANESTHESIA

The procedure is usually performed under a general anesthetic but may be performed under regional or local anesthetic. The patient is placed in the lithotomy position and cleaned and draped. The patient does not require pubic shaving, bladder catheterization, enema or any other special preparation (except preoperative medication with danazol or GnRH analogues as previously described).

A tenaculum is placed on the anterior lip of the cervix and the cavity length determined by sounding. The cervix is dilated to a diameter just sufficient to accommodate the operating hysteroscope. A watertight seal between the cervix and the hysteroscope is the aim. The hysteroscope is assembled with inflow and outflow

fluid channels connected to the infusion pump. A fiber-optic light cable is attached between the light pillar of the hysteroscope and a high-intensity light source and a single or three chip CCD video camera connected **(25.15)**. Good quality optics, light source and video equipment are essential for hysteroscopic surgery **(25.16)**.

Before the laser is activated the patient and the staff in the operating room must put on protective spectacles or goggles. The windows must be covered and warning notices posted and signs illuminated.

With the fluid running, the hysteroscope is inserted under direct vision through the cervix and into the uterine cavity. The endometrial surface is then inspected noting changes suggestive of malignancy, polyps or fibroids or inadequate preoperative endometrial thinning. If endometrial sampling has not been performed previously a full thickness biopsy should be collected under direct vision **(25.17)**.

When everything is ready the laser should be activated at a power of 80 watts. The dragging method of Goldrath should be used. The fiber is first placed on one tubal ostium and the laser activated as the fiber is drawn down towards the cervix **(25.18)**. As the right hand progressively pulls the fiber out, the left hand holding the hysteroscope must move in an arc to ensure the fiber remains

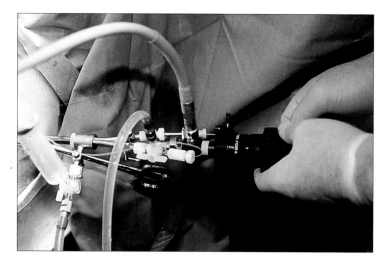

25.15 An operating hysteroscope assembled for ELA. A quartz fiber enters the right-sided channel and fluid and pressure recording catheter enters the left channel. There is a three-way tap on the outflow channel to permit reverse flushing.

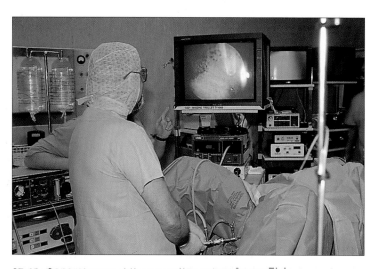

25.16 General view of the operative set up for an ELA.

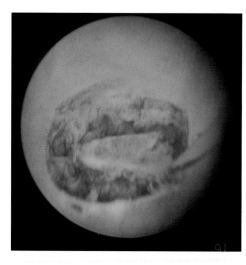

25.17 A full thickness endometrial laser biopsy may be taken under direct vision.

in firm contact with the curved uterine wall. Most beginners underestimate the amount of movement required by the left hand and at first find this action difficult although it soon becomes 'second nature'. Parallel furrows are produced so that the tubal ostial areas are first ablated **(25.19)**. The opposite tubal area is next ablated and then the anterior, posterior, and lateral walls until the whole of the cavity is converted from smooth white or pink endometrium to a brown and furrowed appearance **(25.20–25.22)**. The ablation is extended to the level of the internal os if amenorrhea is the aim of the surgeon **(25.23)**.

The laser should only be activated when the tip of the quartz fiber (which is illuminated with a red HeNe laser) is clearly seen and when the fiber is being moved. Never fire the laser with the fiber stationary and only fire it when drawing towards the operator and never when pushing back towards the fundus of the uterus. If these three 'Golden Rules' of endometrial ablation are followed the laser can only be activated when it is on the surface of the endometrium and cannot perforate the full thickness of the uterus **(25.24)**. We have not had a single case of perforation of the uterus with the laser in our 1000-case series.

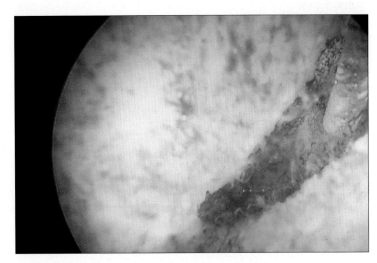

25.18 The first laser furrow of an ELA.

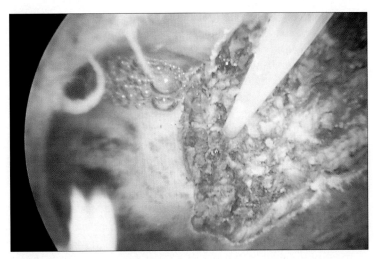

25.19 Progressive ablation of the cavity with parallel furrows.

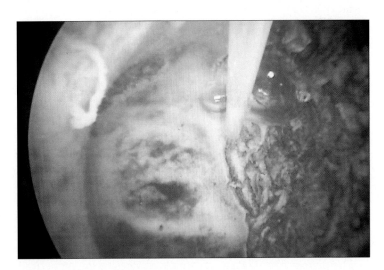

25.20 Progressive ablation of the cavity with parallel furrows.

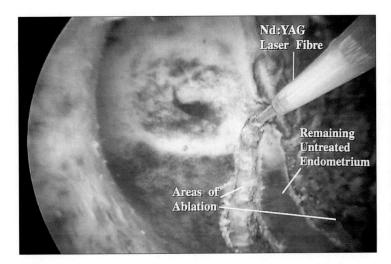

25.21 Progressive ablation of the cavity with parallel furrows.

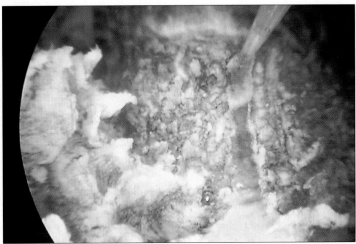

25.22 ELA almost complete with only one strip of endometrium remaining untreated.

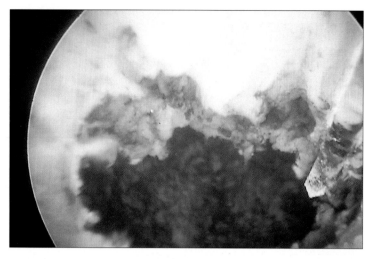

25.23 Ablation extended to the level of the internal os to achieve amenorrhea.

Rule 1:	Only fire laser when illuminated tip of fiber is in view
Rule 2:	Only fire laser when fiber is being drawn towards the surgeon
Rule 3:	Only fire laser when fiber is being moved

25.24 'Golden Rules' of endometrial laser ablation.

POSTOPERATIVE CARE

At the completion of the procedure, which usually takes between 15 and 25 minutes, the laser is turned off and the instruments are removed. A paracervical block with 1% Marcaine (10 mls injected at the 9 and 3 o'clock positions after checking the needle is extravascular) is injected. In my unit, this has been shown to reduce postoperative pain and facilitate early discharge from hospital. The patient usually recovers and is fit to leave hospital within a few hours, but may occasionally stay overnight (less than 5% in our series).

The patient should be given simple analgesics for 'menstrual like' discomfort which continues for 48 hours or so. She must also be advised to anticipate a sero-sanginous vaginal loss of varying intensity for up to six weeks.

Impact of ELA on menstrual loss		
Outcome	Number	%
Amenorrhea	135	28.9
Reduced volume	309	66.2
Same volume	21	4.5
Increased volume	1	0.2
No response	1	0.2

25.25 The results of endometrial laser ablation.

RESULTS

Amenorrhea is the exception (29%) and it may take several months before the maximum reduction in menstrual loss is achieved. Relief of symptoms is, in most cases, maintained although in about 5% of our series to date there has been a secondary relapse. Approximately 95% of our cases report sustained and considerable improvement in the menstrual loss with absent or scanty menstruation sustained for up to five years **(25.25)**.

COMPLICATIONS

ELA should only be performed on patients who have completed their families. It is, however, not a completely effective contraceptive and in our series we have had a pregnancy rate of 0.3% (3/1000). Patients should accordingly be advised of this risk.

The most important feature of any medical treatment is that we should follow the Hippocratic maxim 'First Do No Harm'. Most series using electrosurgical modalities report a 1–2% serious complication rate. Uterine perforation with large vessel, bowel or bladder damage are the most feared complications. Hyponatremia and fluid problems may also occur. In our series of 1000 consecutive cases of Nd:YAG laser ablation we have had no serious complications. There have been no uterine perforations, no cases of hemorrhage or blood transfusions, no laparotomy, no immediate hysterectomy and no cases of major fluid overload. Hyponatraemia is, of course, impossible using normal saline as a distension medium. It is for these reasons that I consider the optimum treatment available for endometrial ablation at the present time is Nd:YAG laser ablation. However, ELA was only performed for the first time in 1979. Long-term follow up data are not yet available. It is essential that audit of this operation continues until long-term risks such as increased uterine malignancy are known.

FURTHER READING

Donnez J, Nisolle M. Laser hysteroscopy in uterine bleeding. Endometrial ablation and polypectomy. In: Donnez J. ed: Laser Operative Laparoscopy and Hysteroscopy. Nauwelaerts Printing, Leuven. 1992

Garry R. Distension media and fluid systems. In: Sutton C. and Diamond M. eds. Endoscopic Surgery for Gynaecologists. WB Saunders Co. Ltd, London 1993, pp282–293

Garry R., Erian J. and Grochmal S. A multi-centre collaborative study into the treatment of menorrhagia by Nd:YAG laser ablation of the endometrium. *Br J Obs Gynae* 1991, **98**: 357

Goldrath M. H., Fuller T. A. and Segal S. Laser photovaporisation of endometrium for the treatment of menorrhagia. *Am J Obs Gyne* 1981, **140**: 14–19

Goldrath M. H. and Garry R. Nd-YAG laser ablation of the endometrium. In: Sutton C. and Diamond M. eds. Endoscopic Surgery for Gynaecologists. WB Saunders Co Ltd, London, 1993, pp317–326

RADIOFREQUENCY ENDOMETRIAL ABLATION

26

Jeffrey H Phipps and B Victor Lewis

INTRODUCTION

It is now over five years since we introduced an alternative method to hysteroscopy of ablating the endometrial cavity in the management of dysfunctional uterine bleeding (DUB): the use of radiofrequency (RF) heating to induce irreversible damage to the basalis layer. The potential advantages of such an approach are that the toxic effects of flushing media – fluid overload and glycine toxicity are avoided, there is no long learning curve for the surgeon, as is the case for hysteroscopic surgery, and the necessary equipment is cheaper than laser systems.

Attempts in the past to use toxic chemicals or physical agents have universally failed. Silver nitrate or fuming nitric acid infused into the uterine cavity was recommended in 1881, but by the turn of the century were no longer used. Quinacrine or urea instillation, cyanoacrylate ester ('superglue') injection, superheated steam and radium packing have all been tried but abandoned. Studies have been carried out on the use of an intracavity cryoprobe for 'congellating' (destroying by freezing) the endometrium, but only partial success was achieved, and the technique has now been abandoned. Hot water has been used to irrigate the uterine cavity either in direct contact with the endometrium or contained within balloons, but recent use of these techniques has led to two consecutive cases of severe intraperitoneal burns, where one patient died.

This chapter describes the investigation and development of the use of RF electromagnetic energy to ablate the endometrium.

PHYSICAL PRINCIPLE

Heating tissue above 43^0 C is referred to as 'hyperthermia', and has been used in the treatment of malignant disease either alone or as an adjunct to radiotherapy for many years. Microwave energy induced hyperthermia has been used in the treatment of both malignant and benign prostatic disease as an alternative to resection. We reported experimental details of the first use of RF induced hyperthermia for treating DUB in 1990.

Human tissues suffer irreversible damage after exposure to temperatures above 42^0 C in a manner which is both time- and temperature-dependent. Cells appear to survive thermal exposure up to approximately 42^0 C, but exposure to 43^0 C for 60 minutes or more causes cell death. For each degree rise, this 'thermotolerance' time is approximately halved. Cell damage occurs because of critical changes in cytoskeletal protein structure, and at higher temperatures because of enzyme denaturation and nuclear damage. Thus heating of the endometrium, including the basalis layer, to a sufficiently high degree for sufficient time, results in endometrial ablation.

The use of simple conductive thermal devices has been tried (heated rods or water-filled balloons), but have proved unsuccessful in the past for various reasons. First, any conductive intrauterine thermal device would have to be of sufficient temperature to drive a thermal gradient such that the basalis layer is heated to histotoxic levels. Blood and protein coagulate above 60^0 C, and this coagulum within the cavity rapidly forms a progressively insulating layer between the device and the endometrium, preventing ther-

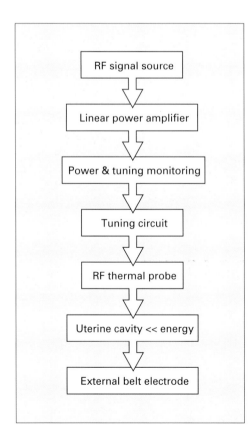

26.1 Block circuit diagram of the radiofrequency generating apparatus.

RF signal source

Linear power amplifier

Power & tuning monitoring

Tuning circuit

RF thermal probe

Uterine cavity << energy

External belt electrode

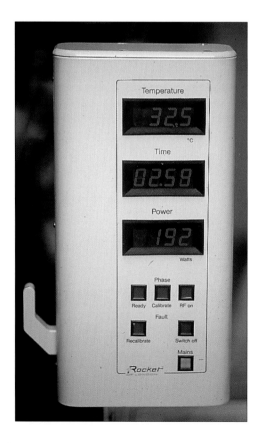

26.2 Detail of 'Menostat' function monitoring display.

mal penetration. Second, tissue heating will depend upon the volume per unit time of local blood flow, since those areas where blood flow is high will be spared due to the cooling effect of perfusing blood. Penetration is therefore erratic. After disappointing initial experimentation with simple conductive techniques, we therefore explored the use of RF energy.

In RF endometrial heating, a conductive angulated probe is placed within the endometrial cavity, and an insulated 'belt' is placed around the patients waist which acts as a ground-plane earth electrode to complete the circuit. A 27.12 MHz signal is applied to the RF thermal probe, and the endometrial surface is heated to between 62° C and 65° C for approximately 15 minutes. Applied power is varied during treatment to maintain therapeutic temperatures. Such temperatures have been experimentally determined (see below).

The electrical load presented by the RF thermal probe, patient and external ground-plane electrode is impedence-matched to the output of a linear-amplified 27.12 MHz signal generator, such that maximum power is deposited as heat within the target tissues (**26.1**).

At this frequency, current flows primarily capacitatively. The tissues act as a 'lossy', or inefficient, capacitor, such that a proportion of the energy transfer across the capacitor is 'lost' as heat. An electric field is thus set up around the active tip of the probe, and tissue lying within the boundary of the field becomes heated. The density of the electric field, and therefore the heating effect, fall off geometrically with distance from the probe surface in an 'inverse square' fashion (although the precise mathematical relationship is more complex than $1/r^2$).

Heating beyond the confines of the endometrial cavity at the powers used clinically is prevented by three major factors. First, the physical attributes of an electric field at this frequency and applied power mean that penetration beyond approximately 5–7 mm is negligible. Second, the uterine blood flow acts as a highly effective heat sink to cool the outer myometrium, and third, the myometrium itself, like all biological tissues, is a poor conductor of heat.

EQUIPMENT

The RF generator is combined with the temperature and power monitoring apparatus, and is now commercially available (Menostat TM, Rocket of London Limited, Watford, UK) (**26.2, 26.3**). The machine is capable of generating up to 400 watts of power at 27.12 MHz, although clinically between 100 and 250 W are generally used. The unit also measures applied power, duration of treatment and intrauterine temperature. The patient application apparatus consists of the thermal probe and vaginal guard (which is a tapered plastic tube in the shape of a frustum of a cone) (**26.4**) inserted into the vagina. The thermal guard is necessary to retract the vagina, particularly the anterior vaginal wall, to protect the bladder from heating. The external ground-plane electrode is an insulated conductive wire mesh 'belt', which is wrapped around the patient's waist before treatment, and is connected at both ends to the generator machine to provide the 'return' arm of the circuit.

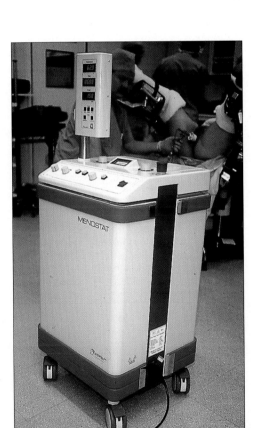

26.3 The 'Menostat' endometrial ablation system.

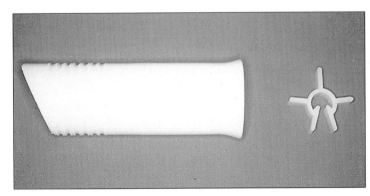

26.4 Vaginal thermal guard and probe location clip.

EXPERIMENTAL STUDIES

Temperatures achieved during treatment were measured in ten volunteers undergoing abdominal hysterectomy, with Ethical Committee approval. Electronic thermometry ('Luxtron' crystal-decay thermography, Luxtron Corporation, California, USA) was used to measure the temperatures during treatment within the uterine cavity, at various distances from the probe within the myometrium, on the surface of the uterus and bowel, and at the base of the bladder. These studies showed that with an intracavity temperature of around 63° C, the surface of the uterus was between 37 and 39° C, and all other tissues remained at normal body temperature (**26.5**).

The heat sink effect of uterine blood flow was demonstrated when RF endometrial heating was performed before and after clamping the uterine arteries on two abdominal hysterectomy patients. The intracavity temperature rose much faster when the uterine vessels were clamped, showing that blood flow has a profound cooling effect (**26.6**).

Systemic venous blood samples were collected before surgery, immediately afterwards, and at one and six weeks. Free hemoglobin, coagulation profiles, and bilirubin levels were all normal and unchanged before and after surgery. Uterine venous blood was sampled from an isolated uterine vein during RF endometrial heating, and examined microscopically. No blood sample showed any red cell crenelation, a sensitive indicator of thermal damage to blood.

PATIENT SELECTION

Patients with dysfunctional uterine bleeding were fully informed of the experimental nature of the surgery, and volunteered to undergo the procedure. They had all completed their families, since the effects of endometrial ablation on fertility are unknown. Permanent sterility after the procedure cannot be guaranteed, and so simultaneous laparoscopic sterilization was offered. Organic dis-

ease is excluded by hysteroscopy, ultrasound scan, and endometrial biopsy. The distance across the cornua (measured ultrasonically) must not exceed 35 mm, because thermal probes currently available are unable to reach the cornual regions in abnormally large uteri.

The uterus must be clinically of normal size and shape, and freely mobile. There must be no suspicion of endometriosis. Patients complaining of cyclic pain or dyspareunia are advised against treatment because of the likelihood of adenomyosis. A history suggestive of significantly heavy menstruation was elicited as follows. Changing pads or towels every one and a half hours or more frequently because of saturation or near saturation, and bleeding heavily for three or more consecutive days.

TREATMENT TECHNIQUE

The patient may be treated under general or regional anesthesia. We have found that a 'single shot' epidural anesthetic is ideal for both intra- and postoperative pain relief.

The external electrode is placed around the patient's waist, and she is positioned in lithotomy. No part of the patient should touch earthed metal such as the operating table or metal stirrups frames, because of the risk of skin burns (as is the case with standard electrosurgery) (**26.7**). The cervix is dilated to size 10 Hegar, and the length of the cavity is measured using a sound. The length of the cervical canal is estimated using a special angulated fine probe to detect the internal os. The estimated length of the cervical canal is subtracted from the total length, and the appropriate probe size selected. This is necessary so that the cervical canal is not heated, which would place the base of the bladder at risk of injury.

The thermal guard is inserted into the vagina until the leading edge is in the fornices with the cervix 'captured' centrally. No vaginal skin should be visible in order that the bladder and rectum are protected. The cervix is held in position using two stay sutures

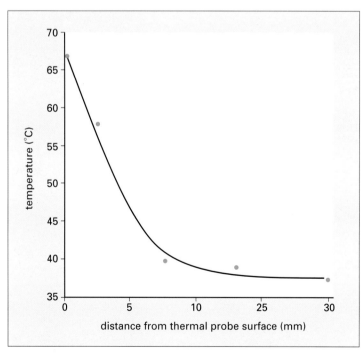

26.5 Temperature as a function of distance from the radiofrequency thermal probe (n – 10, maximum variation between patients 1.2° C).

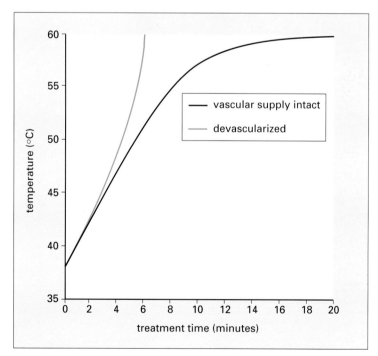

26.6 The effect of devascularization on endometrial cavity temperature rise (n = 2).

placed through the anterior and posterior lips, and passed through the aperture of the guard where they are anchored. The probe is then inserted fully into the cavity of the uterus (**26.8**). If difficulty is encountered in dilating the cervix; if there is any suspicion of perforation; or if rotation is not free, it is essential that the procedure be abandoned because of the risk of perforation of the uterus by the probe. If the probe is placed inappropriately, and the surgeon is unaware, the equipment is capable of detecting the error because circuit tuning occurs outside the normal range for the uterine cavity. If difficulty is experienced in tuning, perforation should be excluded.

A safety check is carried out by the surgeon and the anesthetist before the generator is switched on. There must be no contact by the patient with any metal, and ECG and pulse oximeter must be

filtered and compatible with the RF equipment. Most older monitoring equipment is unstable in the presence of RF energy, and may cause burns at the site of ECG electrodes or pulse oximeter sensors if used without adequate filtering and screening because of earthing. Burns may also occur if monitoring equipment is left connected to the patient but switched off (**26.9**).

The probe and belt electrode are connected to the RF generator/monitor unit, which is switched on and set to the calibration mode. Tuning is achieved by manipulation of the two calibration controls. After tuning, the machine is switched to treat mode, and the power increased to 200 watts. Recent advances in equipment efficiency mean that much lower power levels may be used to produce the same therapeutic effect. Probe temperature is measured every three minutes via a built-in thermistor in the probe tip, and

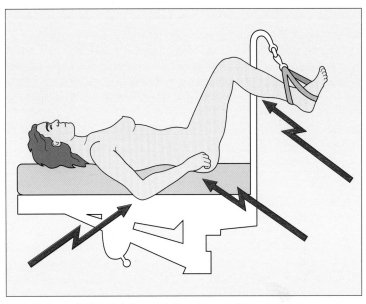

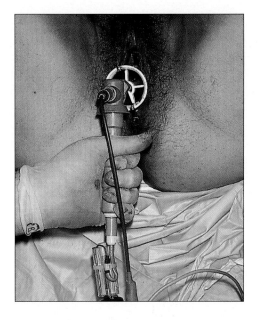

26.8 Thermal probe and vaginal guard in situ.

26.7 Points of high risk for peripheral burns if earth contact occurs.

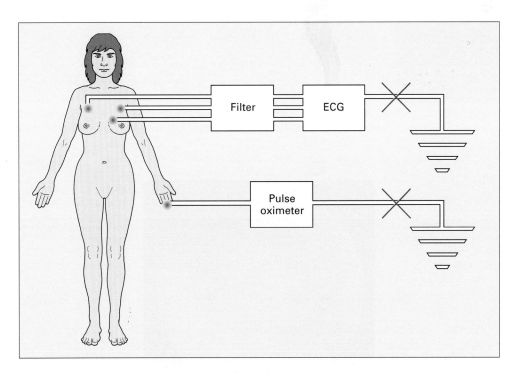

26.9 Potential risks of earth pathways through monitoring equipment which may lead to peripheral burns around ECG electrode pads and pulse oximetry sensors.

power levels are varied so that a probe temperature of 62–65⁰ C is maintained. The uterus is treated for a total of 15 minutes, during which time the probe is rotated through 360 degrees (**26.10**). At the end of the procedure, the probe, guard, clip and external belt are removed.

Postoperative analgesia requirements are very variable. Approximately half the patients treated require narcotics for the first 3–4 hours, but the pain quickly settles thereafter. It may be the case that the pain experienced is mediated by prostaglandin synthesis (many patients complain of 'labour pains'). We have found recently that anti-inflammatory agents such as ketorolac (Toradol, Syntex) injection are highly effective, and usually obviate the need for opiates.

RESULTS

To date, 632 patients have been treated worldwide. Of these, 462 have been treated according to the definitive protocol (62–65 degrees at the endometrial surface for 15 minutes) and have been followed up for between seven and 18 months. Results are shown in **26.11**, and show that using the definitive treatment regime in

patients where the endometrial cavity is ultrasonically and hysteroscopically normal (i.e. where good apposition of the probe with the cavity is achieved) (**26.12**) either amenorrhea or significantly reduced flow was achieved in almost 87% of cases. A cure was judged when patients did not want further treatment, and considered their periods (or absence of bleeding) acceptable.

In 15 patients menstrual loss was recorded over two cycles before and after RaFEA. The radioactive 59Fe iron/whole body gamma counting method was used which is more accurate than, and does not suffer the practical disadvantages of, pad-saving studies. Patients were given radioactive iron before a menstrual period, and whole-body radioactivity measured before and after two cycles. The deficit between the two measurements is directly proportional to blood loss. The pretreatment loss was 97–1330 ml, and after RaFEA was 0–266 ml, with a mean reduction of 195 ml per cycle (74% reduction in loss). It is a feature of the technique that several cycles may elapse before the patient achieves her definitive result. Many patients experience several heavy periods after treatment, which subsequently diminish, presumably because of cavity fibrosis.

The majority of patients are treated as day cases, and in a series of 210 patients treated, only three have required overnight admission for pain relief. All were able to go home the following day. Fifty per cent of cases are able to resume work within ten days, and the

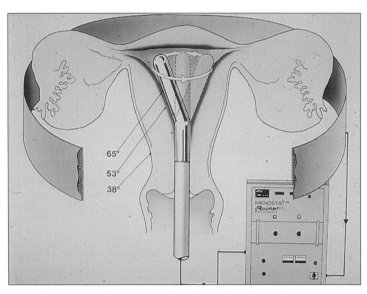

26.10 Schematic diagram showing thermal probe and earth external belt electrode.

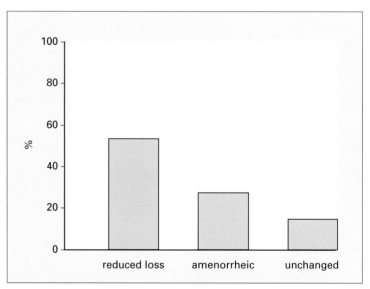

26.11 Results of 462 patients treated with RaFEA, normal uterine cavity, definitive treatment protocol (follow-up period eight months to three years).

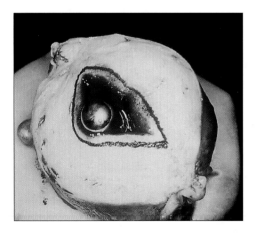

26.12 Thermal probe shown inside hysterectomy specimen, fundus removed, to show apposition to endometrium.

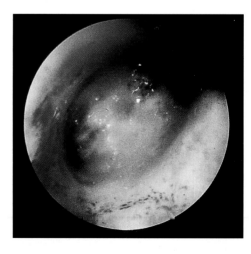

26.13 Hysteroscopic photograph of endometrial cavity six months after RaFEA.

majority of the rest within two weeks. Approximately ten per cent of patients need between two and four weeks recovery. The principle complaint that prevents return to work seems to be a feeling of general malaise and tiredness. This may be because some patients are susceptible to a form of 'burn syndrome', seen in some cases of severe burns, which is presumed to be due to absorption of toxic products from damaged tissue. Patients are told that they should refrain from sexual intercourse and take cephradine 250 mg four times a day for a week as prophylaxis against possible infection. We have yet to ascertain whether or not this precaution is necessary.

Postoperative hysteroscopy at six months after surgery has shown a variable appearance within the uterus. In some cases the cavity is completely stenosed. In others, the endometrium appears to be replaced by fibrous tissue (**26.13**).

COMPLICATIONS

Most patients complain of a varying degree of abdominal pain after RaFEA, which disappears or becomes a dull ache after 4–6 hours. All patients report a blood stained vaginal discharge lasting 1–4 weeks.

Nine patients from the series have complained of protracted cyclical pain. Three of these has settled spontaneously, but the other six continue at the time of writing. Ultrasound scans are unremarkable, but the possibility of small hematometra remains. Seven patients have required hysterectomy for recrudescence of their heavy bleeding, and one for pain, between eight and 24 months after treatment. Histology failed to reveal any significant features to account for their symptoms.

Provided the bladder is fully emptied and the vaginal thermal guard fully engaged such that the cervix is completely isolated, bladder injury is not a problem. If the guard is not properly sited, however, or if the probe is allowed to 'wander' down the cervical canal, such that the canal is heated, the possibility of causing a burn to the bladder, with subsequent vesicovaginal fistula remains. It should be emphasized that in cases where correct vaginal guard insertion proves impossible (usually because of small-bore vagina), the procedure must be abandoned. There have been no cases of bladder injury where the thermal guard has been correctly emplaced.

ECG electrode and a pulse oximeter sensor burn have occurred due to the use of non-compatible equipment. It is vital that only approved monitoring equipment is used. Standard ECG machines are suitable provided a special filter is interposed between the monitor and the patient. Self-powered battery operated pulse oximeter units are also suitable for use provided they have been examined and approved, but a purpose-built combined monitoring unit may also be used. Built-in fuses in the latest monitoring equipment (which may also be used for general theater purposes) mean that even if a fault develops, burns are prevented by stopping current flow.

One case of a skin burn occurred under the external belt electrode. This incident was extensively investigated, and it was discovered that there was a small risk of extraneous heating in very thin or very obese patients. This was because at the two extremes, the belt was at risk of point heating due to inadvertent tuning such that RF nodes occurred. Research has shown that by connecting both ends of the belt to the earth supply cable, such unwanted tuning cannot arise, and the problem has been solved.

Studies have shown that environmental RF electromagnetic energy levels are below the government recommended maximum levels with the equipment operating at power levels in excess of those used clinically. Therefore hazards to theatre staff and patient due to excessive RF exposure are not a problem. The prevention of complications depends upon on the surgeon, the anesthetist and the theatre staff who should be familiar with the safety protocol, with the patient under constant vigilance during treatment. Theater doors should be labelled with appropriate signs stating that RF energy is in use, and entry forbidden by non-authorized staff during surgery.

FUTURE DEVELOPMENT

Currently, a multicentre trial is underway in six centres in the UK and Europe.

RaFEA is particularly suitable for patients with severe cardiopulmonary disease, where the possibility of even a minor degree of fluid intravasation with the hysteroscopic methods might be dangerous. It may be the case that RaFEA has a unique role under these circumstances.

The absence of any need for high technology operating facilities or special training may mean that RaFEA is especially suitable for third world countries, particularly in Moslem communities where hysterectomy is considered culturally unacceptable.

In conclusion, RaFEA offers an alternative to hysterectomy that is simple, effective and relatively inexpensive, and offers potential specific advantages over the hysteroscopic methods of endometrial ablation.

FURTHER READING

Coakley WT. Hyperthermia effects on the cytoskeleton and on cell morphology. *Symp Soc Exp Biol* 1987; **41**:187-211

Droegemueller W, Greer B, Makowski E. Cryosurgery in patients with dysfunctional uterine bleeding. *Obstet Gynecol* 1971; **38**:256-8

Hahn GM. Hyperthermia And Cancer. Publishers SpringerVerlag, New York.1982

Phipps JH, Lewis BV, Roberts T, Prior MV, Hand JW, Field SB, Elder M. Treatment of functional menorrhagia with radiofrequency endometrial ablation. *Lancet* 1990a; **335**:374-6

Phipps JH, Lewis BV, Prior MV, Roberts T. Experimental and clinical studies with radiofrequency induced thermal endometrial ablation. *Obstet Gynecol* 1990b; 76

HYSTEROSCOPIC MYOMECTOMY

27

Jacques Donnez and Michelle Nisolle

MYOMECTOMY

Leiomyomas are the most common benign solid tumors of the genital tract. They can be single but are often multiple and originate from the myometrium.

The major indications for myomectomy include infertility as well as repeated miscarriage, menorrhagia, and pelvic pain with preservation of reproductive function. The location of the myoma determines the symptoms. A submucous myoma may cause menorrhagia or infertility. Hysterography and office hysteroscopy are used to confirm the diagnosis and to evaluate the site and the size of the myoma and its position in the uterine cavity.

Hyteroscopy is useful in the treatment of submucous myomas because the operative hysteroscope allows resection of the fibroid with an electrosurgical loop, scissors and/or neodymium: ytrium-aluminium garnet (Nd:YAG) laser.

INSTRUMENTS

Two main types of endoscopes are used today: the rigid panoramic hysteroscope and the flexible hysteroscope. There are several instruments suitable for endometrial ablation. The continuous flow hysteroscope has an operating channel for a quartz fiber. The double-channel system allows blood, bubbles, and debris, that otherwise would have obscured vision, to be washed out (**27.1**). Aspiration through the catheter is not generally necessary because the pressure of the distending medium washes the debris out through the catheter. There may be cramp-like pains with local anesthesia. We therefore prefer to operate under general anesthesia.

Different distending media are available. A solution of 1.5% glycine solution is used in the operating room, but CO_2 gas is preferable for outpatient diagnostic hysteroscopy. Low-viscosity fluids are less expensive, cause less pain, are readily available, and are relatively safe should intravasation occur.

Both electrosurgery and Nd:YAG laser are effective in performing myoma resection. The resectoscope has a possible disadvantage; the unipolar current means it has the potential to damage the bowel or bladder because the current might be transmitted through the uterine wall. There may be actual penetration of the uterine wall by the cutting loop. The risk of damage by electrosurgical instruments can be reduced by new generators which use a high-frequency current. There is a risk of hemorrhage if major uterine vessels are transected by cutting too deeply into the myometrium. The advantage of the resectoscope over the laser is that it is readily available in most operating rooms and does not require the major capital investment needed for a laser. We prefer laser energy because of its precision.

Uterine distention is obtained by a 3 litre plastic bag of 1.5% glycine solution wrapped in a pressure infusion cuff. Using gravity or a pressure of 100 to 150 mm Hg. When the bag is nearly empty, the nurse should inform the surgeon of the amount of fluid absorbed by the patient. Because fluid overload is a serious problem, the fluid deficit must be closely monitored.

PREOPERATIVE USE OF GONADOTROPHIN RELEASING HORMONE (GNRH) AGONIST THERAPY

Suppression of the hypothalamic-pituitary-ovarian axis with GnRH analogs is used with increasing frequency prior to surgery for fibroids. Continuous administration of this drug results in down-regulation of the hypothalamic–pituitary–ovarian axis which leads to decreased release of the gonadotropin follicle simulating hormone (FSH) and luteinizing hormone (LH). The GnRH agonists administered continuously produce a medical 'oophorectomy' which reduce tumor growth and volume because leiomyomas are estrogen dependent.

GnRH agonists cause a significant reduction in the volume of the uterus and the fibroid as determined by pelvic ultrasound within 6 months of therapy. An average decrease in fibroid volume was 40% most of which occurred within the first 2–3 months of therapy and is related to the level of circulating estrogen. When the GnRH agonist therapy is stopped the fibroids will grow again to their original size within four months. Therefore, these agents cannot be used as definitive medical therapy.

We use GnRH agonist treatment for eight weeks prior to hysteroscopic myomectomy. In a previous study, most of the uterine shrinkage occurred at 8 weeks of treatment and there was no further shrinkage at 12 weeks. The drug is injected subcutaneously at the end of the luteal phase to curtail the initial gonadotropin stimulation phase which is associated with a rise in estrogen. Two further injections were given in four and eight weeks.

The uterine cavity area and the fibroid area were calculated by hysterography using the short-line 'multipurpose text system'. All patients had a pretreatment uterine cavity area of more than 10 cm^2 which decreased by an average of 36%. At eight weeks, hysteroscopic myomectomy was carried out using the Nd:YAG Laser. **27.2** shows the mean fibroid areas in patients with a pretreatment fibroid area of less than 5 cm^2 versus those with an area between 5 cm^2 and 10 cm^2 and those with an area greater than 10 cm^2. In all subgroups, a significant and similar decrease was noted. In patients with menorrhagia, the initial hemoglobin measurement was 11.3 ± 0.9 mg/L. A significant increase (13.8 ± 8 g/100ml; *P=0.005*) was observed by the end of the eight week treatment period.

The advantages of the preoperative use of a GnRH agonist are the significant decrease in the fibroid size, and the restoration of a normal hemoglobin concentration. There should also be decreased fluid absorption during surgery.

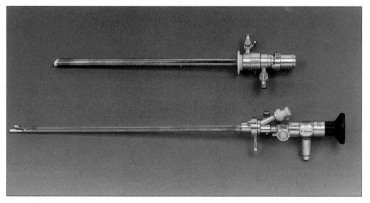

27.1 Continuous flow hysteroscope. The double-channel system permits a continuous in and out flow.

HYSTEROSCOPIC MYOMECTOMY

CLASSIFICATION OF MYOMAS

Hysterosalpingography and hysteroscopy show three different types of submucous fibroids:
1. Submucous fibroids of which the greatest diameter was inside the uterine cavity **(27.3a)**
2. Submucous fibroids in which the greatest diameter was inside the uterine wall and not inside the uterine cavity **(27.3b)**
3. Multiple submucous fibroids with distortion of the uterine cavity in different areas **(27.3c)**. Frequently, these fibroids are associated with multiple intramural myomas diagnosed by ultrasound.

TECHNIQUES

One hundred and sixty-eight patients with submucous fibroids in which the greatest diameter was inside the uterine cavity, underwent myomectomy by hysteroscopy and Nd:YAG laser. In all cases but one, the operation was easily performed. The myometrium overlying the myoma was less vascular and the 'shrinkage' of the uterine cavity may have accounted for the relative ease with which the myoma could be separated from the surrounding myometrium as well as the reduction in perioperative blood loss **(27.4–27.6)**. The decreased vascularity, after treatment with a GnRH agonist, was demonstrated by a reduction in the uterine arterial blood flow as measured by Doppler flow studies. If the diameter was greater than 3 cm the pedicle was divided and the fibroid left inside the uterine cavity. A biopsy was taken from the myoma. No complications such as infection, bleeding, or pain occurred. Subsequent office CO_2 hysteroscopy two to three months later confirmed the disappearance of the myoma, which was probably extruded during the first menstruation after the procedure.

In women with large submucous fibroids in which the largest portion was in the uterine wall and not in the uterine cavity, a two-step operative hysteroscopy is proposed. After preoperative GnRH-agonist therapy for eight weeks, a partial myomectomy is performed by vapourising the protruding portion of the fibroid **(27.7)**. The laser fiber is then directed vertically into the remaining intramural fibroid

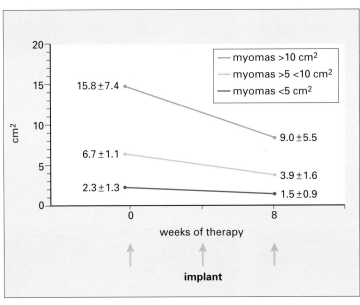

27.2 Mean fibroid area before and after treatment.

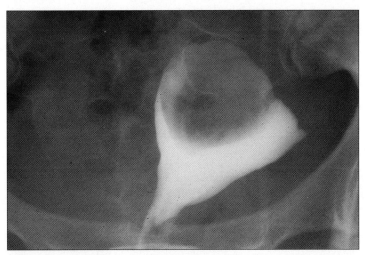

27.3a Submucous fibroid: the greatest diameter is inside the uterine cavity.

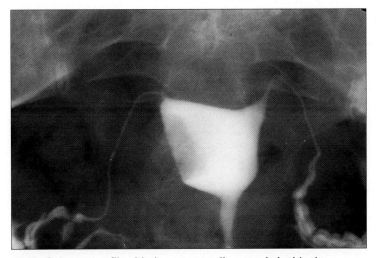

27.3b Submucous fibroid: the greatest diameter is inside the uterine wall.

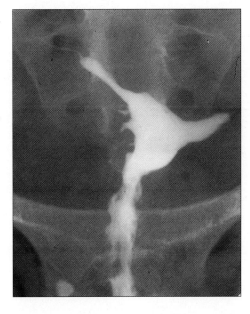

27.3c Multiple submucous fibroids.

to a depth of 5 to 10 mm, depending on the amount of the fibroid remaining. The fiber is slowly withdrawn with the laser activated, vaporizing the tissue as it is removed. This results in multiple 'craters' with brown borders on the surface of the fibroid. The depth of the intramural fibroid portion was estimated by ultrasound prior to surgery.

There is no risk of damage to the bowel or the bladder by the transmural Nd:YAG laser.

The intrapelvic organs are protected from injury because the tip of the fiber is never less than 1.5 cm from the peritoneal surface of the uterus. The fiber can be inserted safely to a depth of 1 cm if the remaining portion of the fibroid is more than 3-4 cm deep.

The aim of this procedure is to decrease the size of the remaining myoma by decreasing its vascularity. GnRH agonist therapy is given for a further eight weeks and repeat hysteroscopy performed. We found that in all cases, the remaining myoma now protruded into the uterine cavity and was white and avascular. **(27.8, 27.9).** Myomectomy can then be carried out as before. The residual myoma is easily separated from the surrounding myometrium. At the end of the procedure, the myoma can be left in the uterine cav-

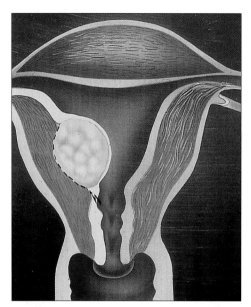

27.4 The greatest diameter of the submucous fibroid is inside the uterine cavity: separation of the myoma from the surrounding myometrium is carried out with the Nd:YAG laser.

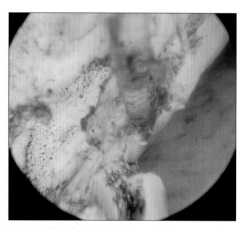

27.5 Nd:YAG laser myomectomy.

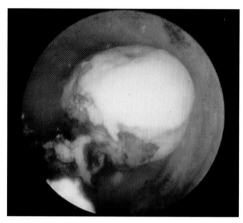

27.6 At the end of the procedure, the fibroid is left in the uterine cavity.

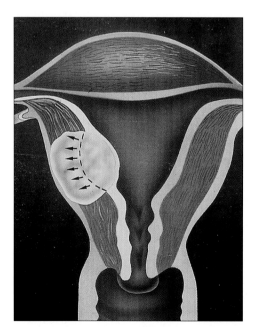

27.7 The greatest diameter of the submucous fibroid is in the uterine wall: partial myomectomy is performed and by introducing the laser fiber into the remaining fibroid portion, coagulation and devascularization of the remaining myoma is carried out.

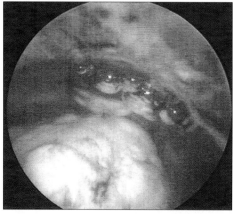

27.8 Second look hysteroscopy. The fibroid appears white and protudes into the uterine cavity.

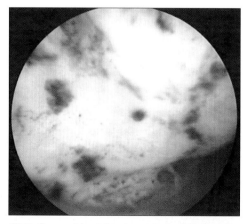

27.9 Second look hysteroscopy. Black areas are clearly visible. They correspond to areas of photocoagulation performed eight weeks earlier.

ity. Concomitant laparoscopy is usually unnecessary but may occasionally be advisable. Hysterography and hysteroscopy carried out two to three months after the second stage myomectomy confirmed the uterine cavity was normal.

In cases of numerous submucous myomas, multiple myomectomy was carried out if possible. In many cases, only partial resection of the myomas could be performed. The protruding portions of all the myomas were resected.

RESULTS

The results are shown in **27.10**. In the first subgroup in which the largest diameter of the fibroid is within the uterine cavity (n=168), the procedure was successfully completed in 167 cases, with one failure. In this case, the myoma was difficult to dissect from the myometrium because the plane of cleavage was not clearly visible. A frozen section revealed a stromal tumour and vaginal hysterectomy was carried out **(27.11)**. It is important to notice that, in this

Surgical procedures and long-term results according to site of myomas			
	Greatest diameter inside the uterine cavity	Largest portion located in the uterine wall	Multiple submucosal myomas (myomectomy and endometrial ablation)
Surgical procedures			
N patients	168	44	32
Successful	168	40	28
Failed	1*	4**	4***
Long-term results			
1 year follow-up			
N patients	92	21	18
Recurrence	1(1%)	1(5%)	4(22%)
2 years follow-up			
N patients	34	11	8
Recurrence	1(3%)	1(9%)	2(25%)

*   Stromal tumor
**   A third look hysteroscopy allowed the myoma to be removed
*** Myomectomy was not totally successful

27.10 The long-term results of hysteroscopic myomectomy according to the site of fibroids.

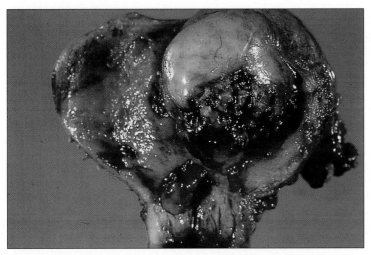

27.11 A stromal tumor must be suspected when there is no decrease in the myoma size after a GnRH agonist therapy.

case, the myoma did not shrink after GnRH agonist therapy. Long-term results are excellent and recurrence of bleeding is infrequent.

In the second subgroup in which the largest diameter of the myoma was in the myometrium, the procedure was successfully carried out in more than 90% of cases. In four cases out of 44, a third-look hysteroscopy enabled the the fibroid to be completely removed. Long term results are similar to those observed in the first subgroup.

In the third subgroup consisting of multiple submucous and intramural myomas, myomectomy and endometrial ablation was carried out. In 12% of cases it was impossible to complete hysteroscopic surgery. The rate of recurrent bleeding was significantly higher (>20%) than that observed in the two other subgroups.

CONCLUSION

Preoperative therapy resulted in the restoration of a normal hemoglobin concentration because of the cessation of uterine bleeding. The risks of transfusion are eliminated. We conclude, that:

- One step hysteroscopic surgery is the optimum treatment for submucous fibroids when the largest diameter is inside the uterine cavity
- Two step hysteroscopic surgery combined with GnRH agonist therapy is the best treatment for large submucous myomas when the largest diameter is in the intramural wall. This decreases the need for myomectomy by laparotomy, which is often accompanied by excessive blood loss and postoperative adhesion formation.
- In multiple submucous myomas, partial hysteroscopic myomectomy with endometrial ablation or hysterectomy must be offered to the patient because of the high rate of recurrent menorrhagia after hysteroscopic myomectomy alone.

FURTHER READING

Donnez J, Schrurs B, Gillerot S, Sandow J, Clerkx-Braun F. Treatment of uterine fibroids with implants of gonadotropin releasing hormone agonist: assessment by hysterography. *Fertil Steril* 1989; **51**:947–50

Donnez J, Schrurs B, Gillertot S, Bourgonjon D, Clerkx-Braun F, Nisolle M. Neodymium: YAG laser hysteroscopy in large submucous fibroids. *Fertil Steril* 1990; **54**:999–103

SEPTA AND SYNECHIAE

Rafael F Valle

INTRODUCTION

Of the many operations that can be performed in the uterus, the surgical treatment of uterine septa, the division of intrauterine adhesions and myomectomy have profited most from the advances introduced in operative hysteroscopy. These procedures require precision, visual guidance, and the least invasive methods to prevent uterine damage and scarring.

In the past hysterotomy, which involves laparotomy to enter the abdominal cavity and division of the uterine corpus were required. Modern hysteroscopic surgery permits transcervical treatment via the endoscope, eliminating entry of the abdominal cavity and bisection of the uterus, both major surgical procedures. In this chapter we will address the evaluation and treatment of symptomatic uterine septa and intrauterine adhesions.

UTERINE ANOMALIES (SEPTA)

Developmental Anatomy

The uterus derives embryologically from the Müllerian ducts, which arise from the urogenital ridge of the embryo as an invagination of the coelomic epithelium, and eventually fuse in the center to form the uterine body. Canalization and reabsorption of the medial septum produces a single cavity early in embryonic life, and failure at different stages in this formation results in a variety of uterine anomalies. The uterine septum is reabsorbed completely by the 19th or 20th week of embryonic life and its persistence results in the division of the uterine corpus either partially or totally. This septum may also involve the cervix and sometimes the vagina as well. Because of the close relationship of this embryologic development with the urinary tract, uterine anomalies, particularly those involving one Mullerian duct, may also result in urinary tract anomalies, particularly in the ipsilateral kidney.

Pregnancy Wastage and Obstetric Complications

While most women with uterine anomalies, specifically uterine septa, do not experience problems with reproduction, about one-fourth of these women may suffer from pregnancy wastage or repeated abortions. This problem seems to correlate with the length of the septum. The more complete the septum, the higher the risk of reproductive failure. Nonetheless, because this anomaly is uncommon, it is important to rule out other possible causes of reproductive failure such as endocrine, genetic, metabolic and/or autoimmune disorders.

Other problems associated with septate uterus include fetal malpresentations, in about 20 to 30% of patients, and dysmenorrhea, in about 20% of patients. A uterine anomaly may be present when termination of an early pregnancy fails or when there is failure to remove products of conception and retained placental fragments.

Diagnosis and Evaluation

While occasional manual exploration of the postpartum uterus, or difficulty in performing a curettage, may arouse suspicion of a uterine anomaly, the best method for its diagnosis is hysterosalpingography. The axis at which the uterus is projected when the radio-opaque material is injected can provide the best assessment of a uterine anomaly and also demonstrates the relationship of the septum with the uterotubal cones and patency of the fallopian tubes. Sonography has also been used for this purpose, but its accuracy and sensitivity are less precise. Magnetic resonance imaging (MRI) can outline the contour of the uterus and determine the endometrial stripes at both sides of the septum. Nonetheless, its expense makes this technique less practical. Because it is difficult to determine consistently and accurately the presence of a uterine septum by hysterosalpingography without confusing some of these anomalies with a bicornuate uterus, laparoscopy is necessary to determine the exact external shape of the uterus to rule out this latter condition. While sonography and MRI are useful for this purpose, laparoscopy is most commonly used for guidance during treatment when the hysteroscopic approach is chosen. Finally, hysteroscopy can determine the actual extent and thickness of the septum and provide a method of surgical treatment.

TREATMENT AND RESULTS

Past Treatments

Since the report in 1884 by Ruge of blind transcervical division of a uterine septum in a patient with pregnancy wastage, the treatment of this condition has been surgical. Attempts were made to divide a uterine septum transcervically followed Ruge's description, but these blind methods were soon abandoned in favor of a direct approach by hysterotomy with excision of the septum, as proposed by Jones, or division without removal of uterine tissue, as outlined by Bret and also by Tompkins. Other modifications of these invasive techniques, such as El Magoub's technique using small, fundal, transverse stab incisions and dividing the septum with long scissors transfundally, did not gain as much acceptance as the classical Jones and Bret–Tompkins techniques.

While these invasive techniques marked the standard of treatment in the 1950's, 1960's and 1970's, and offered good treatment for the symptomatic septate uterus, with results approaching 82% viable pregnancy rates, they required major surgery, including laparotomy and hysterotomy. Therefore, all patients required hospitalization and experienced prolonged postoperative recovery. Furthermore, a significant number of women developed pelvic adhesions and secondary infertility following these procedures. When pregnancy was achieved, a routine Caesarean section was necessary in view of the deep scar left in the uterine body. For these reasons, the surgical approach of the septate uterus was delayed until the patient suffered at least three miscarriages, and on many occasions other adjunctive treatments were used including cerclage, bed rest, and tocolytics to preserve the ongoing pregnancy.

Current Treatment of the Septate Uterus

Following the introduction of modern hysteroscopy by Edstrom in 1970, the possibility of transcervical division of the uterine septum under visual control was initiated. While this procedure began by gradually removing the septum with hysteroscopic biopsy forceps technological advances in operative hysteroscopes and instrumentation allowed the septum to be divided by hysteroscopic scissors. This method proved to be practical, relatively simple, and reproducible. The uterine septum is most suitable for this approach, because its fibrotic component is an embryologic remnant, its poor vascularization, particularly at the nadir of the septum, and its clear visualization when the uterine cavity is distended (**28.1**).

The septum may be divided in several ways; hysteroscopic scissors, fiberoptic lasers, and electrosurgery with the use of a modified loop or knife electrodes.

Hysteroscopic scissors have several advantages, particularly due to the simplicity and quickness in dividing the septum. They can be applied to most septa, including those that are broad. No energy sources are required, and the media used to distend the uterus can

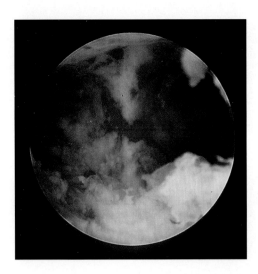

28.1 Hysteroscopic view of thick uterine septum.

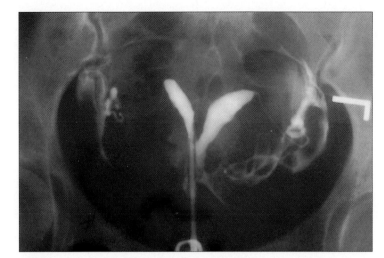

28.2 Hysterosalpingogram showing complete uterine septum.

contain electrolytes, therefore the problems of fluid overload when intravascular absorption occurs are reduced. The division of the septum must remain in the midline to prevent bleeding, which can occur particularly upon reaching the fundal area. The juxtaposed myometrium is an excellent landmark to limit the dissection **(28.2, 28.3)**. It is important to have a laparoscope in place to follow the translucency of the hysteroscopic light. The laparoscope light is switched off to enhance transillumination.

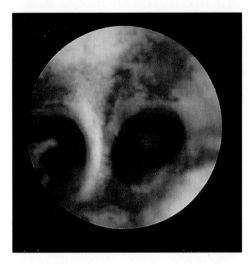

28.3 Hysteroscopic view of complete uterine septum.

The resectoscope can also be used to divide the uterine septum with a knife electrode or a modified loop. This method has the advantage of preventing bleeding. It can cut the septum and, because the resectoscope has a continuous flow system, it provides excellent visibility with a washing effect that removes debris and small clots. Monopolar electrosurgery coagulates the peripheral endometrium which may hamper re-epithelialization of the denuded area. The landmarks of the myometrium are lost while dividing the septum because electrosurgical coagulation prevents bleeding which is usually seen when reaching the myometrium with scissors. Fluids without electrolytes must be used. To avoid fluid overload, meticulous measurement of the inflow and outflow fluids is necessary. Broad septa may be somewhat more difficult to divide using this method.

Finally the fiberoptic lasers (KTP-532, Argon, Neodymium-YAG with extruded or sculptured fibers) may also be used to divide the septum hysteroscopically. The advantages of these methods are that bleeding is prevented; the cutting can be achieved very precisely; and because lasers are not conductive, fluids with electrolytes may be used for uterine distension.

The disadvantages are that lasers are expensive, and special protective glasses are necessary to prevent retinal damage by the backscattering produced by these lasers. Also, the lateral scattering, although reduced by the sculptured fibers, may damage peripheral normal endometrium and hamper re-epithelialization, as happens with electrosurgery. Special maintenance for these units is essential for them to be ready for use when needed.

Whatever the method chosen, the best time for hysteroscopic surgery is in the early follicular phase, so as to avoid the thick endometrium that follows ovulation. While preparing the patient hormonally with Danazol or GnRH analogues is appealing, its cost may be impractical. Hormonal suppression provides an atrophic endometrium and the best field for operative hysteroscopy. The most commonly used pre- and postoperative prophylactic antibiotics are cephalosporins: Kefzol, 1 gram I.V. during surgery, fol-

lowed by Keflex, 500 mgs four times daily for four additional days. Following transection of the septum, hormonal adjuncts may be used to promote re-epithelization. While the use of estrogens and progestogens to promote re-epithelialization may not be necessary, because the endogenous sexual hormones may be sufficient for healing, most practitioners prefer to use exogenous hormones to enhance this effect. Premarin, 2.5 mgs twice daily orally for 30 days with terminal progestogen (medroxyprogesterone acetate) 10 mg a day, added in the last ten days of this artificial cycle is sufficient for this purpose. Following withdrawal bleeding, a hysterosalpingogram should be performed to observe the results of the hysteroscopic division of the septum. If the results are satisfactory, the patient may safely conceive. While office hysteroscopy may be a good alternative for follow-up of these patients, the visualization from the cervical os of any fundal septal remnants may be difficult. Therefore hysterosalpingography approaching the axis of the uterus from a perpendicular angle may be the best method to assure proper treatment.

While most uterine septa encountered in clinical practice are those involving only the uterine corpus, either partially or totally, septa extending to the cervix sometimes require treatment. While the technique of division of the uterine septum is relatively simple, by systematically and serially dividing the septum from side to side, hysteroscopic treatment of a uterine septum that involves the cervix requires some modifications. Usually, this type of anomaly produces two cervical openings. Therefore, a probe is passed through the adjacent cervical canal and a gentle indentation is performed just above the internal cervical os. The hysteroscope is introduced into the opposite cervical canal. Under hysteroscopic view, a small window in the septal wall is created with semi-rigid hysteroscopic scissors. The probe is inserted through this window and then removed. The cervical canal is clamped where the probe has been inserted, and the hysteroscopic division of the septum is performed as it would be for a complete uterine septum **(28.4, 28.5)**.

The results achieved with the hysteroscopic treatment of the septate uterus have not only equalled the results reported with abdominal metroplasties of the Jones and Tompkins type, but have surpassed them, as no cases of secondary infertility have occurred. In patients having this operation because of pregnancy wastage, the viable pregnancy rate following treatment has approached 90%.

Based on the relative simplicity of this method, its minimal invasion, the preservation of the integrity of the uterine walls, and the excellent results achieved by this approach, hysteroscopic division of the symptomatic uterine septum is today the therapeutic method of choice for this uterine anomaly.

INTRAUTERINE ADHESIONS (ASHERMAN'S SYNDROME)

Although intrauterine adhesions were described late in the 19th century, it was Asherman who first outlined and best described adhesions causing menstrual abnormalities following trauma to the endometrium. While his first description in 1948 was that of total amenorrhea secondary to trauma to the uterine cavity in a delayed postpartum period following a delivery, two years later he added partial occlusion of the uterine cavity secondary to adhesions as part of the syndrome which eventually bore his name. The adhesions totally or partially occlude the cavity, causing menstrual abnormalities, and may cause infertility or pregnancy wastage, depending on the extent of occlusion. The problem can be attributed to trauma to the endometrium, particularly the basalis layer, in the vulnerable phase following delivery or abortion.

NORMAL ENDOMETRIUM

The endometrium is an excellent bioassay of the hormonal stimulus of estrogens and progesterone, responding to estrogens with proliferation and to progesterone with maturation. Following pregnancy, and its termination, the endometrium remains in a vulnerable state and can be damaged by any trauma, particularly curettage. The mature endometrium encompasses three distinct layers:
- The endometrium basalis, which is about 25% of the total thickness, represents the non-functional layer
- The functional layer, composed of the compacta, the most superficial portion; the functional layer includes about 50% of the total endometrial thickness
- The spongiosa, or middle layer, comprising 25% of the total thickness.

The two superficial layers comprise the functional endometrial layers, and usually desquamate following menstruation.

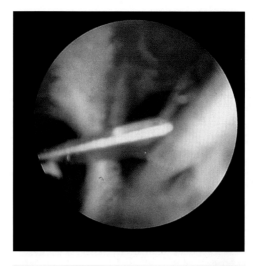

28.4 Hysteroscopic division of uterine septum.

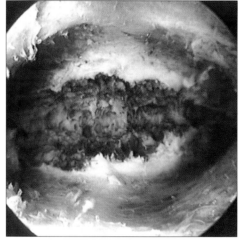

28.5 Hysteroscopic view following division of broad uterine septum with Nd:YAG laser and sculptured fiber.

PATHOPHYSIOLOGY OF INTRAUTERINE ADHESIONS

Many theories have been proposed for the development of intrauterine adhesions. These include infection, trauma, and neurovisceral reflexes. It is clear, however, that mechanical trauma to the endometrium basalis at the vulnerable phase of the postpartum or postabortal period is the main reason for denudation of this area, and the myometrial layers may adhere to one another and originate adhesions. While infection may also play a role in the development of adhesions, it may not be the 'primum movens' of this condition, but rather a secondary and occasional causal factor.

Trauma to this vulnerable phase of the endometrium usually occurs about one to four weeks following delivery or termination of pregnancy. While adhesions may form any time that trauma occurs in the postpartum or postabortal period, including the time of voluntary termination of an early pregnancy, these events are not as common as in those vulnerable phases mentioned.

Trauma to endometrium that has not been recently subjected to pregnancy can occur, but the development of intrauterine adhesions under those conditions is most unusual.

Asherman proposed the theory of a neurovisceral reflex at the internal os and lower uterine segment that produced constriction, and therefore prompted the development of intrauterine adhesions. This theory has never been proved, although it has been revived recently by several authors.

Why some patients develop adhesions and others do not, despite being subjected to similar injuries, is another consideration that points to a subjective and individual vulnerability to this condition.

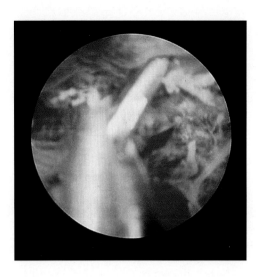

28.6 Completed division of uterine septum close to myometrium.

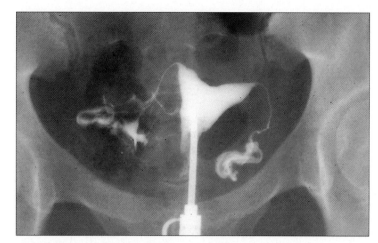

28.7 Follow-up hysterosalpingogram after hysteroscopic treatment of septum, showing normal uterine cavity.

SYMPTOMATOLOGY AND DIAGNOSIS

Women who develop intrauterine adhesions may have menstrual abnormalities, particularly amenorrhea and hypomenorrhea, due to the partial or total destruction of the various layers of the endometrium. The basalis layer is especially vulnerable. Repeated abortions and even infertility may occur when the uterotubal junctions are blocked or the uterine cavity is extensively occluded with intrauterine adhesions. When pregnancies occur, one-third may end in abortion, one-third in premature deliveries and one-third will have placental abnormalities such as placenta accreta, placenta praevia and ectopic pregnancy. Therefore, pregnancies that occur in the presence of intrauterine adhesions should be considered high risk, with a high probability of problems progressing to term and/or placental insertion abnormalities.

While the diagnosis of intrauterine adhesions in the past has been sought by sounding the uterine cavity or by curettage, these methods are not accurate. Sounding the uterine cavity while it is partially occluded may be dangerous because of the risk of uterine perforation. The best screening method for intrauterine adhesions available today is hysterosalpingography, which can outline the areas of occlusion and provide an excellent appraisal of the uterotubal cones, tubal contours and tubal patency. Because hysterosalpingography may produce false-positive results, particularly due to debris, mucus and distortion of the uterine cavity by the technique and the dye used, hysteroscopy becomes mandatory when a hysterosalpingogram is abnormal, to confirm and rectify the abnormality **(28.6–28.9)**.

Ultrasound has been used occasionally to detect intrauterine adhesions due to the echogenicity of adhesions, but is not uniformly accurate and cannot replace the hysterosalpingogram.

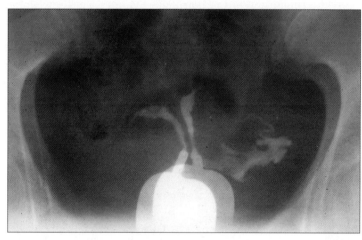

28.8 Hysterosalpingogram shows complete uterine septum with septate cervix.

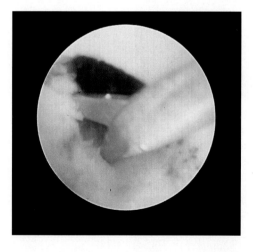

28.9 Hysteroscopic fenestration of septum at level of internal os.

TREATMENT AND RESULTS

Women affected by intrauterine adhesions, and additionally suffering from menstrual abnormalities, pregnancy wastage and/or infertility, usually seek advice for resolution of these problems. Therefore, the aims of treatment should include the restoration of normal menstruation and fertility, and the treatment of dysmenorrhea. The treatment is primarily surgical division of the intrauterine adhesions without trauma to the surrounding remnant endometrium which will be the reservoir for future re-epithelization of the uterine cavity. The best way to achieve this goal is by direct visualization and systematic division of adhesions under visual control. This is achieved best by hysteroscopy. Hysteroscopy is performed in the early follicular phase in those patients who are still menstruating or at any time in patients who are amenorrheic. Based on the extent of uterine cavity occlusion shown by the hysterosalpingogram, laparoscopy is used concomitantly in patients who at hysterosalpingogram demonstrate extensive uterine cavity involvement or tubal occlusion. A 7 mm operating hysteroscope is used, with semi-rigid hysteroscopic scissors to divide the adhesions systematically. When the uterine cavity cannot be completely re-established at one sitting, adjunctive hormonal treatment with estrogens and progestogens are given, and the patient is offered a second hysteroscopic operation after the extent of residual adhesions are demonstrated by hysterosalpingography.

Prophylactic antibiotics are given in the perioperative period depending on whether or not intrauterine splints are used, estrogens, for 30, 40 or 60 days, depending on the severity of the adhesions, and progestogens in the last ten days of the artificial cycle to produce withdrawal bleeding. In more severe cases, intrauterine splints are used, in the form of intrauterine devices (IUDs) or an indwelling catheter, pediatric size 8, which is inflated with 3 to 3.5 ml of fluid and left in place for six to seven days.

At the conclusion of the hormonal therapy, a hysterosalpingogram is performed in patients with severe or moderate adhesions who have extensive uterine cavity occlusion to assess the results of the treatment. In those patients with filmy adhesions that partially occlude the uterine cavity, office hysteroscopy is performed to assess the results. Patients may safely try to conceive after the uterine cavity has been proven normal.

CLASSIFICATION OF INTRAUTERINE ADHESIONS

To assess the results of therapy, it is important to determine the extent of uterine cavity occlusion and the type of adhesions involved. Early adhesions are usually composed of endometrium basalis or the superficial portion of the myometrium, with no thick bands of connective tissue adhesions. Over time, these adhesions become fibromuscular, and eventually, connective tissue invades and bridges walls, making surgical treatment difficult.

Following a similar classification by Sugimoto, we have defined three types of intrauterine adhesions:
1) Mild adhesions: those adhesions that are filmy, usually composed only of basal endometrium; they are usually recent and can also be easily treated; they may occlude the uterine cavity totally or partially;
2) Moderate adhesions: those adhesions composed of fibromuscular tissue usually covered by endometrium, as demonstrated by hysteroscopy; they are composed of bundles of muscle and fibrotic tissue that may bleed when divided; these adhesions occlude the uterine cavity partially or totally;
3) Severe adhesions or connective tissue adhesions: thick adhesions not covered by endometrium, which do not bleed upon division and may partially or totally occlude the uterine cavity; They are usually longstanding and may become thicker and more organized with time. These are the most difficult adhesions to divide hysteroscopically (28.10–28.12).

To standardize the therapeutic outcomes, the American Fertility Society proposed a classification of intrauterine adhesions based on the extent of uterine cavity occlusion, the type of adhesions present, and the menstrual patterns these patients experience. The severity of adhesions (mild, moderate, severe) is determined by a scoring system.

It is clear that the older the adhesions, the thicker they become, and the more likely they are to be composed of connective tissue; these adhesions may recur more frequently following division (28.13–28.27).

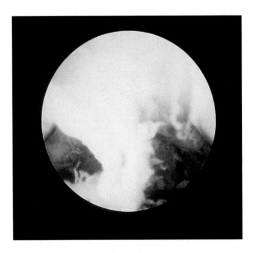

28.10 Fenestration of septum completed showing two cavities divided by medial fibrotic septum.

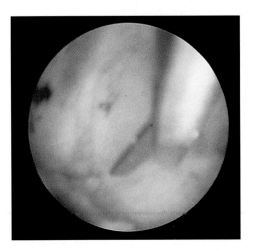

28.11 Division of septum reaching the uterine fundal area.

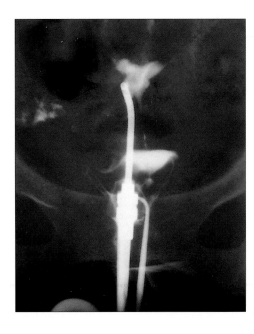

28.12 Follow-up hysterosalpingogram shows the unified uterine cavity.

RESULTS OF TREATMENT ACCORDING TO SEVERITY OF ADHESIONS

The results of hysteroscopic treatment of intrauterine adhesions depends upon the type and the extent of uterine cavity occlusion. The more extensive and severe the adhesions, the more difficult they are to treat and therefore, the more difficult it is to achieve a viable pregnancy. When the adhesions are filmy and recent, the reproductive outcome following treatment is usually successful.

In general, following the division of intrauterine adhesions, menstrual irregularities are cured in over 90% of the patients. Of those women who become pregnant, about 80% will have a normal pregnancy. When the adhesions are severe and extensive the reproductive outcome is markedly impaired. Therefore, it is essential to be aware of the possibility that intrauterine adhesions will develop in patients who have any trauma to the endometrium in the early postpartum or postabortal period and, should menstrual abnormalities result, the diagnosis should be promptly established by a hysterosalpingogram. The best and easiest treatment is early treatment, when the adhesions are filmy and mild. The hysteroscopic treatment of intrauterine adhesions is the standard and there has been a marked improvement in the prognosis and final reproductive outcome.

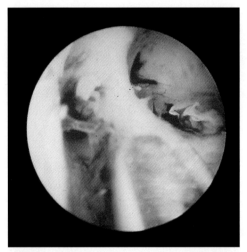

28.13 Hysteroscopic view of adhesion and tip of hysteroscopic scissors.

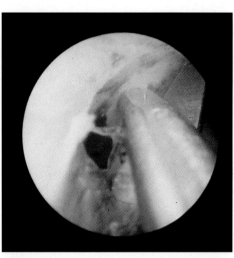

28.14 Hysteroscopic division of adhesion.

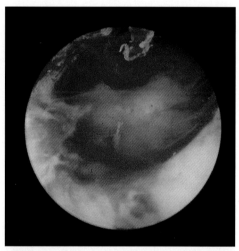

28.15 Uterine cavity's symmetry re-established following division of adhesion.

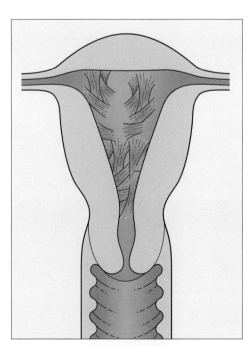

28.16 Isthmic and corporeal adhesions with occlusion of lower portion of uterus.

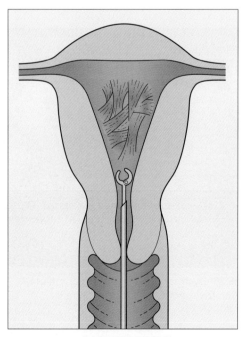

28.17 Extensive, central intrauterine adhesions being treated by hysteroscopy.

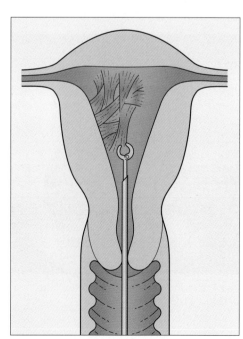

28.18 Hysteroscopic lysis of intrauterine adhesions.

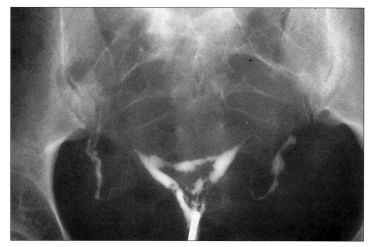

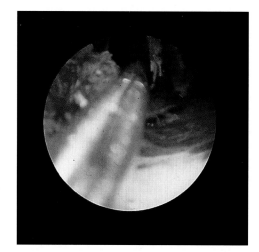

28.20 Hysteroscopic division of adhesions beginning at internal os.

28.19 Hysterosalpingogram showing central uterine cavity occlusion by adhesions.

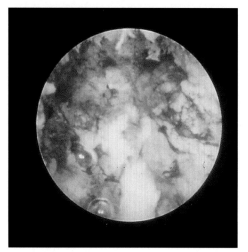

28.21 Hysteroscopic view of uterine cavity following division of adhesions.

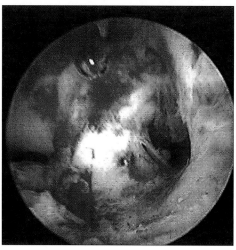

28.22 Central intrauterine adhesion unifying uterine walls.

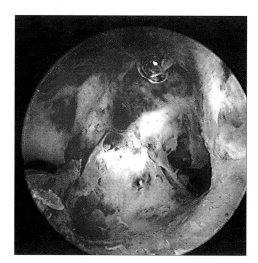

28.23 Closer view of adhesion before division.

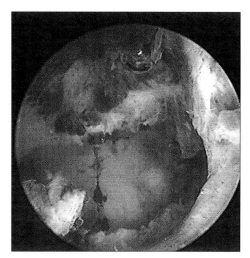

28.24 Uterine walls separate following division of adhesion.

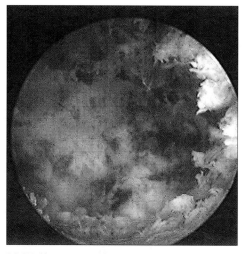

28.25 Hysteroscopic treatment completed, with the uterine cavity's symmetry re-established.

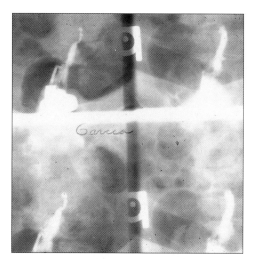

28.26 Hysterosalpingogram showing complete uterine cavity occlusion with central tract only.

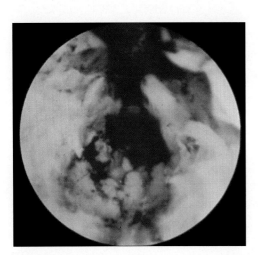

28.27 Hysteroscopic view following division of adhesions. Thick connective tissue stumps can be seen.

CONCLUSION

Uterine septa and intrauterine adhesions are two distinct entities that require intrauterine treatment. While in the past this treatment was not possible without hysterotomy to allow visualization and precision, modern hysteroscopy and its therapeutic applications have made the hysteroscopic approach the gold standard for these conditions. Thus, unnecessary hospitalization is avoided with its concomitant disability and expense, together with invasion of the uterine cavity, and division of the uterine corpus, which may predispose to pelvic adhesions and Caesarean section, should pregnancy occur. Hysteroscopic treatment of these entities can be performed safely, efficiently and expeditiously as ambulatory procedures, with improved reproductive outcome.

FURTHER READING

The American Fertility Society: Classifications of adnexal adhesions, distal tubal occlusion, tubal occlusion secondary to tubal ligation, tubal pregnancies, Müllerian anomalies and intrauterine adhesions. *Fertil Steril* 1988; **49**:944–55

Asherman JG. Traumatic intrauterine adhesions. *J Obstet Gynecol Br Emp* 1950; **57**:892-96

DeCherney AH, Russell, JB Graebe RA, Polan ML. Resectoscopic management of Müllerian fusion defects. *Fertil Steril* 1986; **45**:726–28

Valle RF. Hysteroscopy; diagnostic and therapeutic applications. *J Reprod Med* 1978; **20**:115–18

Valle RF, Sciarra JJ. Hysteroscopic treatment of intrauterine adhesions. In: Hysteroscopy: Principles and Practice, 1984. Eds: Siegler AM, Lindemann HJ. Lippincott, Philadelphia, pp193–97

Valle RF, Sciarra JJ. Intrauterine adhesions: Hysteroscopic diagnosis classification, treatment and reproductive outcome. *Am J Obstet Gynecol* 1988; **158**:1459–470

Wamsteker K. Hysteroscopy in Asherman's syndrome. In: Hysteroscopy: Principles and Practice, 1984. Eds: Siegler AM, Lindemann HJ. Lippincott, Philadelphia, pp198–203

HYSTEROSCOPY AND UTERINE CARCINOMA

29

Raman Labastida, Alicia Ubeda, Santiago Dexeus

INTRODUCTION

Endometrial carcinoma occurs twice as often as carcinoma of the cervix. It is more common in postmenopausal women with a peak incidence in the sixth and seventh decades. Under 3% occur before the age of 40 years. The five-year survival rate is similar to cervical cancer and has not changed in the last two decades even though 70-80% of cases are diagnosed in Stage I. There are four possible reasons for the failure to obtain better results in spite of early diagnosis:

1. Screening programs using endometrial cytology on asymptomatic women over the age of 45 years detected four times the number of endometrial carcinomas than the actual number of women treated for the condition. There may be a four-year occult phase in endometrial carcinoma before abnormal bleeding occurs.
2. Eighty to ninety percent of endometiral carcinomas are diagnosed only after abnormal bleeding occurs. Our own departmental figures confirm this. Of 86 endometrial carcinomas diagnosed hysteroscopically, 69 (80%) had complained of bleeding.
3. There may be two types of endometrial carcinoma. One is related to unopposed and persistent estrogenic effect. The other has no apparent predisposing factor.
4. Screening techniques are uncomfortable and unreliable (**29.1**). Endometrial cytology may give false positive and/or false negative results. In about 10% of biopsies the sample is inadequate for histologic examination.

The American Cancer Society has recommended that certain groups of women who are at high risk of developing endometrial cancer should be screened annually. These include women who are obese, diabetic, hypertensive, are taking unopposed estrogen therapy, have endometrial polyps or have experienced a late menopause in whom we apply the following protocol (**29.2**). It is important to include asymptomatic women in the screening program because of the four-year latent phase.

Experience in our clinic is in accordance with reports in the literature. Histologically confirmed cystic hyperplasia was found in 5–6.5% of pre- and postmenopausal women who complained of abnormal uterine bleeding. Other findings in these patients were adenomatous hyperplasia (2.6%), atypical hyperplasia (1.2%) and endometrial adenocarcinoma (2.6%).

HYSTEROSCOPIC APPEARANCE OF ENDOMETRIAL HYPERPLASIA

SIMPLE ENDOMETRIAL HYPERPLASIA

This is suspected by an increase in the number of glandular dots per field and the disappearance of the normal superficial vascularization. More characteristic features are the appearance of the endometrium which is edematous, avascular, irregular and thick (**29.3**). In more advanced cases the endometrium becomes polypoid, hiding the tubal ostia with straight vertical blood vessels. When this vascularization pattern is excessive it is difficult for the hysteroscopist to distinguish it from well-differentiated endometrial cancer (**29.4**).

CYSTIC ENDOMETRIAL HYPERPLASIA

The diagnosis of cystic hyperplasia becomes unmistakable when there are multiple retention cysts and depressions on a thin and irregular endometrium (**29.5**). This appearance is the result of rupture of deep and superficial vesicles in the thickened endometrium. Typically, blood vessels become scant. Endometrial adhesions are common and occur marginally. Hemorrhagic cysts give a dark color to the uterine cavity (**29.6**).

Diagnostic examination	
	% Inaccuracy
Cervico-vaginal cytology	60%
Endometrial cytology	15–20%
Endometrial biopsy	5–5%
D & C	10%

29.1 Percentage of inaccuracies for diagnostic examinations.

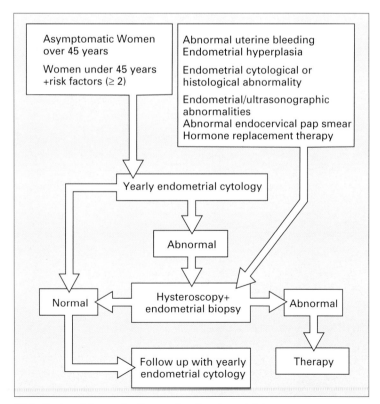

29.2 Protocol for early diagnosis of endometrial cancer.

ADENOMATOUS ENDOMETRIAL HYPERPLASIA

The characteristic feature is of established cystic endometrial hyperplasia (**29.7**) or a polypoid-like endometrial surface (**29.8**) with an increasing number of irregularities (cysts, holes and adhesions). Superficial vascularization appears with hypertrophic vessels (**29.9**).

ATYPICAL ENDOMETRIAL HYPERPLASIA

Although atypical hyperplasia cannot be hysteroscopically distinguished from adenomatous hyperplasia, the vessels show more irregularities in calibre, direction and branching. Special attention must be paid to cancer-like signs, such as necrosis and horns

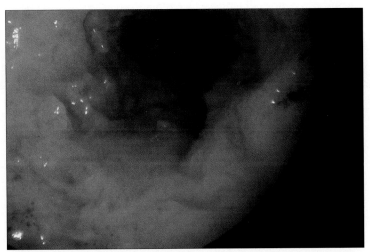

29.3 Hypertrophic, irregular, whitish endometrium in the left cornual region in the established simple endometrial hyperplasia.

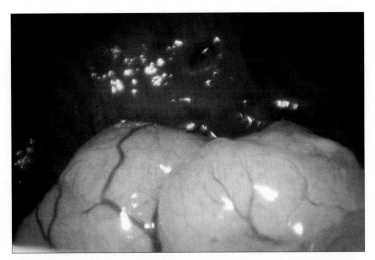

29.4 Increased vascularization in a hypertrophic endometrium of a long-standing simple hyperplasia.

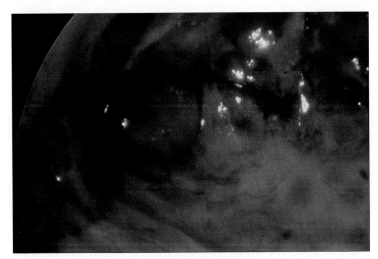

29.5 Cysts and holes in a flat endometrium.

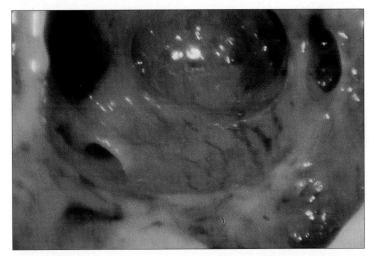

29.6 Adhesions in the uterine cavity in well-established cystic hyperplasia.

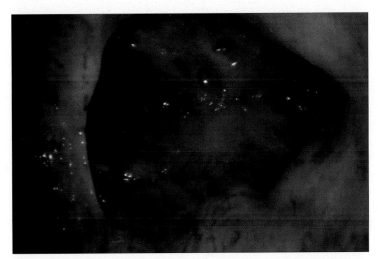

29.7 Adenomatous hyperplasia.

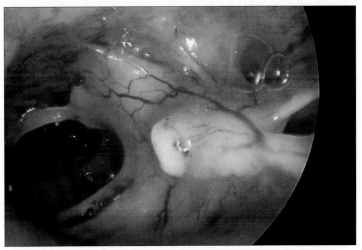

29.8 Polypoid pattern of adenomatous endometrial hyperplasia.

(**29.10**) which may help in localizing the neoplastic changes and guiding the biopsy which should always be taken at the same time as hysteroscopy.

Increased vascularization, superficial growth and hemorrhage, are signs of endometrial activity, and should be specifically examined and biopsied. It should be remembered that treatment of breast cancer with Tamoxifen may lead to endometrial hyperplasia or, rarely, cancer.

DIAGNOSIS OF ENDOMETRIAL CANCER

Hysteroscopy allows the experienced physician to identify two different types of endometrial cancer according to their pathogenesis. An endometrial cancer may develop from preceeding hyperplasia as a result of long-term high estrogen levels. Histologically, this tumor is well differentiated and has a low potential for deep myometrial invasion and metastasis. Many of these women are perimenopausal, nulliparous, obese, diabetic and hypertensive. However, there is an endometrial cancer unrelated to hormonal stimulus which may progress rapidly. It is poorly differentiated and has a worse prognosis. It is frequently found in postmenopausal, thin, multiparous women. The hysteroscopic appearances of the two tumors are also characteristic. While endometrial cancer linked to hyperplasia arises from a hypertrophic endometrium as a polypoid structure with increased and abnormal vessels and areas of necrosis with keratinous horns (**29.11, 29.12**), endometrial cancer unrelated to hyperplasia appears as a single polypoid (**29.13**) or myoma-like tumour (**29.14**) surrounded by an atrophic endometrium in which a few atypical vessels appear. Even though the hysteroscopic diagnosis of endometrial cancer is accurate (94–99%), it is again recommended that endometrial biopsy should be taken to confirm the visual diagnosis (**29.15, 29.16**).

EARLY DIAGNOSIS OF ENDOMETRIAL CANCER

The general view that there is a progression from simple glandular proliferation to cancer, with intermediate endometrial hyperplasia, is now being challenged. Progression from hyperplasia to endometrial carcinoma occurs in 1–2% of cases. 75% of non-atypical hyperplasias revert to normal with progesterone. This suggests that hyperplasia and carcinoma may have a different pathogenesis.

Thus the diagnosis and treatment of endometrial hyperplasia becomes simplified, but the diagnosis of endometrial cancer becomes

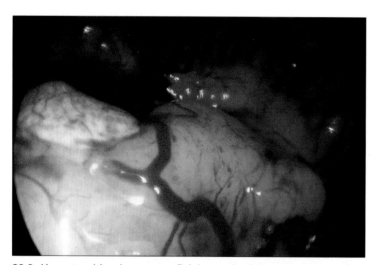

29.9 Hypertrophic, short, superficial vessels. Adenomatous endometrial hyperplasia in detail.

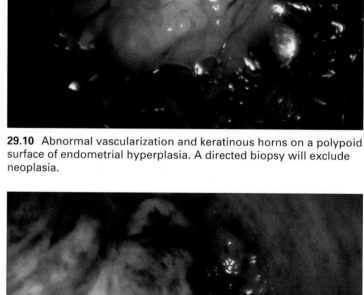

29.10 Abnormal vascularization and keratinous horns on a polypoid surface of endometrial hyperplasia. A directed biopsy will exclude neoplasia.

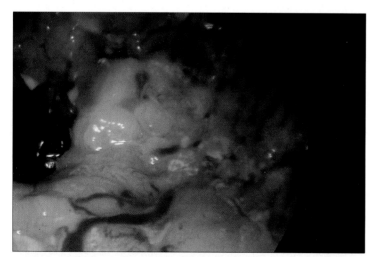

29.11 Endometrial cancer associated with hyperplasia. Polypoid surface with beds of necrosis and keratinous horns.

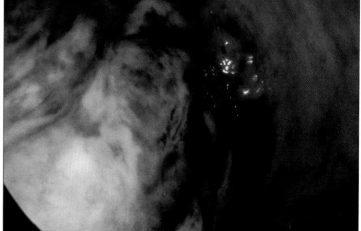

29.12 Endometrial cancer without hyperplasia. Detailed anomalous superficial vessels.

more complicated because it can be found in women with minimal endometrial proliferation without clinical hyperplasia (**29.17**).

The prevalence of malignant degeneration in endometrial polyps is low. The incidence of polyps and hyperplasia in pre- and postmenopausal women is given in **29.18**. Since both conditions have a low rate of progression to malignancy it is possible to give a good prognosis, when they are detected early.

DETERMINATION OF LOCAL PROGNOSTIC FACTORS

Once the diagnosis of endometrial cancer is established, hysteroscopy can help to determine local factors, which indicate the prognosis and help the decision as to the best therapeutic regime.

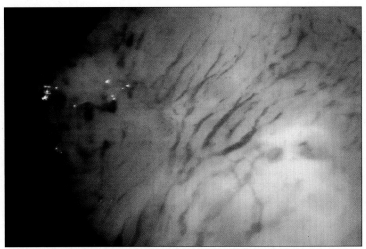

29.13 Polyp-like endometrial cancer unrelated to hyperplasia. Basal growth on an atrophic endometrium.

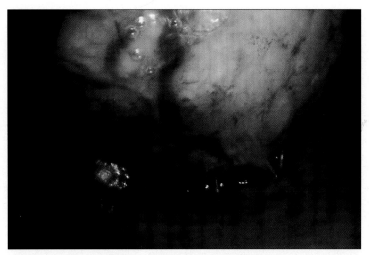

29.14 Myoma-like endometrial cancer unrelated to hyperplasia.

Reliability of hysteroscopy for cancer. Statistical analysis (5059 patients). Endometrial cancer		
Hysteroscopy	Histology	
	Cancer	No cancer
Cancer (n=86)	66	20
No cancer (n=4973)	12	4961

29.15 Reliability of hysteroscopy for diagnosis of endometrial cancer.

Reliability of hysteroscopy for endometrial cancer	
Sensitivity	99.56%
Specificity	84.61%
Positive predictive value	76.74%
Negative predictive value	97.76%
Accuracy	99.37%

29.16 Reliability hysteroscopy for cancer statistical analysis (5059 patients – endometrial cancer).

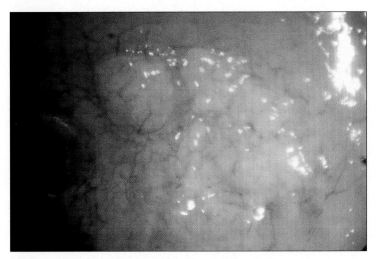

29.17 Suspicious right cornual endometrial growths.

Diagnostic hysteroscopy (n=5059) Hysteroscopic findings in abnormal uterine bleeding (n=2046)					
	Premenopause (n=1483)		Postmenopause (n=563)		Total (n=2046)
Polyps	179	12.1%	114	20.2%	293	14.32%
Hyperplasia	75	5.06%	37	6.57%	112	5.47%
Cancer	20	1.4%	49	8.7%	69	3.37%

29.18 Diagnostic hysteroscopy. Hysteroscopic findings in 2046 cases of DUB.

ACCURATE UTERINE SIZE MEASUREMENT

Even though uterine size is no longer in the F.I.G.O. classification of uterine cancer, several authors have shown a strong relationship between uterine length and metastatic lymph gland involvement. The prognosis appears to be worse when the uterus is over 10 cm long.

CORRECT CLASSIFICATION OF STAGE II

Endocervical involvement (**29.19**), occurs in about 9% of endometrial cancers and reduces the prognosis from 75% stage I five-years survival rate to 57.8% in stage II. A F.I.G.O. report in 1985 showed that stromal involvement reduces the five-years survival rate from 74% to 47% and there is a difference between survival rate in stage IIA (0% recurrence) and stage IIB (57% recurrence). In spite of the above, it seems there is no significant difference in five-year survival rate in cases of gross cervical involvement and occult cervical disease. Hysteroscopy helps to distinguish isthmic and intracavi-

tary tumor spread down to the inner third of the cervical canal and is more accurate than endocervical curettage which has 50% false positive rate. Cervical stromal involvement (**29.20**) has a worse prognosis and should be diagnosed by a skilled hyperoscopist. Little craters, hypertrophic vessels with anomalous branches and deep necrosis at the level of the endocervical canal constitute the first warning signs. In those patients a visually directed endocervical biopsy is precise.

DETERMINATION OF TUMOR ORIGIN

Some doubts may arise about the origin of the tumor if there is endocervical canal involvement. Endometrial cancer typically grows into the endocervical canal without a break in continuity (**29.21**) and the lower end of the endocervical canal is free of tumor (**29.22**). If the origin of the cancer is from the endocervix, neoplastic tissue encircles the whole endocervical canal (**29.23**) and the endometrial cavity beyond the isthmus is atrophic.

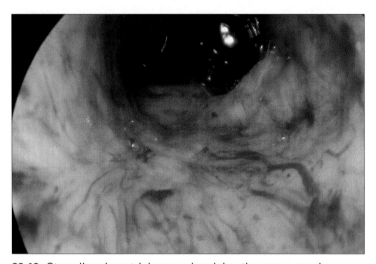

29.19 Stage II endometrial cancer involving the upper canal.

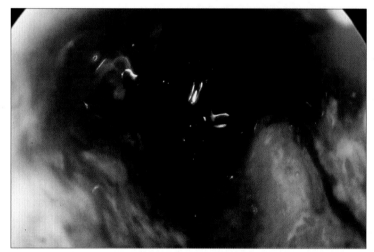

29.20 Bleeding, loss of tissue due to necrosis and superficial irregularity in suspected stromal neoplastic involvement.

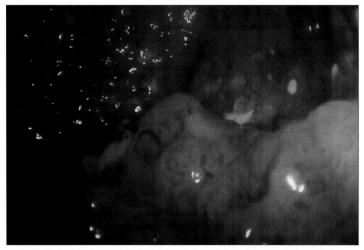

29.21 Endometrial cancer involving the whole uterine cavity.

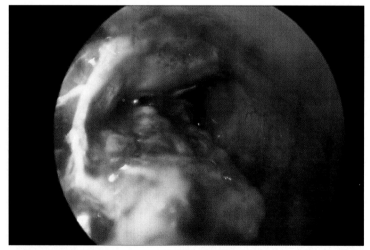

29.22 Endometrial cancer spreading to the endocervical canal.

DETERMINATION OF TUMOR SIZE

Tumour size is important in prognosis. It has been reported that nearly 80% of lymph nodes were positive when the tumor involved more than one-third of the uterine cavity whereas under 10% were positive when the cancer was smaller. A larger mass implies either that the tumour has been present a long time or is faster growing. Deep myometrial invasion, lymphatic or blood borne metastases are related to a poor final prognosis. Fundal cancers involving the cornua may spread through the tubal ostia to the peritoneal cavity. Tumors in the lower part of the cavity grow towards the cervical canal and the cervical lymphatic chain. Hysteroscopy, more than ultrasonography or hysterosalpingography, can diagnose the tumor size more accurately. The hysteroscopist should establish whether endometrial cancer involves one-, two- or three-thirds of the uterine cavity.

DETERMINATION OF ISTHMICAL INVOLVEMENT

Endocervical involvement behaves like cervical cancer and spreads laterally to the cervical and obturator lymph nodes (**29.24**).

DETERMINATION OF CORNUAL INVOLVEMENT

The thin cornual area with its extensive vascularization, uterine contractility and the proximity of the tubal ostia allows early dissemination of the cancer (**29.25, 29.26**). When cancer develops in the cornua the peritoneal surface is involved in nearly 10% of cases and peritoneal washings are positive in 15% of stage I, which would explain local relapses.

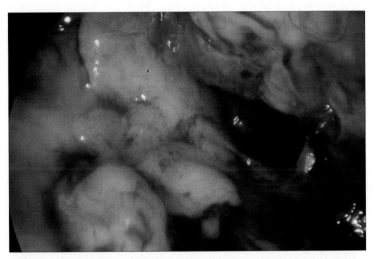

29.23 Endometrial cancer involving the whole surface of the canal.

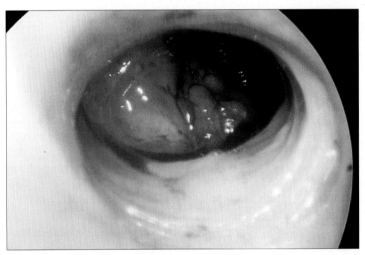

29.24 Isthmical involvement of an endometrial malignant tumor.

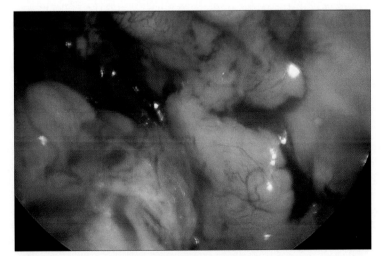

29.25 Right cornual and tubal ostium involvement of an endometrial cancer related to hyperplasia.

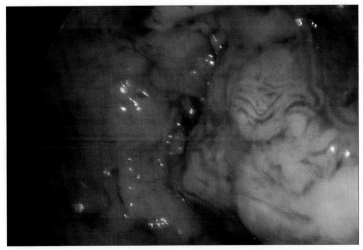

29.26 Right cornual endometrial cancer which leaves the tubal ostium free.

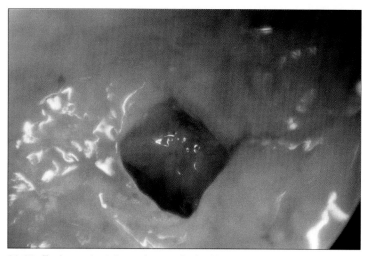

29.27 Endocervical tissue hyperplasia. Hypertrophic surface with disappearance of papilla, crypts and folds.

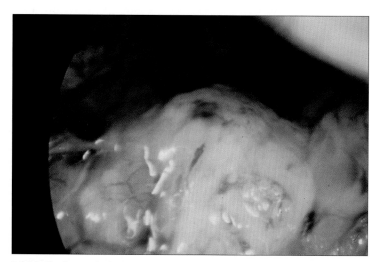

29.28 Endocervical cancer in the upper half of the canal.

DIAGNOSIS OF ENDOCERVICAL CANCER

Endocervical carcinoma arising from cervical glandular cells, causes 10-30% of primary carcinoma of the cervix. The incidence has increased in line with the steady decrease in the number of new squamous epithelial cancers. Its importance lies in the difficulty of early diagnosis and rapid progression and poor prognosis.

In order to differentiate between primarily endocervical glandular cancer and endometrial cancer spread to the endocervical canal, there has to be an endocervical cancer with normal endometrium or both endometrial and endocervical cancers separated by normal tissue. There are problems in early diagnosis by cytology, colposcopy and curettage because of the special characteristics of this cancer. These are:

1. It usually arises from the upper endocervical canal.
2. There is rapid growth and it is highly malignant.
3. The tumor grows deeply in 30% of cases and an obvious cervical ulcer occurs in only 20% of cases.
4. 20% women are asymptomatic until they present with metastases and they are often younger women.
5. As a result routine gynecologic examination may fail to detect the tumor.

Cytologic screening may not detect premalignant stages of endocervical cancer, and only a small minority are diagnosed while still *in situ*. Hysteroscopy is useful for exploring the endocervical canal and taking directed biopsies in women with cytologic abnormalities in their cervical smear, abnormal bleeding, persistent discharge without a proven cause, morphologic cervical abnormalities and risk factors for endometrial cancer.

In early well-differentiated tumors, the endocervical tissue maintains its normal pattern with some papillae, crypts and hypertrophic folds. They also have a pale appearance because the number of blood vessels is decreased (**29.27**). Later the tissue becomes hypertrophic, more vascular and bleeds readily on contact.

In poorly differentiated or slow growing cancers, hypertrophic growths surrounded by ulceration and necrosis are the rule (**29.28**). Cancer growing deeply into the endocervix may show craters with profuse bleeding.

CONCLUSION

Any method of detecting early cancer or its precursors will reduce mortality. Women can be examined with the hysteroscope in the outpatient department without the need for an anesthetic. Hysteroscopy explores both the whole endometrial cavity and the endocervical canal. With skilled endoscopy and directed endometrial biopsy, it gives a high diagnostic accuracy for uterine carcinoma.

FURTHER READING

Eifel PJ, Morris M, Oswald MJ, Wharton JT, Delclos L. Adenocarcinoma of the uterine cervix: Prognosis and patterns of failure in 367 cases. *Cancer* 1990; **65**:2507–14

Fanning J, Alvarez PM, Tsukada Y, Plver MS. Prognostic Significance of the Extent of Cervical Involvement by Endometrial Cancer. *Gynecol Oncol* 1991; **40**:46–7

Ferenczy A, Gelfand MM. Outpatient endometrial sampling with endocyte: comparative study of its effectiveness with endometrial biopsy. *Obstet Gynecol* 1984; **63**:295–332

Greenwood SM, Wright DJ. Evaluation of the office endometrial biopsy In the detection of endometrial carcinoma and atypical hyperplasia. *Cancer* 1979, **43**.1474–8

Hendrickson MR, Kempson RL. Surgical Pathology of the uterine corpus. LUB. Londers, Philadelphia,1980

Kaunitz AM, Masciello A, Ostrowski M, Rovira EZ. Comparison of Endometrial Biopsy with the Endometrial Pipelle and Vabra Aspirator. *J Reprod Med* 1988; **5**:427–431

Novak ER, Yui E. Relation of endometrial hyperplasia to adenocarcinoma of the uterus. *Am J Obstet Gynecol* 1936; **32**:674

Te Linde RW, Jones HW, Galvin GA. What are the earliest changes to justify diagnosis of endometrial cancer? *AM J Obstet Gynecol* 1953; **66**:953

ASSISTED CONCEPTION

Jose Balmaceda, Ediberto Araujo and C Terence Lee

INTRODUCTION

Hysteroscopy has many uses in the management of infertility. In addition to the diagnosis and treatment of intrauterine pathology, hysteroscopy can also be used to catheterize the proximal ends of the fallopian tubes. Developments in falloposcopy have made possible attempts to visualize and assess the lumen of the tubes. More recently in assisted reproductive techniques, methods have been developed to use the hysteroscope to place gametes or zygotes directly into the fallopian tubal lumen.

ANATOMY OF THE FALLOPIAN TUBE

In order to better understand the techniques, it is helpful to review the surgical anatomy of the fallopian tube. The human tube is divided into four segments: fimbriae, ampulla, isthmus and intramural segment.

The fimbriae are at the distal end of the tube. They have many folds, but few muscle fibers. The longest of the fimbrae is the fimbria ovaricae and is attached to the ovary. The ciliated epithelium of the fimbriae sweep unidirectionally towards the uterus and help to perform its principal function of transporting the ovum into the fallopian tube.

The ampulla is the longest part of the tube and is the site of fertilization. The zygote spends several days here prior to entering the uterus. The muscle fibers are arranged in three layers, a longitudinal inner layer, a circular middle layer and a longitudinal outer layer.

Proximally, the next segment is the isthmus, which is muscular. Ciliated cells represent only a quarter of all the epithelium. The isthmus leads to the proximal cornual or intramural segment.

The cornual segment can be straight, curved or convoluted. The richness of its blood and nerve supply suggests it can function as an autonomically controlled sphincter.

CATHETERIZATION EQUIPMENT AND METHODS

Many methods have been invented to cannulate the fallopian tubes, with reports of ultrasonic, hysteroscopic and fluoroscopic guidance as well as blind catheterization.

The catheters used in hysteroscopic cannulation are similar to those used in ultrasonically guided catheterization. In 1987, Jansen and Anderson described the technique of ultrasound-guided trans-vaginal catheterization of the fallopian tubes using a flexible catheter. The original equipment consisted of a set of concentric catheters. The outer 5-Fr Teflon catheter was designed to reach the uterotubal junction. Next, the inner soft 3-Fr catheter, reduced to 2-Fr in the last 5cm, allowed entry to the isthmus. A separate metal obturator was used to guide the entire system through the cervix, into the uterus. Later modifications were made to the equipment to improve sonographic visualization of the inner catheter.

The development of fine, flexible fiber optic systems has allowed hysteroscopic imaging of the lumen of the tubes. The advantage of hysteroscopy over ultrasound guidance is the ability to see the ostia and tubes which improves the accuracy of threading the catheter into the tube. Also, hysteroscopy allows the uterine cavity to be seen for diagnostic purposes.

Using a standard operating hysteroscope, various catheters have been passed through the operating channel, including urologic catheters, balloon catheters and epidural catheters. The ideal catheter for tubal transfer should have a diameter between 0.8 and 1.00 mm with sufficient rigidity to allow nontraumatic tubal cannulization. Coaxial catheters allow easier loading and insertion of games or embryos. The outer 1mm catheter cannulates the ostium while the inner one is loaded with the gametes or embryos (**30.1**).

For gamete intrafallopian transfer (GIFT), a specimen of semen is prepared with the standard wash and swim-up technique using human tubal fluid (HTF) media. About 100,000 to 300,000 capacitated sperm are placed in 50 to 70 microliters of buffered solution. One to three oocytes are usually inserted into the catheter.

It is important to fill the dead space of the catheter with culture medium as the intrauterine pressure tends to push the gametes and embryos back into the catheter (**30.2**).

The medium used to distend the uterine cavity for hysteroscopic visualization differs depending on the application. 32% dextran-70 (Hyskon) is often used for diagnostic hyperoscopy and treatment of proximal tubal obstruction.

Carbon dioxide is used as the distending medium in cases of embryo or gamete tubal transfer. Pressures are maintained at 40-50 mmHg until the catheter reaches the ostium. At this time, the CO_2 is shut off to avoid blowing the gametes through the tube into the peritoneal cavity. After a few minutes, the intrauterine pressure will have fallen and it is safe to inject. Only one tube is catheterized, because the gametes could be pushed out during catheterization of the other tube.

One other important technical consideration is the volume of the transferred material. Jansen and Anderson have reported radiographic studies showing that a volume of 10-20ml is enough to

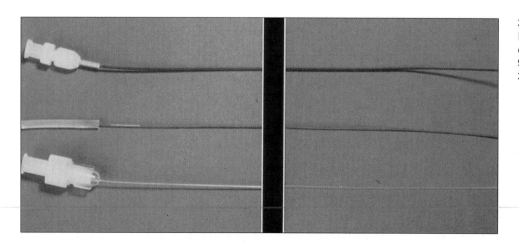

30.1 Coaxial catheter systems used for hysteroscopic fallopian tube cannulation. Length: black, 69 cm, wire 92 cm, clear, 67 cm. Diameter: black 3.5–2.5 Fr, wire 2 Fr, clear 2 Fr.

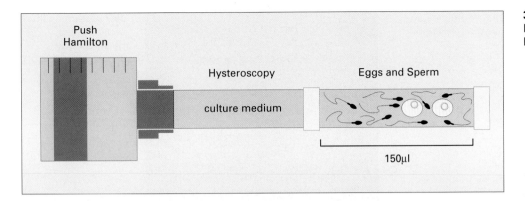

30.2 Loading scheme for laparoscopic GIFT versus hysteroscopic GIFT.

reach the ampulla, while 60–100ml is enough to spill out of the fimbriae. Our figures show significantly larger amounts are required to reach the ampullary–isthmic junction assessed by concomitant radioscopy. The amount required for peritoneal spill was confirmed by laparoscopy. **30.3** summarizes the volume necessary to spill into the abdominal cavity.

PROXIMAL TUBAL OBSTRUCTION

A basic part of standard infertility investigation includes a hysterosalpingogram to assess the condition of the uterine cavity and the status of the fallopian tubes. However, there is evidence that up to 50% of cases of proximal tubal obstruction diagnosed by HSG turn out to be wrong when reassessed laparoscopy or laparotomy. An HSG showing a block cannot distinguish between a true anatomical obstruction and transient muscular spasm. Also, it cannot elucidate the etiology.

Microsurgical resection has been performed on tubal segments which were diagnosed by HSG and laparoscopic chromopertubation as being obstructed. Surprisingly, examination of these segments under the microscope often revealed no histologic abnormalities. This suggests that a proportion of tubal obstructions may represent mild filmy adhesions or soft intraluminal debris which can be cleared by passing a catheter or injecting a liquid medium. This explains the observation that the pregnancy rate is increased immediately following HSG or laparoscopy.

Since 1987, several authors have reported successful treatment of proximal tubal obstruction with hysteroscopic cannulation of the fallopian tubes, resulting in relief of obstruction and pregnancy. Selective hydrotubation has also been described, in which the fallopian tubes were cannulated under hysteroscopic guidance and flushed with a mixture of hydrocortisone, gentamicin and procaine in 50 women, resulting in seven pregnancies. One study described the use of a balloon device to help open proximal tubal obstruction using a principal similar to angioplasty **(30.4–30.7)**.

Catheter	Number of cases	Volume (microliters)
2.5–3.0	6	175
3.0–3.5	5	140
3.5–4.0	4	170
4.0–4.5	2	155

30.3 Volume of fluid injected to produce peritoneal space.

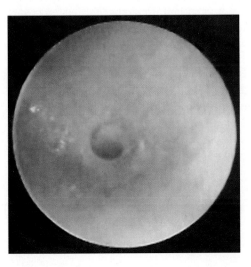

30.4 Hysteroscopic view of tubal ostium.

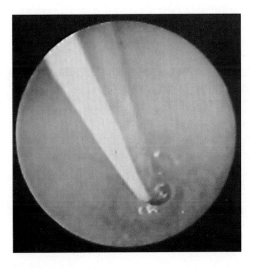

30.5 Catheter approaching ostium.

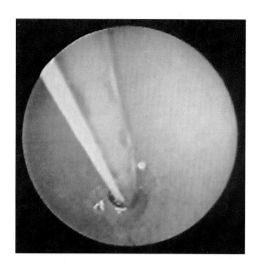

30.6 Multiple views of catheterization

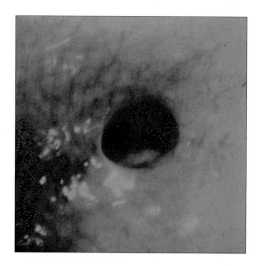

30.7 Ostium with benign polyp. Hysteroscopy allows diagnosis of uterine lesions such as these.

ADVANTAGES OF HYSTEROSCOPIC EMBRYO TRANSFER OVER LAPAROSCOPY

Tubal cannulation has been employed for ease of assisted reproductive techniques. Tubal insemination, gamete transfer and embryo transfer have all been reported. The main advantage of doing this through tubal cannulation is to avoid the risks of laparoscopy.

Another advantage of hysteroscopy over laparoscopy is the opportunity to identify uterine pathology, such as polyps or septae, which can adversely affect pregnancy rates.

Patients with serious medical conditions or who have had anesthetic complications or psychological aversion to surgery will also benefit from the avoidance of surgery.

There are also some women with pelvic adhesions which makes access to the tubes difficult, despite their patency. These patients and those with distal tubal obstruction could benefit from transcervical intratubal transfer. In these cases a hysteroscopic approach is the only option.

Overall, the present studies of hysteroscopic GIFT show lower pregnancy rates as compared with current techniques of laparoscopy or minilaparotomy. Possible reasons for this include an adverse environment created by the CO_2. Subtle endometrial and tubal trauma caused by the catheterization process may also play a role.

INSEMINATION

Reports of hysteroscopic insemination have not demonstrated any advantage over intrauterine insemination, so it is not worth the additional technical difficulty and expense to perform hysteroscopic intratubal insemination.

GAMETE INTRAFALLOPIAN TRANSFER

After the initial success of *in vitro* fertilization embryo transfer (IVF-ET), further advances resulted in GIFT, in which the sperm and oocytes are placed together in the fallopian tube without prior culturing *in vitro*. The key advantage over IVF-ET is that by allowing the gametes to meet and fertilize under more physiological conditions, better pregnancy rates were obtained. Furthermore, there was less need for extensive laboratory manipulation because the oocytes were immediately returned instead of being incubated.

However, there are some disadvantages of GIFT over IVF-ET, most notably the need for laparoscopy or laparotomy to introduce the oocytes into the fallopian tube. This becomes especially important when oocytes are collected transvaginally under ultrasound guidance, thereby avoiding the need for surgery and general anesthesia.

Hysteroscopic tubal cannulation for GIFT can reduce the cost and risks associated with laparoscopic GIFT while theoretically having the same success rate. Unfortunately, there are few reports of good pregnancy rates with hysteroscopic GIFT, but one group reported twenty-seven hysteroscopic GIFT procedures resulting in seven clinical pregnancies. Two aborted, while two delivered healthy twins and one a healthy singleton baby. Two pregnancies were still ongoing at the time of publication.

The technique involved loading the catheter with sperm, oocytes, more sperm and then human tubal fluid with no air or medium separating the gametes. A flexible endoscopic catheter (Teflon-Katheter 1.15 ¥ 1.60 mm: Wisap, Sauerlach, Germany) was threaded into the operating port of a 30-degree chorionhysteroscope with a 4 mm outer sheath (Storz, Tuttlingen, Germany). The catheter was advanced 2–4 cm into the tubal lumen and after stopping the flow of CO_2 for one minute, the gametes were gently injected using a 1cc syringe. Approximately 100,000 to 200,000 motile sperm and two to five mature oocytes in 60 to 100 cc of fluid were transferred per tube.

The same authors performed an unrandomized comparison between laparoscopic GIFT and hysteroscopic GIFT. The group of patients who underwent hysteroscopy were all patients who for various reasons were not good laparoscopic GIFT candidates. These included poor ovarian response (two or fewer follicles), pelvic adhesions, unavailability of operating room, extensive distal tubal damage, refusal of anesthesia and patient preference for hysteroscopy. These patients would otherwise have been candidates for IVF-ET.

The 50 hysteroscopic GIFT patients who underwent 49 retrievals were compared with 81 patients who underwent laparoscopic GIFT and had 73 retrievals. There was no statistical difference in pregnancy rate per retrieval (26.5% in the hysteroscopy group vs 30.1% in the laparoscopy group), abortion rate (23.0% vs 22.7%) nor implantation rate (7.8% vs 7.9%). However, there was a difference in mean oocytes recovered per retrieval (5.0 ± 3.1 vs 6.8 ± 3.4) and mean oocytes transferred per patient (3.9 ± 2.0 vs 4.7 ± 1.3). No ectopic pregnancies were observed in either group.

It is especially interesting that the populations of patients in each group were not identical, with the hysteroscopy group having the apparent poorer prognosis because of the lower numbers of oocytes per transfer and the inclusion of ten patients with a poor ovarian response. Yet, despite this, the decreased pregnancy rate did not reach statistical significance.

Our experience has been different. Our unpublished data shows nine transfers using hysteroscopic GIFT with no pregnancies.

There are several theories as to why hysteroscopic GIFT may not be as successful as laparoscopic GIFT. The first question is the final location of the transferred gametes. Although our volumetric studies provide information that should allow us to place gametes in the ampulla, there is always the possibility that the gametes enter the peritoneal cavity because of the high intrauterine pressure caused by the CO_2. In addition, CO_2 itself has been shown to adversely affect cleavage and fertilization of mouse and human oocytes. Also there is the possibility of minor damage to the tubal epithelium and endometrium during the hysteroscopy.

Further refinements in equipment and technique are necessary before hysteroscopic GIFT becomes comparable to laparoscopic GIFT or IVF-ET.

EMBRYO TRANSFER

Embryo production during an IVF-ET cycle often exceeds the number needed for that cycle. This results in excess embryos that can be cryopreserved.

Also, when a male infertility factor is present it is helpful to ensure that all transferred ova have been successfully fertilized. In these situations, it would be preferable to combine the ova and sperm *in vitro*, as in IVF-ET, and allow embryo development to occur before transfer. In both of these situations involving embryos rather than gametes, the tube can still be used for transfer. It is still debatable whether the tube is a better transfer site for zygotes as for gametes.

Using a Storz office hysteroscope and a coaxial catheter kit (Cook Co,. Bloomington, IN. USA) we placed three cryopreserved embryos into a fallopian tube 1.5cm distal to the ostium. This resulted in a term delivery of a healthy infant.

CONCLUSION

Hysteroscopic GIFT, although still in the early stages of development, holds promise for the future in reducing the costs and risks involved in GIFT.

FURTHER READING

Breckenridge JW, Schinfeld JS: Technique for US-guided fallopian tube catheterization. *Radiology* **180**:2569, 1991

Thurmond AS, Novy M, Uchida BT, et al: Fallopian tube obstruction: Selective salpingography and recanalization. *Radiology* **163**:511–514, 1987

Jansen RPS & Anderson JC: Catheterization of the fallopian tubes. *Lancet*, **ii**:309–310 1987

Balmaceda JP, Alam V, Borini A: Fallopian tube catheterization. *Infertility Rep Med Clinics of NA* **24**:783–797, 1991

Daniell JF and Miller W: Hysteroscopic correction of cornual occlusion with resultant term pregnancy. *Fertil Steril* **48**:490, 1987

Deaton JL, Gibson M et al: Diagnosis and treatment of cornual obstruction using a flexible tip guidewire. *Fertil Steril* **53**:2, 1990

Asch RH, Ellsworth LR, Balmaceda JP, Wong PC: Pregnancy after translaparoscopic gamete intrafallopian transfer. *Lancet* **2**:1034, 1984

Possati G, Seracchioli R et al: Gamete intrafallopian transfer by hysteroscopy as an alternative treatment for infertility. *Fertil Steril* **56**:3, 1991

COMPLICATIONS OF HYSTEROSCOPY   31

B Victor Lewis and Alan G Gordon

INTRODUCTION

Diagnostic hysteroscopy is a safe procedure with very few complications. Operative hysteroscopy is associated with more complications because sharp instruments, monopolar electric current or laser are used.

Training in diagnostic and operative hysteroscopy is essential. Attendance at courses where there are formal lectures and practical instruction on models is invaluable. Animal tissues are helpful but no animal model has a uterus similar to the human organ. The bovine uterus or porcine bladder make satisfactory models but nothing can replace practical instruction in the operating room and supervision by an expert in the early learning curve.

The British Royal College of Obstetricians and Gynecologists and the British Society for Gynaecological Endoscopy have recently published Guidelines on Training in Endoscopic Surgery. This recommends three levels of difficulty of hysteroscopic surgery be recognised. Levels 1 and 2 can be achieved during routine residency training. Level 3 techniques require attendance at courses followed by assisting and being assisted until certified as competent by the trainer (**31.1**).

Complications may occur during hysteroscopy, shortly after or some time after the operation is completed.

INTRAOPERATIVE COMPLICATIONS

UTERINE PERFORATION

One of the main dangers associated with hysteroscopy is uterine perforation. Perforation may occur during diagnostic or operative hysteroscopy. The factors which predispose to perforation during diagnostic hysteroscopy are failure to recognize a sharply retroverted uterus, insertion of the telescope without clear vision, a recent pregnancy, the presence of endometrial carcinoma or pymometra in a postmenopausal woman.

Simple perforation of the fundus can be made with a dilator or the hysteroscope (**31.2**) . Perforation should be suspected if the dilator passes to a greater depth than expected. The hysteroscope should always be passed under constant visual control. Perforation may be recognized by the sight of loops of bowel where the uterine fundus should be. This event rarely causes damage to an intra-abdominal organ and can be treated conservatively. A lateral perforation, which is uncommon, may cause a broad ligament hematoma and require laparotomy.

Complex perforations are made with forceps, scissors, the resectoscope or laser. It is unusual for forceps or scissors to damage an internal organ although bowel or an appendix epiploica may be pulled down inadvertently. Scissors are commonly used to resect septa or synechiae. It is during the latter procedure that the risk is greatest because it is difficult to recognize anatomical landmarks in advanced Asherman's syndrome. This is the only condition where concomitent laparoscopy is mandatory to prevent or immediately detect perforation with scissors. Transillumination of the fundus allows an assistant to recognize when the dissection is approaching the fundus before perforation occurs.

Perforation with a cutting loop or rollerball may occur if ablation is attempted without clear vision, the same area is resected more than once, the loop is activated and advanced instead of being withdrawn or when the thin area around the cornu is being resected.

Perforation of the uterus during operative hysteroscopy is usually recognized easily because the intra-uterine pressure drops, and the flow of distending fluid and fluid deficit increase rapidly as the fluid enters the peritoneal cavity and previous clear vision is lost. The action taken depends on whether or not the electrode was activated at the time of perforation. If the surgeon is absolutely sure that the electrode was not activated, the operation should be abandoned and the patient observed for signs of intra-abdominal bleeding. If the perforation is not recognized and the surgeon continues to resect there is danger that the electrode may enter the peritoneal cavity and injure an intra-abdominal organ.

Uterine perforation seems to be less frequent when Nd:YAG laser is used. The penetration of the beam is limited to 4–6 mm so, provided the same area has not been treated more than once, perforation is unlikely except at the cornua where the myometrium may be only 4 mm in thickness.

Perforation can be prevented by gentle cervical dilatation, introduction of the hysteroscope under direct visual control, resection or ablation from the fundus towards the cervix where feasible and discontinuing division of a septum if bleeding occurs. Extreme care should be taken when resecting a deep intramural fibroid. If there is suspicion that the uterine wall may be at risk from perforation, the operation should be abandoned, the patient given suppressive therapy with GnRH analogues for 3–4 months and the operation

Hysteroscopic procedures by levels of training	
Level 1	**Diagnostic procedures**
	Diagnostic hysteroscopy Removal of simple polyps Removal of non-imbedded IUCDs
Level 2	**Minor operative procedures**
	Proximal fallopian tube cannulation Minor synechiotomy Removal of pedunculated fibroid or large polyp
Level 3	**More complex procedures requiring additional training**
	Division/resection of septum Endometrial resection/ablation Resection of submucous myoma Surgery for advanced Asherman's syndrome Repeat endometrial resection/ablation

31.1 Hysteroscopic procedures by level of training.

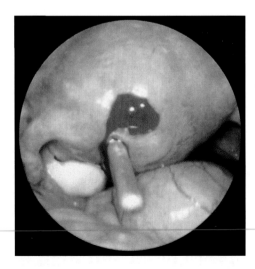

31.2 Perforation of the uterine fundus with the sound.

repeated. At the second hysteroscopy the fibroid will nearly always be found to be avascular and extruding into the uterine cavity. The myomectomy is then easy to perform. Always remember that the part of the uterus at greatest risk is the cornual area and patients with adhesions or deep intramural fibroids are also at increased risk.

INJURY TO INTRA-ABDOMINAL VISCERA OR VESSELS

The main danger of perforation is when it is produced by an activated loop or ball. If the perforation is not recognized and the surgeon continues to resect, the loop or rollerball may enter the peritoneal cavity and damage intraperitoneal organs. These injuries are life threatening. The activated loop may burn and perforate the bowel resulting in the development of peritonitis.

The flow of fluid should be stopped, the electricity turned off and the hysteroscope left *in situ*. If laparoscopic monitoring has been in progress, the nature of the defect can be immediately assessed. Otherwise laparotomy is mandatory.

Manipulation of the uterus may cause the fundus to lie high or laterally in the pelvis and bring it into close contact with the aorta, common iliac vessels, ureter or sacral plexus. There have been reports of all these structures being injured by an activated resectosocope loop or rollerball. Injury to these organs may cause catastrophic hemorrhage, ureteric fistula or paralysis.

If perforation does occur, the bowel, ureter and great vessels must be inspected in detail to ensure that they have not been damaged. This cannot normally be done by laparoscopy. The assistance of a general, urologic or vascular surgeon should be sought as appropriate.

Although perforation with laser is less common than with electrosurgery, laser imposes an exceptional hazard of its own. If the myometrium is perforated, the laser will vaporize the next structure in its path which may be the bowel or, indeed, any intra-abdominal organ. Even if the bowel is displaced into the upper abdomen, it remains at risk of thermal injury by the laser beam.

FLUID OVERLOAD

Infusion of fluid into the circulation through open uterine veins can occur during Nd:YAG laser ablation or electroresection. It is less likely to occur during rollerball ablation. Predisposing factors include prolonged operations or resection of a submucous fibroid where large uterine vascular sinuses may be opened. A large volume of fluid may then enter the circulation within a few minutes leading to pulmonary edema. This occurs in about 1% of operations. It is essential that the inflow and outflow is measured at frequent intervals throughout the procedure. If the deficit rises above one litre, the operation should be rapidly completed. If the deficit is in excess of 1500–2000 ml the procedure should be abandoned, diuretics administered, a bladder catheter inserted and urinary output measured. The patient should be observed both clinically and radiologically for signs of pulmonary edema. If glycine has been infused there is a risk of hyponatremia which may produce cerebral edema. If the serum sodium concentration falls below 120 mmol/l agitation, vomiting and headache occur and may be followed by fits, coma, respiratory arrest and death. Whenever fluid overload is suspected it is important to measure the serum sodium concentration and administer an osmotic diuretic to minimize the risk of cerebral edema. This risk has been recognized for some years and, as a result, glycine is banned in some countries.

PRIMARY HEMORRHAGE

The major causes of primary hemorrhage during resection or ablation are operating on an intra-mural fibroid, resecting too deeply into the myometrium and resecting close to the endocervix. The pseudocapsule of deep intramural fibroids, especially those situated on the lateral uterine wall, may lie close to the uterine artery. There is considerable risk of injuring the artery when resecting or ablating in this area. Any technique which causes destruction of the myometrium 4–6 mm deep to the endometrium may involve a plexus of large vessels and produce significant bleeding. Branches of the uterine artery which run downwards at the level of the internal cervical os may be encountered by resection close to the endocervix and bleeding may follow.

If vision is obscured by hemorrhage, the flow of infusing fluid should be increased until vision is restored and individual bleeding vessels coagulated separately. If, in spite of this manoeuvre, vision is still obscured by blood, the operation should be abandoned and a Foley catheter inserted into the cavity of the uterus and inflated. The pressure of the inflated balloon usually controls bleeding within a few hours. The catheter can safely be removed in six hours. Very occasionally the hemorhage may be so severe that it is safer for the surgeon to proceed to hysterectomy. Patients should be warned of this possibility when they sign the consent form for endometrial ablation.

GAS EMBOLISM

Deaths have been reported from CO_2 embolism. These tragedies occur because CO_2 is insufflated from a high-flow gas insufflator instead of insufflating with a hysteroflator. Laparoflators can deliver over 3000 ml per minute whereas the hysteroflator has a limit of 100 ml per minute. It is unusual for more than 400 ml of gas to be used during diagnostic hysteroscopy so embolism should not occur during a competently performed examination.

In the past, laser fibers were used with a coaxial cooling system using high flow CO_2. These systems have now been abandoned because of deaths due to gas embolism.

Gas embolism can be recognized by the patient's blood pressure falling and the development of cyanosis caused by a drop in blood oxygen saturation. Auscultation over the praecordiium reveals a typical machinery or mill wheel murmur. If this potentially disastrous complication is recognized the procedure should be stopped, the patient turned on her left side and, if necessary, cardiac aspiration performed to remove the gas bubbles.

ANAPHYLAXIS

This is a complication of the high molecular weight fluid dextran-70 ('Hyskon'). This was popular for diagnostic hysteroscopy particularly in North America but has largely been abandoned because of its viscosity and the rare but significant risk of anaphylactic shock.

Intravasation of dextran-70, even in small volumes, has a powerful osmotic effect which draws extracellular fluid into the circulation and may produce pulmonary edema.

EARLY POSTOPERATIVE COMPLICATIONS

Complications may arise during the first few hours or days after hysteroscopy.

INFECTION

Infection after diagnostic hysteroscopy is uncommon but the operation should be avoided in the presence of sexually transmitted disease, vaginal discharge or recent acute pelvic inflammatory disease (PID). Endometritis caused by a misplaced intrauterine contraceptive device (IUCD) is not a contraindication to hysteroscopy. Management includes admission to hospital, the administration of fluids and analgesics, taking appropriate specimens for bacteriological culture and prescribing antibiotics.

The use of prophylactic antibiotics after endometrial ablation or resection is controversial. Intrauterine infection, localized peritonitis and deaths from septicemia have all been reported so it is probably wise to give a broad spectrum antibiotic combined with metronidazole for a few days.

There is nearly always a vaginal discharge for 2-4 weeks after hysterosopic surgery as fragments of excised tissue are passed. No treatment is necessary but the patient should be warned to expect this discharge.

SECONDARY HEMORRHAGE

Hemorrhage may occur during the few days following hysteroscopic surgery. The treatment may be conservative initially with uterine tamponade with a Foley catheter if appropriate. Occasionally hysterectomy or even ligation of the uterine or internal iliac artery is necessary

HEMATOMETRA

One of the theoretical risks, which fortunately is uncommon, is the production of intrauterine adhesions behind which there is active endometrium which undergoes cyclical bleeding producing a small localized hematometra. This presents as cyclical pain and may be diagnosed by transvaginal ultrasound scans. Drainage may be performed either under hysteroscopic or sonar control. A further possibility is the late development of malignant change in an area of hidden endometrium. There is as yet no evidence this occurs but long term follow-up is required to confirm or refute the possibility.

Resection of the endometrium down to the cervix may result in the production of scar tissue and cervical stenosis. This may produce a hematometra with cryptomenorrhea and cyclical pain. Treatment is by probing and dilating the cervix to relieve the stenosis.

CYCLICAL PAIN

Cyclical pain may be caused by cryptomenorrhea following low endometrial resection but some women with no obvious pathology present with cyclical pain which on occasion can only be cured by hysterectomy.

TREATMENT FAILURE

The procedure may fail to cure the symptoms. The definition of failure depends to a large extent on the patient's expectations. She should be counselled in detail preoperatively and should understand that the amenorrhea rate is usually 30% or below and a further 50% of women can expect to be relieved of their menorrhagia. The disatisfied patients are usually those whose expectation has been too high and who may not have been properly counselled.

It is common for the blood loss following ablation to improve for up to six months. Early postoperative assessment may be misleading.

LATE POSTOPERATIVE COMPLICATIONS

Complications may arise some months or years after endometrial ablation.

RECURRENCE OF SYMPTOMS

In about 5% of patients who have had satisfactory relief from menorrhagia or even amenorrhea, symptoms may recur after 1–3 years. This is more likely to happen in younger women in whom there is more time for the endometrium to regenerate. The situation should be carefully assessed and a decision made to repeat the ablation or to perform a hysterectomy. Repeat ablation may be difficult because the uterine cavity is small and the myometrium thin making access difficult and perforation more likely.

Fibroids may grow again if they have not been completely resected or new ones may form and produce symptoms some years after the operation. There is insufficient data at the moment to estimate the risk.

PREGNANCY

Pregnancies have been reported after endometrial ablation. The placentation may be abnormal and the patient may have a placenta accreta and there may also be intrauterine growth retardation.

UTERINE MALIGNANCY

The risk of malignant change in an area of hidden endometrium cannot be quantified at present. In general terms, one would expect the risk of endometrial carcinoma to be reduced because a large proportion of the endometrium has been removed but such statements are pure conjecture at present.

CONCLUSION

Complications of hysteroscopic surgery can, and will arise. Only careful case selection and efficient safe surgery will reduce their incidence.

FURTHER READING

Corfman RS, Diamond MP and DeCherney AH. *Complications of Laparoscopy and Hysteroscopy.* Blackwell Scientific Publications, Oxford, 1993

Lewis BV and Magos AL. *Endometrial Ablation.* Churchill Livingstone, Edinburgh, 1993

Sutton C and Diamond MP. *Endoscopic Surgery for Gynaecologists.* WB Saunders, London, 1993

Taylor PJ and Gordon AG. *Practical Hysteroscopy.* Blackwell Scientific Publications, Oxford, 1993

ANESTHESIA AND ANALGESIA FOR GYNECOLOGIC ENDOSCOPY

Ian F Russell

INTRODUCTION

The anesthetic techniques required for endoscopic gynecologic procedures are relatively simple, irrespective of the complexity or duration of the surgery. Nevertheless, even for very short procedures, a fully equipped operating theatre is required so that complications, both surgical and anesthetic, can be detected readily and treated as they occur.

Some endoscopic techniques can be performed under local infiltration, with or without sedation, but in these cases the surgeon must bear in mind not only the possible surgical complications but also the potential dangers of the analgesic and other adjuvant drugs. There should be a clear understanding of the toxic dose limits of local anesthetics (with and without adrenaline), the dangers of accidental intravenous injection of local anesthetics and the consequences of over sedation with intravenous agents (respiratory depression, respiratory obstruction, aspiration of gastric contents). In these situations, in the absence of an anesthetist, it is incumbent on the surgeon to be proficient in cardiorespiratory resuscitation.

Many endoscopic procedures are suitable for performing on a day care basis and experience has shown that with the appropriate community facilities even prolonged surgery (> 2 hours) can be performed on an ambulatory basis. However, in these longer cases it is important that appropriate short-acting anesthetic agents be used. Some anesthetic techniques which are acceptable for short (< 30 minutes) procedures may result in significant post-operative sedation if they are used inappropriately. Other important considerations to take into account when assessing a patient's suitability for day treatment are the distance she lives from hospital (some feel that the patient's journey home from hospital should not exceed about 60 minutes), home circumstances, the availability of responsible adult assistance at home, the level of postoperative pain to be expected and the existence of an adequate method of pain relief for the patient to use at home.

The prevention and treatment of postoperative pain is challenging and methods include local infiltration of the abdominal wall and mesosalpinx, prophylactic antiprostaglandin drugs (e.g. ibuprofen) and various oral and intra-muscular non-steroidal drug regimens. However, it must be accepted that some women will experience significant postoperative pain and may require intramuscular narcotics. Apart from pain, the patient may be unfit to go home for other reasons and so facility must always be available for an overnight stay.

GENERAL ANESTHESIA

Despite the simplicity of the general anesthetic techniques, the patients should be monitored according to the recommended criteria for any anesthetic. The proposed duration of an endoscopic procedure and whether it is intraperitoneal or intrauterine are two of the principal factors governing the choice of anesthetic.

INTRAUTERINE PROCEDURES

While many short intrauterine procedures (e.g. hysteroscopy) can be performed on an 'office' basis, some patients will still require general anesthesia. In these cases the technique should be kept simple. In the United Kingdom this would entail intravenous or inhalational anesthesia with the patient breathing spontaneously through a face mask. A laryngeal mask airway (LMA) could also be used. Endotracheal intubation, when used routinely for such simple short procedures, introduces an increased risk of unnecessary complications.

For longer procedures (>15–20 minutes) endotracheal intubation and mechanical ventilation are used widely, although as experience is obtained by both anesthetists and surgeons it is likely that a LMA and spontaneous respiration will become equally acceptable. The final choice is likely to depend upon factors other than the intrauterine surgical procedure (e.g. expensive dental bridgework).

Endometrial resection presents particular problems for the anesthetist, not so much with the anesthetic technique but rather with the difficulties inherent in estimating blood loss and fluid balance. The surgical technique for endometrial resection, described in detail elsewhere, depends on distending the uterine cavity with fluid under pressure. The inevitable consequence of this for the patient is that when the endometrium is resected fluid may be absorbed into the vascular system.

It is incumbent upon the anesthetist to maintain an input and output balance of the irrigation fluid, and to keep the operator appraised of the situation when certain limits are approached. While recommendations vary, it is suggested that an irrigation fluid deficit (i.e. a gain by the patient) of 1000 ml should be drawn to the attention of the operator so that surgery can be completed as expeditiously as possible. Until further evidence has been obtained it may be advisable to stop surgery when the fluid deficit reaches 2000 ml. These limits may be conservative when one considers that the majority of patients having endometrial resection are young fit women with good cardiac and renal reserves, factors that are in contrast to the elderly population undergoing transurethral resection of the prostate (TURP).

Under general anesthesia signs of excessive fluid absorbtion (TURP syndrome) are difficult to detect until pulmonary edema occurs. When the patient is awake signs of cerebral irritability may be observed (restlessness, confusion, headache, ultimately leading to convulsions) and some suggest that the ability to observe these signs of cerebral irritability is a valid reason for using epidural or spinal anesthesia for endometrial resection. In these fit patients the hyponatremia (secondary to the fluid overload) should be treated conservatively: fluid removal with diuretics should only be considered if there are frank symptoms of cerebral irritation or pulmonary edema. In the latter case cardiac support may be necessary. Apart from the difficulty of estimating blood loss, another complication of endometrial resection is uterine perforation. This could result in damage to major pelvic blood vessels, resulting in catastrophic hemorrhage unknown to the surgeon: the first warning of anything untoward may be the patient's sudden cardiovascular collapse.

INTRAPERITONEAL ENDOSCOPIC PROCEDURES

Short Laparoscopic Procedures

The anesthetic technique of choice for short laparoscopic procedures is the subject of much debate. Conventionally, general anesthesia for laparoscopy entails the use of muscle relaxants, endotracheal intubation and assisted ventilation of the lungs. However, a growing number of experienced anesthetists do not intubate, as a routine, patients for such short procedures. General anesthesia is provided as described above for hysteroscopy. **32.1** indicates the advantages and disadvantages of the two techniques.

The advantages of intubation and controlled ventilation are essentially surgical, and include a lax abdominal wall and the ability to use a steep Trendelenburg position while the respiratory effects of this position and the pneumoperitoneum are minimized. The anesthetist is also free to respond immediately to any complication which might arise. Conversely, the disadvantages of the technique are mostly anesthetic. These include a higher morbidity related to the use of muscle relaxants and intubation: sore throat; cardiac arrhythmias; potential trauma to the larynx, lips, teeth and gums; a high incidence of muscle pains if suxamethomium has been used (prolonged apnea, and malignant hyperpyrexia are other rare risk factors associated with the use of suxamethonium); difficulty reversing the effects of intubating doses of 'short-acting' non-depolarising muscle relaxants (vecuronium and atracurium) within 15–20 minutes; the potantially fatal effects of failed intubation (aspiration of gastric contents into the lungs, cerebral hypoxia, cardiac arrest). Intubation and ventilation is a time consuming technique which can double the total procedure time of a short laparoscopy. If it is felt that intubation and ventilation provide the ideal operating conditions then the extra anesthetic time must be taken into account when organizing a busy operating schedule: four such 'short' procedures may require an extra hour of 'non-productive' anesthetic time.

With increasing operator experience and with the volume of gas insufflated kept to a minimum there is less respiratory embarrassment. This reduces the need for controlled ventilation.

Assisted versus spontaneous respiration in general anesthesia for laparoscopy	
Advantages	Disadvantages
Intubation and assisted respiration	
Secure airway and mechanical ventilation allows mobility for anesthetist	Cardiac arrhythmias associated with intubation
Abdominal wall relaxed	Potential trauma to lips teeth, pharynx, larynx
Steep Trendelenburg position possible	Failed intubation and aspiration of gastric contents
Better surgical conditions	Longer induction and recovery time
Duration of surgery not limited	Greater post-operative morbidity
Spontaneous respiration	
Reduced patient morbidity	Less abdominal muscle relaxation
Simple induction and maintenance of anesthesia	Possible limited Trendelenburg position and duration
Rapid 'turnaround' between cases	Anesthetist mobility restricted use of LMA overcomes this
	Possible restriction on the use of halothane and carbon dioxide pneumoperitoneum

32.1

Furthermore, if nitrous oxide is used for the pneumoperitoneum in these short 'non-operative' laparoscopies then the deleterious metabolic, respiratory and cardiac effects of carbon dioxide are avoided. If halothane is avoided the risk of cardiac arrhythmias, even in spontaneously breathing patients with a carbon dioxide pneumoperitoneum, is negligible.

Consequently, many short laparoscopies are now being performed with patients breathing spontaneously through a mask. With or without halothane, the author has not seen a clinically significant arrhythmia in 12 years experience of a busy gynecologic anesthetic practice and rarely intubates patients for short laparoscopic procedures. However, it must be accepted that there will be poorer abdominal relaxation (this conveys a different 'feel' to the operator during instrumentation), there may be a restriction on the degree and duration of Trendelenburg position and intraperitoneal pressures may be higher.

If the LMA is used for short laparoscopies then muscle relaxants are not required. The LMA removes the need for the anesthetist to maintain an airway with a face mask, but apart from 'freeing' the anesthetist, and on occasions permitting better airway control, the LMA should not be regarded as a substitute for endotracheal intubation where paralysis and mechanical ventilation are indicated.

Prolonged Laparoscopic Procedures

For more prolonged laparoscopic surgery intubation with controlled ventilation is required. In these circumstances, because of the use of lasers or electro-surgery, carbon dioxide should always be used to distend the peritoneal cavity. If the procedure is very prolonged then care should be taken to maintain both the patient's fluid balance and central body temperature. Prolonged laparoscopic surgery may involve considerable irrigation and it is essential that this fluid should be warmed to 40°C. Unless special precautions are taken the washout fluid will cool down to room temperature and continued irrigation with this cold fluid will augment the usual drop in central body temperature observed with prolonged anesthesia.

REGIONAL ANESTHESIA

Epidural anesthesia has been used for most gynecologic endoscopic procedures, but is more time consuming than general anesthesia. The advent of small (26 gauge or smaller) or non-cutting pencil point spinal needles enables spinal anesthesia to be considered as a realistic alternative to both epidural and general anesthesia without an undue risk of spinal headache. With the appropriate use of short-acting drugs regional techniques may be used for day case surgery. However, the correct use of epidural or spinal catheters will enable the duration of analgesia to be extended to accommodate even the most protracted procedure, while very light sedation or hypnosis is provided by another route.

LOCAL ANESTHESIA

Local anesthesia for hysteroscopy is usually unnecessary if the cervix is patulous, but can be provided by bilateral cervical block when the cervix is closed. It is advisable, on safety grounds, that an intravenous cannula should be in place before starting the block. A low concentration of local anesthetic, such as 0.5% lignocaine in a dose of 5–8ml, should be injected into the vaginal fornix on each side at the 4 and 8 o'clock positions. This blocks the pain fibers, innervating both the uterus and the cervix, from T10, T11, T12 and L1.

Local anesthesia is suitable for a large proportion of patients having laparoscopic sterilization and for a small number undergoing other operations of short duration, such as investigation of pain or the suitability of the tubes for reversal of sterilization, but not for the investigation of infertility which demands a much more detailed examination of the pelvis. The patient should be counselled preoperatively and given appropriate premedication and/or sedation.

Many drugs and combinations of drugs are used for sedation, but because of the potential medico-legal consequences, if sedation is being used by a single handed 'operator/anesthetist', it is as well to remember one of its accepted definitions. 'Sedation is: 'A carefully controlled technique in which a single intravenous drug, or a combination of oxygen and nitrous oxide, is used to reinforce hypnotic suggestion and reassurance in a way which allows treatment to be performed with minimal physiological and psychological stress, but which allows verbal contact with the patient to be maintained at all times. The technique must carry a margin of safety wide enough to render unintended loss of consciousness unlikely'.

Since the patient is awake, the standard operating technique must be modified. It is easier to insert the cervical tenaculum using a Weisman-Graves speculum (**32.2**), the speculum being subsequently removed. The uterus can then be freely manipulated by the tenaculum without producing discomfort.

The umbilicus and the site of the second incision are each infiltrated with 20 ml 0.5% lignocaine, ensuring that the full depth of the abdominal wall is anesthetized. While the local anesthetic needle is being introduced and again while the Veress' needle and other instruments are being inserted, the patient is asked to push out her abdominal wall (**32.3, 32.4**). This gives a firm platform for the surgeon to push against. This manoeuver also ensures that the abdominal wall is lifted away from the underlying major blood vessels and pelvic organs. While inserting the trocar of the laparoscope (**32.5**) it is important to hold one hand underneath the pushing hand to prevent sudden penetration and possible trauma to underlying structures. If the second puncture is made laterally through the rectus sheath, care must be taken to prevent the trocar skidding caudally on the surface of the sheath and penetrating the peritoneum at a distance from the site of the anesthetic.

Whenever procedures are performed under local anesthesia the operating room staff must learn to work quietly and without verbal instructions. A dialogue is conducted between the surgeon and patient as each step of the operation is explained. An assistant should always be assigned to the patient to reassure her and help her to relax.

Laparoscopy under local anesthesia should not be considered if the patient has undue fears about the operation. Obesity is not a contraindication provided the abdominal wall is not too thick, but any suspicion of intra-abdominal adhesions should be an indication for general anesthesia.

In the majority of patients the operation is completely acceptable. Some pain occurs in about 3% of patients but it is rarely severe. Pain may be caused by the pneumoperitoneum, or may be due to incomplete anesthesia of the abdominal wall. Compression of the tubes by clips or rings also produces pain, but rarely interferes with the successful completion of the operation.

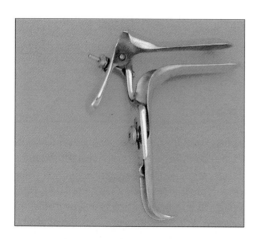

32.2 Weissman Graves speculum.

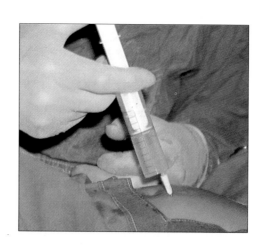

32.3 Anesthetizing the abdominal wall.

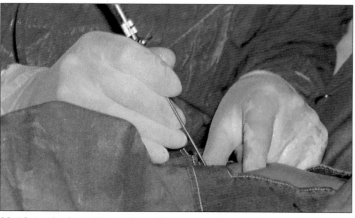

32.4 Introducing a Veress' needle.

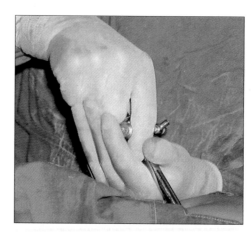

32.5 Introducing a laparoscopic trochar.

DOCUMENTATION OF
ENDOSCOPIC SURGICAL PROCEDURES 33

John M Leventhal

INTRODUCTION

'One picture is worth ten-thousand words'
Chinese Proverb

The documentation of endoscopic procedures, as of other surgical operations, is not only mandated by law, but is an essential element to optimal surgical care. Although the dictated operative summary and written operative note remain the accepted standard for documentation, rapidly evolving visual techniques, with their inherent inflexible objectivity may soon replace the subjective written chronicle.

The advent of electronic micro-circuitry has made possible rapid, accurate imaging of almost every portion of any endoscopic operation, and has thus made the details of the operative procedure available to a wide variety of secondary observers.

WHY DOCUMENT?

Recording the details and/or important aspects of an endoscopic operation serves a number of purposes and people. Among these are:
- Patient information and education, health professional education and teaching
- Review by the surgical team
- Communication with referring and other physicians
- Documentation for the patient record
- Follow-up review
- Possible medico-legal documentation

The obvious regulatory reasons aside, the first of these is perhaps the most significant. It can be argued that the most important person other than the surgeon to have full understanding of the problem and the proposed surgical procedure is the patient herself. The use of photographs or videotapes before the proposed surgery is an outstanding method of achieving truly informed consent, and serves to give the patient (and perhaps her family as well) a real basis for understanding her own operation **(33.1)**. Similar documentary material, from the case itself, used *after* the procedure can be utilized for a number of educational and diagnostic purposes. The patient can learn from her surgeon through the viewing of even an unedited videotape, the conditions existing in her pelvis and abdomen at the time of surgery, and can visualize directly the operative procedures undertaken to address them. In the case of videotape, a permanent 'dynamic' record of the operation can be stored with the medical record and thus be available to others involved in her care.

Documentary material, either static (still pictures or slides) or dynamic (videotape) is of great value in resident and postgraduate teaching, and is widely used as such. In the future, with the development of virtual reality systems, it may be possible to use interactive three-dimensional video representations to allow 'hands-on' training of physicians in laparoscopic procedures.

Lastly, visual documents obtained at surgery, are especially useful for reporting to referring physicians and for review by the operating team at in-service teaching sessions.

WHAT IS VISUAL DOCUMENTATION?

A working definition, as well as the established objective of visual documentation might be simply stated as the 'optical recording of observed phenomena in a form available for secondary observers'.

Most forms of traditional documentation are, to some degree subjective. By the very fact that they arise from the initial observer's concept of what was viewed at the time of the operative procedure, they often reflect as much the background and bias of the observer as they do the properties of the objects under scrutiny. The written progress note or operative dictation is then at best an interpretation, and in the modern lexicon, not transportable. In its attempt to accurately record the findings of a surgical procedure, even the most detailed operative dictation falls short of being truly objective. It must always be a document created out of the mind of the initial observer, and therefore a version of what was observed. The subsequent reader (the secondary observer) has no recourse to the original 'data', and for better or worse, must draw conclusions or base actions on the original observer's subjective documentation.

Modern visual documentation can therefore provide every secondary observer with a fresh opportunity to draw conclusions based upon original 'data'. In this context, visual documentation techniques provide for a much closer subsequent evaluation of the initial operative findings, and are to be preferred over older traditional methods of documentation.

TECHNICAL REQUIREMENTS

Visual imaging can be thought of as either dynamic or static. Dynamic imaging in surgical documentation usually refers to video imaging, but can also encompass cinematography as well. Static imaging refers to the recording of portions of surgical procedures onto slides or print material, either by photographic (silver halide) or electronic (digital) techniques **(33.2)**. Both types of imaging have a place in endoscopic surgery and conform to the objectives of visual documentation.

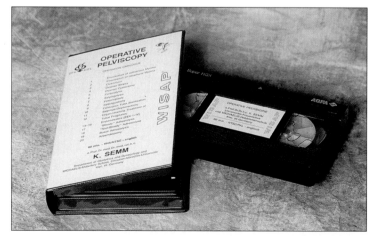

33.1 A videotape of the proposed operation serves to explain the procedure to the patient, and make the postoperative expectations realistic.

In order to render usable and accurate documentation, all visual recording systems depend upon sufficient illumination of the subject matter. This illumination in turn can be thought of as being dependent upon four variable factors: (1) the sensitivity of the recording system, (2) the transmission efficiency of the lens system used with the recording equipment, (3) the illuminating power of the light source, and (4) the size of the image to be recorded.

SENSITIVITY OF THE RECORDING SYSTEM

Photographic still imaging, which currently translates as color transparency (35 mm slide) photography involves the use of color slide film which is balanced for electronic flash illumination. So-called 'daylight' film with color temperatures in the range of 5,000°K to 6,000°K (e.g. Ektachrome® daylight) should be used. Film sensitivity is designated by the ASA (American Standards Association), DIN (German), or ISO (comparable to ASA) rating. The higher the rating, the more sensitive the film is to light. For most endoscopic applications utilizing synchronized electronic flash, film with ASA ratings of 200 or 400 is appropriate. Until about an hour before use, film storage should be at about 13°C (an ordinary refrigerator). These films are of the type utilizing E-6 processing which is widely available and can be accomplished in a matter of hours in most cities. Processing should be done promptly after exposure to ensure the best image quality.

The sensitivity of the recording system used for electronically obtained still (static) images is identical with that of the video system employed, from which the images are 'frame grabbed' (*see below*).

TRANSMISSION EFFICIENCY OF THE LENS SYSTEM

Most endoscopes are essentially tubes filled with a series of lenses comprising a lens system. The design of the system is such as to provide for some calculated degree of magnification and optimum light transmission. Both are dependent on the design, the light transmitting properties of the lens material itself, and the distance over which the light must travel. Recently, with the advent of high sensitivity, high resolution microprocessor chips, the lens-filled endoscope has begun to share the stage with a whole generation of entirely new instruments which employ a solid state microchip mounted at the distal end of a solid 'endoscope'. When conventional lenses are employed with these latter systems they are for focus and magnification and have little influence on the light transmission characteristics of the system.

THE ILLUMINATING POWER OF THE LIGHT SOURCE

Since all visual documentation requires the recording on light sensitive media, sufficient illumination of the recorded object is essential. The medium itself may be sensitive to light directly (e.g. silver-halide film), or indirectly as transmitted from light sensitive electronic sensors (microprocessor chips). It is usually necessary to provide greater intensity light for photographic imaging than for electronic recording. This correctly implies that even very fast (high ASA rating) film is usually not as sensitive as the electronic light sensors of a microprocessor chip. The desired end product of every recording is an image recognizable to the eye and accurately representative of the original object of observation. Therefore the illumination of the object must be matched to the sensitivity of the primary recording medium.

Sufficient light critically depends on the source of illumination. Virtually all light sources for endoscopy utilize a metallic arc bulb which produces light in the 'daylight film' range of 5,000°K–6,000°K and is capable of producing brighter illumination (more lumens) than the old incandescent sources. It is important to remember that the intensity of a metallic arc source can only be varied over a relatively small range, unlike an incandescent source which can vary infinitely. This property becomes an important consideration in the design of video cameras requiring illumination intensity to vary over a wide range of endoscopic applications **(33.3)**.

THE SIZE OF THE RECORDED IMAGE

The amount of light necessary for successful imaging on film is inversely proportional to the required size of the recorded image. It therefore requires more light for a 35 mm image for a slide than it does for a 16 mm frame of a movie film. This principle is less important in the case of electronic imaging where the light gathering properties of the microprocessor chip is dependent upon the sensitivities of the individual units (pixels), their density in the electronic chip array, and the total surface area of the chip is small.

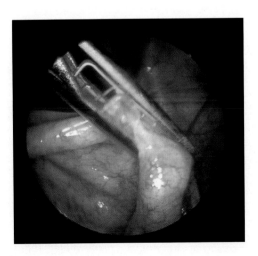

33.2 An example of a static image is a 35 mm color slide of a part of the procedure.

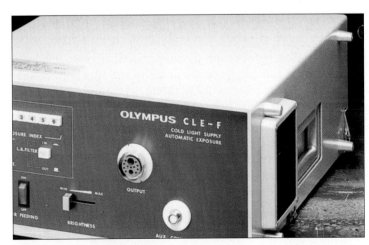

33.3 A typical light metallic arc light source used for laparoscopy. (By courtesy of Olympus Corporation).

PHOTOGRAPHIC DOCUMENTATION

Until the past decade, the recording of gynecologic endoscopic operative procedures has been traditionally on photographic film. The development and almost explosive refinement of electronic imaging, however, has made the video camera and its ability to register a real-time record, the optimal method of endoscopic documentation.

STILL PHOTOGRAPHY

For almost three decades 35 mm color transparencies have been the stock in trade for teaching and illustration of various aspects of endoscopic surgery. Slides remain valuable for the same purposes today, and are easily obtained with a wide variety of automated camera systems. Most manufacturers supply 35 mm documentation systems utilizing synchronized electronic flash with a diversity of single-lens reflex cameras. **(33.4.)** Although accurate and relatively inexpensive, taking 35 mm pictures during a procedure is disturbing and time-consuming. If the procedure is being performed under video camera-monitor control, the video camera must be detached from the endoscope and the relatively heavy and bulky 35mm camera attached, The surgeon must view the field through the camera and often obtain the desired images only by being forced into an awkward and uncomfortable position. Rapid developing with the E-6 system can yield mounted slides in a matter of an hour or so if desired.

CINEMATOGRAPHIC PHOTOGRAPHY

Cinematographic documentation with endoscopy has had less application, and has been generally confined to the creation of professionally produced films for teaching or patient education. Formats have been 8 mm, 16 mm, and even 35 mm, and in almost all cases have required the use of heavy, bulky equipment, not well suited for routine documentation purposes. Today, with the possible exception of the large professional film production, dynamic documentation of surgical endoscopy is exclusively the province of the video camera and electronic imaging. Even this exception may soon vanish with the advent of extremely high resolution video cameras and high quality recording media.

ELECTRONIC DOCUMENTATION

To the endoscopist, electronic documentation requires the use of a video system consisting of a video camera and monitor, videotape and video cassette recorder (VCR) **(33.5)**. In the near future, optical laser disks and video frame grabbers will become additional routine components. Video has become not only the vehicle for recording endoscopic procedures, but also the means of visualizing the field as well. The arthroscopist has depended upon the video system for years, and the general surgeon, more recently introduced to the laparoscopic approach, has learned to be totally dependent upon it. The surgeon's eye has been removed from the endoscopic eyepiece and onto the color video monitor, thus bringing the pre-

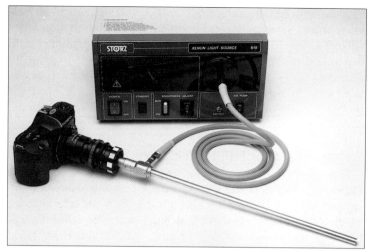

33.4 A single-lens reflex 35 mm still photography system for endoscopic documentation.

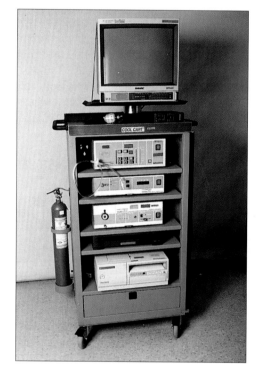

33.5 An endoscopic video system consisting of camera, monitor and video cassette recorder.

viously concealed procedure into the immediate visual realm of the entire operating team. This has allowed for more efficient utilization of assistants and instrumentation, and significantly, a much more comfortable position for the surgeon. **33.6** illustrates a useful positioning scheme for video documentation during a laparoscopic procedure. The applications of the video recorded image are no different than those for any other visual documentation method. However, the video image is an easily obtained dynamic, real-time moving record, of the procedure, and therefore the best approximation to the procedure itself.

VIDEO FORMATS

The ideal electronic format for video recording equipment does not exist, but has been the subject of numerous international meetings over many years. No universal format has yet emerged. In North America, parts of South America, Japan and parts of Asia, the National Television Standards Committee (NTSC) is in general use. In most of Europe and Australia the Phase Alteration Line (PAL) format is the usual standard, although in France Sequence de Couleurs Avec Memoire (SECAM) format is used. Other standards exist and newer ones arise at an alarming rate. Each has its advantages and disadvantages with respect to image quality, and if is unfortunately probable that no universal format will arise for a number of years to come. From the practical standpoint, the difference in formats causes considerable inconvenience to the physician transporting videotapes overseas for lectures or meetings. Conversion facilities exist, but represent an added cost.

VIDEO SYSTEMS

Continuing miniaturization and microcircuitry are the key words of modern video imaging in endoscopic surgery. In less than a decade the video camera for use in the operating room has gone from a two pound box the size of a flashlight to a half-ounce cylinder the size of a the surgeons finger. And while growing smaller and lighter, the resolution and light sensitivity has increased enormously. With greater camera resolution has come also higher density, high resolution videotapes, allowing for even small VCR equipment.

The video documentation system can be considered to consist of five essential components:

- The video camera
- The camera controller and video recorder (VCR)
- The monitor
- The light source
- The endoscope

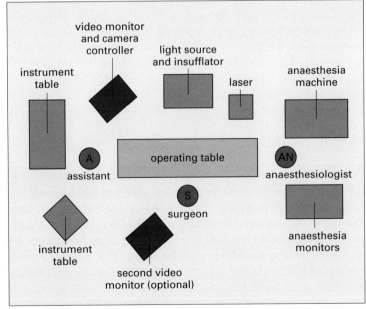

33.6 Schematic diagram of the positioning of documentation equipment in a typical laparoscopic procedure.

THE VIDEO CAMERA

Today the vacuum tube video camera continues to provide (by the smallest of margins) the highest image resolution. For medical applications, however, it has been replaced, in almost all instances, by the solid state single microprocessor 'chip' camera. Tube cameras are still used for commercial television, but even this application is slowly giving way to the three-chip camera with high resolution. Advances in solid state camera technology have been extremely rapid, until today these units are capable of resolution and light sensitivity almost indistinguishable from those of larger, bulky camreas.

There are currently two basic types of microprocessors used in solid state video cameras: (1) the charge-coupled device (CCD) chip and, (2) the metal oxide semiconductor (MOS) diode chip. As a general statement, the CCD chip has greater light sensitivity, but somewhat less resolution capability than the MOS chip. Improvements in both types of chips, however, have moved quickly. The addition of a negative charge to the MOS chip, creating the Negative MOS diode chip has resulted in a marked increase in light sensitivity for this device. In its present form the MOS or NMOS diode chip camera strikes a state-of-the-art compromise between sensitivity, dynamic range, noise, and what is termed 'lag' (the effect of light 'contaminating' the image before it can be moved from the collecting diode to the storage register). Even greater improvements in CCD technology, such as the hole accumulator diode (HAD) sensor and the frame interline transfer CCD (FIT CCD) by Sony, have given this technology some outstanding advantages over the older conventional CCD or MOS sensors.

Both the CCD and MOS microprocessors are integrated circuit devices which utilize the principle of changes in electrical resistance of a metallic or silicon oxide in response to varying intensities of light striking its surface. The part of the chip facing the object being recorded is divided into an array of PICture ELementS called 'PIXELS' which are arranged along horizontal scanning lines. One of the major factors in determining the resolution of a chip is the number of horizontal lines. Therefore the greater the number of lines in a particular camera, the greater is its power of resolution. The NTSC format contains 700 pixels per line, whereas the PAL and SECAM formats contain 833 pixels per line. The latter formats therefore have inherently better resolution per line that the NTSC format used in the USA.

Although application requirements will vary from institution to institution, today's endoscopic video camera should have all or most of the following features (**33.7**):

- Horizontal resolution of at least 500 lines – preferably more
- Automatic light intensity control or controllable form camera head
- Simple one-hand focusing at the camera head
- Automatic and continuous white balancing
- Recorder on-off control at the camera head
- NTSC format (PAL or SECAM where appropriate)

The Camera Controller and Recorder

Light striking a pixel induces changes in resistance which are stored in what is called the 'image register'. The electronic circuitry controlling the microprocessor chip allows for rapid sequential 'sweeping', or transfer of the information stored in the image register to temporary storage in the 'storage register', thus freeing the image elements (pixels) for the next fragment of light stimulation. The rate at which this transfer occurs is known as the 'frame rate' and is

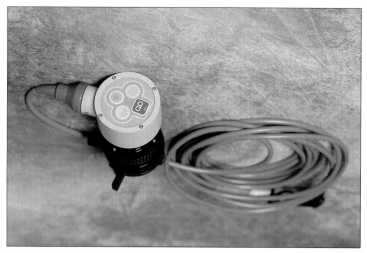

33.7 Typical endoscopic camera with controls at the camera head easily available to the surgeon.

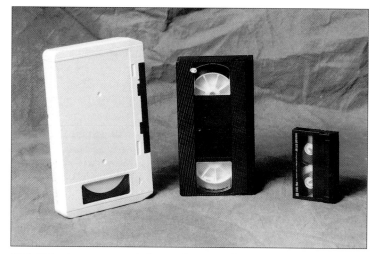

33.8 Videotapes currently in use for recording endoscopic procedures (3/4" U-matic, 1/2" VHS, and 8 mm).

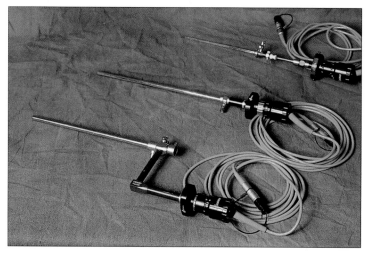

33.9 A 10 mm diagnostic laparoscope and a 12 mm operating laser laparoscope fitted with video cameras.

measured in images per second. The frame rate varies with different electronic formats (*see below*). For NTSC format, used in the USA, the frame rate is 30 per second, while for PAL and SECAM the rate is 25 frames per second.

The Recording Medium

Today magnetic videotape (analog data) remains the most widely used medium for recording, primarily because of its low cost and compatability with most video systems. It is no longer necessary to employ three-quarter inch U-Matic tapes for top quality imaging. Half-inch VHS tapes (200 horizontal lines), Super VHS tapes (400 horizontal lines), and now 8 mm tapes of equal image quality are in common use, and are perfectly satisfactory **(33.8)**. However, video recording has begun to move significantly into the digital age to accommodate the use of the computer and the laser compact disk for archiving and fast retrieval of information. Videotape has the inherent disadvantages of the physical bulk and inefficient access to specific images.

The Monitor

Two types of monitors are available: analog and digital. Most video monitors in current use in operating rooms are of the analog type (like a home television set) and are usualy capable of higher resolution than that of the camera employed. Because the original signal is customarily acquired as digital data, a digital-analog converter is a common component of the camera controller. Digital monitors are in increasing use, and offer some advantages in clarity and resolution. At least two monitors should be available in the operating room for easy vision of the surgeon and the assistant **(33.6)**.

The Light Source

A wide variety of light sources for endoscopy are available. For the surgeon desiring both photographic and video capability, a metallic arc light with built-in synchronized electronic flash, and automatic light control is basic.

The Endoscope

It should be remembered that the smaller the diameter of the endoscope, the less the light transmissibility. It is therefore appropriate to good endoscopic documentation to use an endoscope with the largest size available for the particular requirements of the case. In the case of laparoscopy, this should be 10 mm for a diagnostic laparoscope and 12 mm for an operating scope with an instrument or CO_2 laser channel **(33.9)**.

FRAME GRABBING (STILL VIDEO)

The electronic approach to still images in endoscopic documentation is what is termed 'frame grabbing'. The process involves the capture, in digital form of a single frame of a videotape or real-time image and the subsequent printing out to hard copy material such as paper or transparency film. The process requires a computer for storage of the acquired frame and for output to a suitable printer to produce the 'hard copy' or picture. A number of color printers are available, and, depending upon the system used, both prints and slides can be produced. The quality of the final image obtained, utilizing the newest equipment on the market, is little different than a still photograph. This approach to static images has proved to be valuable for recording important parts of the operation for inserting into the patient's hospital or office chart. The process of frame grabbing combined with the operative dictation is available commercially (Med Images Inc.©)

ARCHIVING

Ideally, appropriate archiving of visual documentation material should require little space and should allow rapid and accurate retrieval of information. The endoscopic surgeon with two or three years of videotapes may wonder whether the ideal has been achieved. Unfortunately, it is not attainable with videotape, which over time even in the 8mm format, begins to occupy enormous amounts of physical space. It is possible to transfer video images from videotape, or directly from the camera controller at the time of surgery, to optical laser discs which are similar to the compact disks used in the home for music. These disks are capable of extremely large storage capacities measured in gigabytes, and will allow almost instant retrieval of specific information. Identification of interesting segments of a procedure, for instance, are coded digitally on the optical disk, and retrieved in milliseconds by barcode reader or database search on a computer. Whole segments of video imaging can be archived on a single disk, and with the advent of advanced data compression techniques now in use, many videotape equivalents can be stored on a single disk. Color transparency slides can also be scanned, digitized and stored in quantities of many thousand on a single disk. Since this archived visual documentation data is stored in digital form, it can be transmitted over long distances by telephone or satellite, and thus can be available for viewing in widely separated geographic locations simultaneously and at any time.

THE FUTURE

There are few fields of information management changing more rapidly than that of imaging technology. Endoscopic documentation is no exception. The optical lens endoscope will soon be replaced by the electronic endoscope with the camera chip imbedded into the distal end of the instrument. It will not be long before the surgeon will not be able to look through the endoscope. High resolution scanners (2,000+ lines) are even today capable of resolutions finer than the grain in conventional films, and camera resolution improves with each passing month.

Three-dimensional recording and viewing is in its infancy, but is already being applied to endoscopy in some crude ways. The whole world of virtual reality is just beginning to open possibilities almost impossible to imagine. A virtual reality trainer for laparoscopic cholecystectomy, which allows the surgeon to minipulate the operative field in a way which is completely interactive and realistic, has already been introduced. The computer generated organs displayed are, at this point still largely diagrammatic, but their replacement with video images of live structures is under serious developement.

CONCLUSION

The documentation of endoscopic procedures is presently the province of the video camera, and its many peripheral devices. For reasons of education of both patient and medical team, referral, and legal considerations, it is fair to state that all endoscopic surgery should be documented. When there is a choice of methods, dynamic documentation should be employed, so that a real-time recording of the operative findings is available for all those with immediate and long-term interest in the diagnosis, treatment, and follow-up of the patient.

THE FUTURE OF ENDOSCOPIC SURGERY   34

Alan De Cherney

INTRODUCTION

Gynecologic surgery has undergone dramatic changes in the last two decades. Procedures which were once considered to be possible only by laparotomy are performed routinely by laparoscopy. Advances in hysteroscopy have made the diagnosis of uterine pathology easier and more accurate and have made possible the resection of polyps and fibroids. Endometrial ablation is now commonly performed as an organ preserving alternative to hysterectomy for abnormal bleeding.

LAPAROSCOPY

The most radical change in endoscopic surgery in recent years has been the introduction of video cameras in the operating room. The practice of occular observation which permits only one physician to view the operative field has been replaced by microchip cameras and video monitors allowing operating room staff to participate and accurate recordings of the procedure to be made on video recorders. With the introduction of digital recording technology, the clarity of these images will continue to improve.

One of the major problems which must be faced is the adequate training and certification of the gynecologic endoscopist. Virtual reality is an advancing field in computer technology that creates a visual and tactile experience for the user based on anatomical and pathological images created from computer designed pictures. The trainee may then participate in a 'hands-on' mock operation in the laboratory before proceding to live surgery. There are already available interactive programs where disection and surgical procedures are simulated on a television screen with computer enhancement. This can help to overcome some of the complications associated with the 'learning curve' that are experienced when any new surgical procedure is introduced.

If we can create a virtual reality image for physician training, one may postulate that similar images can be used for robotics. It will then be possible to design surgical situations which will then be applied to a robotic technique in which automated instrumentation will rehearse the procedure. This requires precision in every aspect of the operation, but the installation of this precision into any procedure will certainly enhance the outcome from the patient's perspective.

Another application of computer technology to laparoscopic surgery may involve the use of interactive networks. The information highway will enable us to record images and transmit them to other terminals to allow intraoperative consultation with colleagues in different centers or, indeed, different countries. A dream of every aggressive surgeon has been to perform three or four procedures at the same time, something which may one day be possible with today's technology of interactive computerization.

In addition, this technology will allow impeccable record keeping. Images created can be stored on small chips or discs which have a greater capacity for memory than was previously thought possible. The operative note of the future will be a stored re-enactment of the procedure on file.

Other technological advances may seem retrogressive in that they combine components of both laparotomy and laparoscopy. Gasless endoscopy, using a device which lifts the peritoneum, enables the surgeon to perform minimal access gynecologic surgery (MAGS) with conventional surgical instruments. This would broaden the range of MAGS to include operations such as tubal anastomosis which is extremely difficult using current laparoscopic techniques. Operations may be carried out by instruments introduced through flexible auxillary cannulae and observed through a fiberoptic laparoscope without the difficulties experienced by present day surgeons by loss of the pneumoperitoneum.

Suturing techniques can often be difficult in endoscopic surgery. The large gauge of suture that has to be used may create considerable tissue reaction and consequent adhesion formation. Gasless surgery is one approach which may overcome this problem because it allows microsurgical techniques and materials to be used. New advances in surgical clips and staples and also tissue glues may ultimately replace older techniques.

Laparoscopic surgery has a clear advantage over traditional laparotomy in the prevention of adhesion formation. Major advances will be made that will continue this trend. New barrier materials which produce minimal tissue reaction will give the surgeon the abilty to reform peritoneal surfaces accurately.

Ancillary technology will improve and introduce new possiblities. This includes the development of new lasers that are more specific in their application and less destructive of normal tissue while being easier to control. An element of precision will be added that is beyond today's imagination. Photo-activation of specific tissues by injected agents may make them more sensitive to specific laser wave-lengths. The application of dyes may also assist in defing the border between normal and abnormal tissue.

The advances in endoscopic surgery will bring the fields of oncology and urology within its scope. MAGS will allow malignancies to be detected and treated earlier. The continued development of advanced laparoscopic surgery will permit radical procedures to be performed with faster recuperation and earlier introduction of adjuvent therapy. Correction of urinary incontinence is currently being performed laparoscopically in some centers and one can envision a day when a woman will undergo her urodynamic study and treatment in a single visit to the physician's office.

The two most rapidly growing areas of surgery today are fetal surgery and transplant surgery. It is difficult to imagine how laparoscopic surgery will be applied to the latter because we have found a convenient way in most instances to substitute an *in vitro* method for an *in vivo* method but endoscopic fetal surgery is burgeoning at this time. These procedures will be done primarily by pediatric surgeons but undoubtedly this will influence techniques applied to our discipline.

HYSTEROSCOPY

Many of the dramatic changes in laparoscopy will also be applied to hysteroscopic procedures. Improvements in the design of hysteroscopes and ancillary instruments will allow safer entry into the uterine cavity and improved visualization. New distension media with fewer side effects will soon be developed and will enhance safety. With medical economics currently dictating a more cost-effective approach to endoscopy, the objective will be to take hysteroscopic procedures out of the operating room and into the physician's office with smaller, more flexible instruments and improved distension media.

Computer technology will be applied in the same three areas: training, robotics, and documentation. Training techniques will be similar to those employed in laparoscopy in that students of surgery will learn by computer interactive programs and be able to practice them in the laboratory before performing them *de facto*. Robotic surgery will be applied to hysteroscopic procedures in the same manner in which it will be applied to laparoscopic surgery. The images of the procedure will be created through a combination of prior documentation and virtual reality and will allow the operation to be carried out with greater precision because it has been rehearsed beforehand. It is difficult to imagine many new procedures being developed in hysteroscopy since this an already limited field, yet current procedures will be dramatically improved upon. The less than perfect results obtained today from ablation of the endometrium and endoscopic removal of intracavitary lesions demand that progress be made.

Endometrial ablation currently has a significant failure rate. By applying more precise destruction of the endometrial cavity with the use of improved lasers and photoactivation of certain tissue, it should be possible to achieve a 100% rate of post-operative menorrhea. This procedure is currently performed in the operating room, often under general anesthesia. Technological advances may soon make this a routine procedure completed under office anesthesia.

A thermal technique of endometrial destruction has recently been developed in which a balloon is introduced into the uterine cavity and filled with boiling water. Like the laprolift, this technique, although appearing primitive, may be found to hold advantages in the near future.

Current methods of achieving tubal occlusion by hysteroscopy such as the application of chemicals or silastic plugs have not proved as effective as originally hoped. New techniques will be developed which will allow effective effective occlusion at a single visit to the physician's office. Contraceptive technology will combine with office hysteroscopic technique to allow tubal occlusion in a single visit to the gynecologist. This is potentially an area of patient care that desperately needs to be developed and exploited since it represents such a large problem for the population in general. The technology would not only make sterilization simpler and more cost-effective in the developed world but would also be applicable in third-world countries in need of population control without the resources to provide universal access to laparoscopic methods.

Possibilities for advancing hysteroscopic technology in the treatment of gynecologic malignancy certainly exist. One can only hypothesize about a better ablative approach combined with the application of growth or anti-growth factors and chemotherapy. The day may come when carcinoma of the endometrium is treated purely in an ablative manner leaving much of the uterus intact.

CONCLUSION

To put things into perspective, it is helpful to dream about what the operating room of the future will look like. The majority of procedures will be done in the office with very small instruments including laparoscopes that require very little in the way of anesthesia for the patient. The room will be filled with television screens, computers, and robotic devices to the point where there is very little room for anyone but the patient. The clarity of reproduction of the pictures produced will be stunning. The operative techniques will be more precise, and they will be done with minimal upset to the patient and less cost to the health-care provider. Outcomes will be markedly improved and recovery time will be minimal. Complications will be diminished as surgeons train and rehearse procedures with the use of virtual reality.

A common scenario could be a patient comes into the office with an ovarian cyst picked up at routine ultrasound examination of the pelvis. An endoscope is introduced before the patient gets off the table. The cyst is vaporized with the laser. Biopsies are taken and read immediately and the patient is discharged to return to work that same day. A digitally produced record of the procedure is sent through the computer network to the patient's medical record and the referring physician. Another scenario is the patient who presents with peri-menopausal bleeding that is diagnosed and treated with an office microhysteroscopic procedure that is also used to completely ablate the endometrium.

Let us hope that the gynecologic endoscopic surgeons of the future do no look back on us too harshly and realize that we were captives of the times in which we practiced.

INDEX